The Role of the Clinical Nurse Specialist
in Cancer Care

The Role of the Clinical Nurse Specialist in Cancer Care

Edited by

Dr Helen Kerr PhD, RN
Queen's University Belfast

Foreword by
Johan De Munter
President of the European Oncology Nursing Society

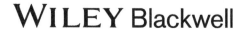

This edition first published 2024
© 2024 John Wiley & Sons Ltd

The right of Helen Kerr to be identified as the author of the editorial material in this work has been asserted in accordance with law.

Registered Offices
John Wiley & Sons, Inc., 111 River Street, Hoboken, NJ 07030, USA
John Wiley & Sons Ltd, The Atrium, Southern Gate, Chichester, West Sussex, PO19 8SQ, UK

For details of our global editorial offices, customer services, and more information about Wiley products visit us at www.wiley.com.

Wiley also publishes its books in a variety of electronic formats and by print-on-demand. Some content that appears in standard print versions of this book may not be available in other formats.

Library of Congress Cataloging-in-Publication Data
Names: Kerr, Helen, editor.
Title: The role of the clinical nurse specialist in cancer care / edited by Helen Kerr.
Description: Hoboken, NJ : Wiley-Blackwell, 2023. | Includes bibliographical references and index.
Identifiers: LCCN 2023023154 (print) | LCCN 2023023155 (ebook) | ISBN 9781119866992 (paperback) | ISBN 9781119867005 (adobe pdf) | ISBN 9781119867012 (epub)
Subjects: MESH: Neoplasms–nursing | Nurse Clinicians | Nurse's Role
Classification: LCC RC266 (print) | LCC RC266 (ebook) | NLM WY 156 | DDC 616.99/40231–dc23/eng/20230626
LC record available at https://lccn.loc.gov/2023023154
LC ebook record available at https://lccn.loc.gov/2023023155

Cover Design: Wiley
Cover Image: © Israel Sebastian/Getty Images

Set in 9.5/12.5pt STIXTwoText by Straive, Pondicherry, India
Printed and bound by CPI Group (UK) Ltd, Croydon, CR0 4YY

C9781119866992_130324

To my mother, Meta Bell, whose career as a Marie Curie nurse inspired me and many others to compassionately care for others.

To my partner, Sharon Kerr, who believes in me.

Helen Kerr

Contents

List of Contributors

Karen Armstrong, BSc (Hons), PGDip, RN
Northern Ireland Cancer Centre
Belfast, Northern Ireland
United Kingdom

Edel Aughey, MSc, BSc, PGCE, RN
Belfast City Hospital and School of
Nursing and Midwifery
Queen's University Belfast
Belfast, Northern Ireland
United Kingdom

Ruth Boyd, MSc, BN, RGN, DN
Northern Ireland Cancer
Trials Network
Belfast Health and Social Care Trust
Belfast, Northern Ireland
United Kingdom

Laura Croan, MSc, RN
Haematology
Belfast Health and Social Care Trust
Belfast, Northern Ireland
United Kingdom

Monica Donovan, MSc, RN
School of Nursing and Midwifery
Queen's University Belfast
Belfast, Northern Ireland
United Kingdom

*Sarah Hanbridge, RN, RNT, FNF Digital
Scholar, MA, PCGE, BA (Hons)
Dip Nursing*
Digital Informatics Team
Leeds Teaching Hospital
Yorkshire, England
United Kingdom

Michelle Keenan, MSc, BSc, RN
Belfast Health and Social Care Trust
Belfast, Northern Ireland
United Kingdom

Helen Kerr, PhD, RN, Dip Counselling
School of Nursing and Midwifery
Queen's University
Belfast, Northern Ireland
United Kingdom

Caroline McCaughey, MSc, PGCE, RN
School of Nursing and Midwifery
Queen's University Belfast and
Oncology/Haematology
Belfast City Hospital
Lisburn Road
Belfast, Northern Ireland
United Kingdom

Johanna McMullan, RN, MSc, MEd
School of Nursing and Midwifery
Queen's University
Belfast, Northern Ireland
United Kingdom

Oonagh McSorley, PhD, RN
School of Nursing and Midwifery
Queen's University Belfast
Belfast, Northern Ireland
United Kingdom

Clare McVeigh, PhD, RN
School of Nursing and Midwifery
Queen's University Belfast
Belfast, Northern Ireland
United Kingdom

Shelley Mooney, MSc, RN
Belfast Health and Social Care Trust
Belfast, Northern Ireland
United Kingdom

**Adrina O'Donnell, MSc, BSc (Hons)
RN, DipN**
Northern Ireland Cancer Centre
Belfast Health and Social Care Trust
Belfast, Northern Ireland
United Kingdom

Hinal Patel, MSc, RN
University College London
Hospitals NHS Foundation Trust
London, England
United Kingdom

Barry Quinn, PhD, RN
School of Nursing and Midwifery
Queen's University Belfast
Belfast, Northern Ireland
United Kingdom

Susan Smyth, MSc, RN
Macmillan Unit
Ulster Hospital
Upper Newtownards Road
Belfast, Northern Ireland
United Kingdom

Kerrie Sweeney
Cancer Services
Antrim Area Hospital
Northern Health and Social
Care Trust
Northern Ireland
United Kingdom

Ruth Thompson, MSc, RN
Nursing Policy and Practice
Royal College of Nursing
Belfast, Northern Ireland
United Kingdom

**Stephanie Todd, BSc(Hons)
Postgrad Dip, RN**
Belfast Health and Social Care Trust
Belfast, Northern Ireland
United Kingdom

Amy Vercell, MSc, RN
Digital Services
The Christie NHS Foundation Trust
Manchester, England
United Kingdom

Trevor Wightman
Northern Ireland
United Kingdom

Foreword

Today, it is recognised that the burden of cancer in the population lies across the whole lifespan and that innovation in cancer care is crucial to tackling the cancer burden across the globe. Apart from the imperative of ensuring that every person with cancer has the best possible chance to receive treatment and survive cancer, the potential for the best outcome demands an interprofessional collaboration among all stakeholders in cancer care. Cancer nurses are key healthcare providers who contribute to innovative, qualitative and safe cancer care, from prevention to survivorship and end-of-life care. As forefront healthcare providers, they have a great responsibility and, at the same time, a great opportunity to contribute to the success of the provided care. However, developments in healthcare are not remaining constant, as great leaps continue to be taken to meet the current needs of those who need care.

To meet this modern standard of care, the development and implementation of lead roles such as clinical nurse specialists (CNS) are crucial in supporting person-centred care and health outcomes. CNS are advanced practice nurses who have completed advanced education programmes and clinical training in a specific area of healthcare. In the field of cancer care, the CNS plays a vital role in improving patient outcomes and providing high-quality care. A CNS works closely with patients, families and other healthcare professionals to coordinate and deliver cancer care that is tailored to the unique holistic needs of each individual. They are skilled in conducting comprehensive assessments, developing care plans, and providing education and support to patients and families.

The CNS also has a strong understanding of the various innovative cancer treatment modalities, including chemotherapy, radiation therapy, immunotherapy, hormonal therapies and surgery and is able to provide expert guidance and support to patients undergoing these treatments. They often care for patients throughout all stages of cancer, from diagnosis and treatment to post-treatment follow-up and survivorship.

In addition to their direct patient care responsibilities, CNS also serve as leaders within the healthcare community. They may act as consultants to other healthcare professionals, providing expert advice and guidance on cancer care and treatment. CNS may also serve as educators, teaching other healthcare professionals about the latest research and best practices in cancer care. Next to education is research, an important aspect of the work of a CNS in cancer care. The CNS may conduct research studies or participate in clinical trials to advance the field of cancer care and improve patient outcomes. They may also work to identify and address care gaps, developing innovative treatments, care and support approaches.

As advocates for patients, CNS work to ensure that individuals with cancer and their families and carers receive the best possible care and support. They may also advocate for policies and practices that promote cancer prevention and early detection, contributing to reducing the burden of cancer on individuals and society as a whole. Overall, the work of a CNS in cancer care is multifaceted and vital in improving the lives of patients and their families affected by cancer.

For those interested in pursuing a career as a CNS in cancer care, it is important to have a strong foundation in nursing and a passion for cancer care. CNS must also be willing to continue learning and staying up-to-date on the latest research and best practices in cancer care.

If you are a CNS, a nurse seeking to specialise in cancer care, or simply interested in learning more about this important area of cancer nursing, this book is an invaluable resource. It provides a comprehensive look at the work of CNS in cancer care and their vital role in improving patient outcomes and advancing the field. As a cancer nurse whose own ventures into cancer care were encouraged and supported by talented and inspirational national and international nursing colleagues, I warmly welcome this book. Finally, to all readers, I want to thank you for recognising the important role of the CNS. When going through this book, you will notice that many chapters are written by clinical nurse specialists for clinical nurse specialists. As a result of this comprehensive collaboration, the book provides important, reflective depth with an honest and current perspective of the CNS role. We hope that you will enjoy reading this book and that it will inspire you to embrace the full potential of the CNS role in cancer care.

Johan De Munter
Cancer Nurse Manager
Cancer Center, University Hospital Ghent, Belgium
President, European Oncology Nursing Society

Introduction

Helen Kerr

From nursing's inception as a profession, there has been a continual evaluation of the profession in response to changing health and societal needs (International Council of Nursing 2020). One aspect of this relates to the growing global interest in extending nursing practice beyond the level of initial registration (East et al. 2015) in response to changing demographics (Holloway et al. 2009), greater user involvement and rising expectations (Por 2008). One component of advanced nursing practice is advanced nursing roles, with up to 52 different roles in 26 countries reported in one study (Heale and Buckley 2015). The clinical nurse specialist (CNS) is one advanced nursing role.

The CNS's role within cancer services significantly contributes to providing high-quality care delivery. In cancer care, the role is reported to contribute to improvements in psychological outcomes for patients; increased patient satisfaction; improvements in patient knowledge; enhanced clinical outcomes, particularly in relation to symptom management; and enhanced service delivery outcomes, such as increased access to services (Kerr et al. 2021). Understanding and appreciating the specific components of the role has been outlined by various authors and includes broad categories of direct patient care and other aspects such as administration, research, education and leadership. This book further delineates the various components of the CNS role to provide clear insights into the contribution of this role in improving patient outcomes and supporting the development of these aspects within current roles.

This book is in four sections. The first section has two chapters that relate to the emergence and evolvement of advanced nursing practice with a focus on one specific component: advanced nursing roles. Chapter 1 focuses on the historical context of advancing nursing practice and advanced practice nurse roles. Chapter 2 outlines the historical and current context of the CNS role, providing a background for the book.

Section two has two chapters that provide a patient and carer perspective of the CNS role. Chapter 3 is written by Johanna, who shares her experiences of being diagnosed with breast cancer and reflects on the CNS's role in her care. Chapter 4 is written by Trevor, a carer of an individual who had cancer; he shares his experience of being a carer and the impact the CNS had in their care.

The third section has nine chapters, and each is co-authored by a CNS along with an academic with a clinical background in cancer services. Each chapter focuses on a different component of the CNS role. Chapter 5 provides an overview of the operationalisation of the *key worker role* and a discussion of how challenges associated with this role could be effectively managed. Chapter 6 focuses on the skills required by the CNS in providing *psychological support* to individuals with a cancer diagnosis and their carers. There is also a discussion of the importance of self-care for nurses working in cancer services. Chapter 7 focuses on how *research and evidence-based practice* must be integrated into the CNS role, discussing the importance of cancer clinical trials. Chapter 8 focuses on *symptom management*. There is an outline of the presentation, assessment and management of gastro-intestinal symptoms associated with a diagnosis of cancer and treatment interventions, along with a focus on pain assessment and management. Chapter 9 focuses on the CNS's important contribution to *the multi-disciplinary team* and how to integrate this role within an established interdisciplinary team. Chapter 10 provides a clinical approach to developing the *leadership* aspect of the CNS role in managing patient care to optimise services. Chapter 11 focuses on the steps involved in introducing and establishing *nurse-led clinics* in cancer services. Chapter 12 outlines the historical context of the *non-medical prescribing role* and the contribution this role has for the CNS in enhancing patient care. Chapter 13 focuses specifically on the role of the CNS for *adolescents and young adults with cancer*, identifying the skills required to provide care for these individuals and their families and carers.

Section four considers the future direction of the CNS role and has three chapters. Chapter 14 explores the impact the *COVID-19 global pandemic* had on the role of the CNS in cancer services, including a discussion on the introduction and evolvement of approaches adopted for patient safety. There is an exploration of how the CNS can contribute to reviewing the sustainability of some of these approaches. This is followed by Chapter 15, which provides an overview of the historical evolvement of *digital health* and how the CNS can contribute to addressing the challenges of moving aspects of care delivery to a virtual environment, particularly in the context of the COVID-19 global pandemic. Chapter 16, the final chapter, examines the *future direction* and possible trends in practice and care delivery for CNS working in cancer services. There is an emphasis on the continuing central role of delivering person-centred care within this specialist role.

The book should be of interest to nurses considering the CNS role as part of their career trajectory, as it delineates some of the various components of the role. The book will also be of interest to those currently in CNS roles, as it identifies aspects of the role that could be developed, such as nurse-led clinics and non-medical prescribing. Finally, those who work alongside CNS or are in strategic leadership roles will appreciate the significant contribution the CNS role makes to improving patient outcomes and delivering healthcare in the cancer context.

Twenty-two authors contributed to this book, providing their perspectives on the significant and valuable contribution the CNS role makes to enhancing patient care. We invite you to explore, reflect on and enjoy engaging with this book and consider how you and others can develop the CNS role so as to improve outcomes for individuals with cancer and their families and carers.

References

East, L., Knowles, K., Pettman, M., and Fisher, L. (2015). Advanced level nursing in England: organisation challenges and opportunities. *Journal of Nursing Management* 23: 1011–1019.

Heale, R. and Buckley, C. (2015). An international perspective of advanced practice nursing regulation. *International Nursing Review* 62: 421–429.

Holloway, K., Baker, J., and Lumby, J. (2009). Specialist nursing framework for New Zealand: a missing link in workforce planning. *Policy Politics and Nursing Practice* 10 (4): 269–275.

International Council of Nurses (ICN) (2020). *Guidelines on Advanced Practice Nursing*. Geneva: ICN.

Kerr, H., Donovan, M., and McSorley, O. (2021). Evaluation of the role of the clinical Nurse Specialist in cancer care: an integrative literature review. *European Journal of Cancer Care* 30 (3): 1–13.

Por, J. (2008). A critical engagement with the concept of advanced nursing practice. *Journal of Nursing Management* 16: 84–90.

About the Companion Website

Don't forget to access the accompanying podcasts, which are hosted on the companion website:

www.wiley.com/go/kerr

1

Evolvement of Advanced Nursing Practice

Helen Kerr

Abstract

This chapter will focus on the emergence and evolvement of advanced nursing practice. The historical context of the inauguration of nursing as a profession and the subsequent regulation of nursing will be outlined. The rationale for the development of advanced nursing practice will be explored, leading to a focus on one component of this concept: advanced practice nurse roles. The nomenclature associated with advanced practice nurse roles will be outlined, leading to an introduction to the emergence of the specialist nursing workforce, specifically the clinical nurse specialist, which will be the focus of Chapter 2.

1.1 Introduction

This chapter will focus on the emergence and evolvement of advanced nursing practice. The historical context of the inauguration of nursing as a profession and the subsequent regulation of nursing will be outlined. The rationale for the development of advanced nursing practice will be explored, leading to a focus on one component of this concept: advanced practice nurse (APN) roles. The nomenclature associated with APN roles will be outlined, leading to an introduction to the emergence of the specialist nursing workforce, the focus of Chapter 2.

1.2 Evolvement of Nursing as a Profession

It is well-recognised that modern nursing, as it is currently delivered, is accredited to the influence of Florence Nightingale (World Health Organization [WHO] 2020), who introduced the idea that nursing was a profession that required education

The Role of the Clinical Nurse Specialist in Cancer Care, First Edition. Edited by Helen Kerr.
© 2024 John Wiley & Sons Ltd. Published 2024 by John Wiley & Sons Ltd.
Companion website: www.wiley.com/go/kerr

(Wilson 2005). Glasper and Carpenter (2019) report that prior to these influences, nurses were considered incompetent. In the 1850s, when Florence Nightingale was in her 30s, she was internationally renowned for her services in Turkey as part of the British Army's employment of female nurses during the Crimean War (National Council of State Boards of Nursing 2020). Florence Nightingale subsequently developed a Nightingale Training School on the grounds of St Thomas's Hospital, London, United Kingdom (UK), in the 1860s. Despite reports that medicine was unsupportive of Nightingale's attempts to introduce formal education and training for nursing, training schools were developed across England (Glasper and Carpenter 2019).

In the late nineteenth and early twentieth centuries, Ethel Bedford Fenwick lobbied for a nursing register and, in December 1921, became the first nurse to register with the newly formed General Nursing Council (GNC) (Glasper and Carpenter 2019). In 1943, the responsibilities of the GNC were extended by a Nurses Act to include *assistant nurses*, renamed *state enrolled nurses* by the Nurses (Amendment) Act in 1961 (Glasper and Carpenter 2019). The Nurses, Midwives and Health Visitors Act was passed in 1979, effective from 1983, and replaced the GNC with the United Kingdom Central Council (UKCC) and four national boards for nursing, midwifery, and health visitors in each of the four countries of the UK: England, Northern Ireland, Scotland and Wales.

Project 2000 was introduced in the late 1980s and moved nurse education and training into higher education. In 2001, under the Nursing and Midwifery Order, the Nursing and Midwifery Council (NMC) was established in the context of the UK. In many countries across the globe, a similar trajectory regarding the professionalisation and regulation of nursing emerged, albeit on a different timeline, with most countries around the world now regulating and governing nursing practice through regulatory bodies (National Council of State Boards of Nursing 2020). The WHO (2020) reported that 86% of countries now have a body responsible for the regulation of nursing, and most countries also have a statute of law that regulates nurses (National Council of State Boards of Nursing 2020).

Nursing has evolved to become the largest staff group in healthcare globally, accounting for approximately 59% of the workforce and a reported 27.9 million nurses worldwide, of which 19.3 million are categorised as professional nurses (WHO 2020). Nursing does not have a set of international standards, which means nurses are educated, regulated and disciplined in a variety of ways across the globe (Stievano et al. 2019). Despite these geographical variations, a series of recommendations for nursing for all countries was published by the WHO in 2020. These relate to increasing funding to educate and employ nurses, establishing leadership positions, equipping nurses in primary healthcare to work to their full potential including prevention and management of noncommunicable disease, implementing gender-sensitive workforce policies and modernising nursing regulation by harmonising education and practice standards (WHO 2020). The WHO recommendations demonstrate the continuing development of the nursing profession at a time when the regulation of nursing marked a centenary in the UK in December 2021.

1.3 Advanced Nursing Practice

From nursing's inception as a profession, the profession has been continually evaluated in response to health, societal and person-centred care challenges (International Council of Nurses (ICN) 2020). One aspect of the evaluation is the growing global interest in extending nursing practice beyond the level of initial registration (East et al. 2015). The need to extend nursing practice is attributed to multiple rationales. There has been an increasing demand for healthcare due to changing demographics and new government strategies (Holloway et al. 2009). Nursing has also evolved in response to greater user involvement and rising expectations, with service users requiring greater choice (Por 2008). There has also been a suggestion that nurses advancing their practice was due to changes in the field of medicine, such as shortages in physicians (Por 2008); however, this is refuted by Hamric and Tracy (2019), who state that advanced nursing practice is not a substitute for medical practice. Although the origins of advanced nursing practice date back about a century (Hamric and Tracy 2019), advanced practice nursing has only existed in the United States of America (USA) since the 1960s and the UK since the 1980s (Callaghan 2008). This supports Barton's (2012) assertion that the evolution of advancing nursing practice has been protracted.

There is contention about the accepted terminology for nurses developing their practice beyond the level of registration. In general, the literature reports two similar terms: *advanced practice nursing* and *advanced nursing practice*. Although these terms are used interchangeably in the literature, Hamric and Tracy (2019) argue that they are different, so it is important to explore the differences.

Although Jamieson (2002) stated that there is no singular definition for *advanced practice nursing*, there have been recent attempts to clarify this concept. The ICN (2020, p. 6) states that advanced practice nursing 'is viewed as advanced nursing interventions that influence clinical healthcare outcomes for individuals, families, and diverse populations'. This highlights a definition with a narrower emphasis on nursing interventions rather than a broader focus on expanded practice. In contrast, Sheer and Wong (2008) argue that *advanced practice nursing* is an umbrella term for nurses practising at a higher level. 'Advanced practice nursing is the patient-focused application of an expanded range of competencies to improve health outcomes for patients and populations in a specialised clinical area of the larger discipline of nursing' (Hamric and Tracy 2019, p. 213).

The second term, *advanced nursing practice*, appears to be used more frequently in the literature with a definition similar to that of *advanced practice nursing* previously outlined by Hamric and Tracy (2019). *Advanced nursing practice* is 'an umbrella term describing an advanced level of clinical nursing practice that maximises the use of graduate educational preparation, in-depth nursing knowledge and expertise in meeting the health needs of individuals, families, groups, communities and populations. It involves analysing and synthesising knowledge, understanding, interpreting, and applying nursing theory and research; and developing and advancing nursing knowledge and the profession as a whole' (Canadian Nurses Association 2010, p. 14). Por (2008) states that advancing nursing practice is an 'ongoing process in nursing practice using expanded knowledge, clinical expertise and research to further the scope of nursing practice' (p. 84). The Registered Nurses Association of British Columbia Policy Statement (2001, cited in ICN 2020, p. 6) provides a similar definition, stating that 'advanced nursing practice is a field of nursing that extends and expands the boundaries of nursing's scope of practice, contributes to nursing knowledge and promotes advancement of the profession'. The American Association of Colleges of Nursing (2004, p. 3, cited in Hamric and Tracy 2019) provide an alternative definition for advanced nursing practice as 'any form of nursing intervention that influences healthcare outcomes for individuals or populations, including the direct care of individual patients, management of care for individuals and populations, administration of nursing and healthcare organisations and the development and implementation of health policy'. These terms appear to be used interchangeably, so the confusion and debates continue. This book will use the term *advanced nursing practice* and borrow the definition published by the ICN in 2020, outlined in the previous paragraph.

A further area of confusion regarding this concept relates to the criteria associated with advanced nursing practice. Understanding how advanced nursing practice differs from a registered nurse at the point of initial registration regarding the broad skills, attributes and competencies will help to demystify advanced nursing practice. A simple distinction made by Calkin (1984) between basic or advanced practitioners relates to the latter associated with expertise being gained through education and experience. However, there is no universal understanding of the attributes or competencies associated with advanced nursing practice.

1.3.1 Criteria Associated with Advanced Nursing Practice

In attempting to delineate the criteria related to advanced nursing practice, which may include identifying the level of skills, attributes and competencies, it is important to recognise the geographical variations that have an impact, such as policy development, regulation and healthcare demands, as the evolution of advanced practice nursing has differed in each nation (Sheer and Wong 2008).

Two decades ago, Castledine (2001) suggested the introduction of levels of nursing, with level one commencing at registration, recognising the anticipated development of expertise as nurses develop through experience and education. A starting point to understanding the criteria associated with advanced nursing practice is the recognition that advanced nursing practice involves advanced nursing knowledge and skills (Hamric and Tracy 2019). This identifies the higher platform of expertise in both knowledge and skills related to advanced nursing practice. Dowling et al. (2013) identify what they describe as four attributes related to advanced nursing practice, which include clinical expertise, leadership, autonomy and role development. These overarching components identify the areas in which advanced knowledge and skills should be demonstrated.

Hamric and Tracy (2019) state that there is a growing consensus on the core competencies related to advanced practice nursing (these authors use this terminology rather than advanced nursing practice). This work significantly contributes to understanding the competencies related to advanced nursing practice by identifying seven core competencies. The first competency is central and relates to providing direct clinical practice. The additional six competencies are guidance and coaching, consultation, evidence-based practice, leadership, collaboration and ethical decision-making. An enhanced level of knowledge, skill, and expertise should be exercised within the seven competencies when practising at an advanced level. Although there have been attempts to provide transparency, practices related to advanced nursing are often invisible (Por 2008), providing a strong argument for the need for further clarification.

There have been attempts to clarify advanced nursing practice in different geographical locations from a policy and strategic perspective. In the context of Northern Ireland, an Advanced Nursing Practice Framework Department of Health, Social Services and Public Safety (2016) identifies four core competencies and also four components associated with advanced nursing practice. The four competencies are direct clinical practice, leadership and collaborative practice, education and learning, and research and evidence-based practice. The first of the four components relates to clinical practice and the scope of the role. This includes an ability to work autonomously, undertaking comprehensive health assessments; an ability to diagnosis, prescribing care and treatment; providing complex care; acting as an educator, leader and innovator; and contributing to research. The second component is a supervision requirement relevant to the area of practice. The third component is service improvement and an ability to influence policy development and lead service improvement initiatives. The final component relates to an education requirement: a masters-level qualification and completion of the Nursing and Midwifery recordable Non-Medical Prescribing V300 qualification.

Although these competencies and components are a very useful attempt at delineating advanced nursing practice, the specific level at which the nurse should demonstrate the four components is unclear. The identification of a specific level in this continuum in each of the components outlined by the Department of Health, Social Services and Public Safety (2016) would provide some further guidance on a flexible threshold for advanced nursing practice. Jamieson (2002) states that advanced practice could be considered part of a continuum with the development of expertise. This aligns with Benner's seminal work on the development of a taxonomy, first published in 1982 which is a model related to the stages of clinical competence. Five levels are identified, from level one, novice, to advanced beginner, competent, proficient and finally level five, expert (Benner 1984). This also supports Calkin's (1984) philosophy that nurses become experts through experience.

Despite the progression in achieving a level of clarity on the terminology of advanced nursing practice and the associated attributes and competencies, it continues to be poorly articulated (MacDonald et al. 2006), and conceptual confusion remains (Arslanian-Engoren 2019). Hamric and Tracy (2019) argue that full clarity on advanced practice nursing is yet to be achieved. *Advanced nursing practice* is a broad concept that captures nurses extending their practice through an expanded range of attributes and competencies with an advanced level of skills and knowledge. *Advanced-level nursing* is generic in that it applies to all clinical nurses working at an advanced level regardless of area of practice, setting or client group. It describes a level of practice, not a specialty or role that should be evident as being beyond that of first-level registration (Department of Health 2010; Hamric and Tracy 2019). In practice, this means nurses can demonstrate advanced nursing practice but not be in an APN role. The APN role will be explored in the next part of this chapter.

1.3.2 Advanced Practice Nurse Roles

Reviewing roles and responsibilities has provided opportunities for the nursing profession to create new roles (Por 2008) and improve efficiency in healthcare delivery (Delamaire and Lafortune 2010). 'An Advanced Practice Nurse (APN) is one who has acquired, through additional education, the expert knowledge base, complex decision-making skills and clinical competencies for expanded nursing practice, the characteristics of which are shaped by the context in which they are credentialed to practice' (ICN 2008, cited in ICN 2020, p. 9).

Similar to the rationale for the development of advanced nursing practice as a concept, the rationale for the development of advanced practice nursing roles includes changes in the developing health needs of society, advances in healthcare systems, government policy, workforce supply and advances in nurse education (Canada Nurses Association 2010). Chang et al. (2011) suggest that the APN role initially emerged to meet the evolving needs of healthcare. Delamaire and

Lafortune (2010) suggest that the rationale includes improving access to care, promoting higher quality of care, improvements in costs and enhancing career prospects. Woo et al. (2017) state that the APN role was introduced as a solution to the lack of primary care physicians and subsequently extended into other healthcare settings.

An estimated 40 countries have now established or are in the process of developing APN roles, with different timelines for the emergence of APN roles globally. These countries include Canada, the USA, Australia, New Zealand, the UK, Switzerland, Japan, Spain and Botswana (Oulton and Cardwell 2016). In the USA, APN roles emerged in the 1940s and are now well-established (MacDonald et al. 2006). These roles include nurse anaesthetists and nurse midwives. The first APN programme commenced in Australia in 1990 (Sheer and Wong 2008), and the development of advanced practice in the UK was pioneered in 1970s. However, it was 1990 when Barbara Stilwell led the establishment of the first advanced nursing practice course at the Royal College of Nursing Institute (Leary and MacLaine 2019).

Although APN roles have provided opportunities for nurses to develop their practice and improve patient care, there is confusion about the nomenclature related to advanced practice nursing roles (Gardner et al. 2009). Stasa et al. (2014) state that there is a lack of clarity on key terms related to advanced nursing positions, with Jokiniemi et al. (2021) stating 'the common feature in international literature on advanced practice nursing and its subroles, is ambiguity!' (p. 422). Internationally, a range of terms are used to describe advanced practice nursing roles, which is argued to have hindered developments in the roles (Dowling et al. 2013). There is an assumption that the term *advanced practice nurse* is homogenous, but in reality, it covers multiple roles (Ketefian et al. 2001).

Advanced practice nursing is associated with a range of titles (Por 2008). One study identified 13 titles beyond basic registered nurse titles (Pulcini et al. 2010); and an international study identified 52 different advanced practice nursing roles in 26 countries (Heale and Buckley 2015). WHO (2020) reported that 53% of countries that provided data for a report had advanced practice nursing roles, with the number of nurses holding advanced practice nursing positions increasing (Stasa et al. 2014). APNs can be generalists or specialists (Sheer and Wong 2008), as reflected in some of the following advanced practice nursing role titles: clinical nurse specialist, advanced nurse practitioner, nurse practitioner, higher level practitioner, nurse consultant, specialist practitioner, nurse therapist and physician's assistant (Daly and Carnwell 2003). There are four established advanced practice roles in the USA: certified registered nurse anaesthetist, certified nurse midwife, nurse practitioner and clinical nurse specialist (Hamric and Tracy 2019). Dowling et al. (2013) state that the two most common advanced practice roles are the clinical nurse specialist and nurse practitioner.

1.3.3 Regulation

There is wide variation in the regulation of APN roles globally (Heale and Buckley 2015). In the USA, an educational and regulatory framework is administered by the American Association of Nurse Practitioners (Leary and MacLaine 2019). A similar framework exists in Australia (Leary and MacLaine 2019). Guidance has been developed, but as yet there is no regulatory or legal framework for advanced practice in the UK (Leary and MacLaine 2019). As an example, the advanced nurse practitioner role is currently not regulated in the UK by the NMC, but this is currently under review (NMC 2020–2025). Although nursing is a regulated profession, advanced practice is not regulated in most countries globally, with the Republic of Ireland being in the minority in regulating advanced practice at a national level (Carney 2016).

1.3.4 Components of Advanced Practice Nurse Roles

Although the role responsibilities and components for each APN role vary, there is also a common identity (MacDonald et al. 2006). One commonality is that most APN roles involve direct patient care. Direct care in APN roles includes assessment, investigations, procedures, and counselling patients and families (Chang et al. 2011). Kleinpell et al. (2014) suggest eight global characteristics of an APN role: the right to diagnose, authority to prescribe medication, authority to prescribe treatment, authority to refer clients to other professionals, authority to admit patients to hospital, legislation to promote the role title, legislation or other forms of regulation mechanism specific to the role and recognition of the APN role. These universal components are a useful template for various countries in developing advanced nurse practice roles regarding education and clinical standards.

1.3.5 Education Requirements

Education is a crucial component in developing knowledge and skills related to APN roles and is often linked to regulation (Heale and Buckley 2015). In an international survey, 42 of 52 APN roles had a minimum level of education requirement; education requirements for each role varied widely (Heale and Buckley 2015) and differed across the globe. Hamric and Tracy (2019) state that all advanced practice registered nurse roles should require at least a master's education, and this is a requirement in many (but not all) countries. In Canada and the USA, each province or state is a separate jurisdiction for the regulation of nursing, resulting in a patchwork of legislations and regulations related to advanced nursing practice (MacDonald et al. 2006). The American Academy of Nurse Practitioners (2019) state that the entry-level qualification for nurse practitioners is the master's, post-master's or doctoral level. In the USA and Canada, nursing leaders have proposed a doctor of nursing practice as the entry level for APN roles (Apold 2008). In the UK, the Royal College of Nursing (RCN) state that advanced nurse practitioners should be educated to the masters level (RCN 2018). In summary, there appears to be a consensus that the minimum level of education required for an APN roles is a master's qualification; however, as countries are at different levels of development, this is currently not applied globally.

1.3.6 Outcomes Associated with Advanced Practice Nurse Roles

There are reported benefits associated with APNs in terms of safety, quality and efficiency to patients and services (Leary and MacLaine 2019). Engaging APN roles has the potential to improve access to care, promote higher quality of care and reduce waiting times (Delamaire and Lafortune 2010). Htay and Whitehead (2021) found that advanced nurse practitioners were associated with improved service provision outcomes such as improved patient satisfaction and reductions in waiting times and costs. Nurses in advanced practice in emergency and critical care improved the length of stay, time to consultation/treatment, mortality, patient satisfaction and cost savings (Woo et al. 2017).

A range of studies report on the outcomes associated with individual advanced nurse practice roles, such as an integrative review related to the role of the clinical nurse specialist in cancer care (Kerr et al. 2021). Positive outcomes were reported related to this role, including improvements in psychological support, information provision, symptom management, service coordination and patient satisfaction. However, there are challenges in measuring the outcomes associated with APN roles. This is due to team-based care being provided and collaborative models of care (Kapu et al. 2017), resulting in challenges in determining if the outcomes are attributed specifically to the APN role. A wide range of outcomes may potentially be impacted by the input of an APN role, and some of these outcome metrics measure patient's length of stay, costs of care, adverse events, patient and family knowledge, staff nurse knowledge, readmission rates and hand hygiene compliance (Kapu et al. 2017). It is the responsibility of organisations to ensure that these outcomes are measured and disseminated, as doing so will enhance public confidence in the investment in advanced nurse practice roles.

1.3.7 Barriers to Advanced Practice Nursing Roles

It is well-recognised that barriers exist to APNs practising to their full extent (Kleinpell et al. 2014). Heale and Buckley (2015) report on findings from an international survey of 38 countries, with most countries not reporting any barriers. However, for those that did report barriers, they related to physicians and medical organisations, legislative limitations, low nursing representation in policy development and lack of regulation. Delamaire and Lafortune (2010) report on four barriers that can also act as facilitators, which relate to professional interests such as potential opposition by the medical profession regarding the development of advanced nursing practice, the organisation of care and funding mechanisms, the impact of legislation and regulation of health professional activities on the development of new roles and the capacity of the education and training system to provide nurses with higher skills. Barriers to APNs practising to their full potential can have a significant negative impact on health services (Heale and Buckley 2015). Kleinpell et al. (2014) suggest approaches to overcoming barriers that include communicating the value of the role to stakeholders, including patients; media campaigns on the role in patient care; lobbying to change restrictive APN role regulations; demonstrating the outcomes related to the role; and disseminating exemplars of collaborative models of quality and safety improvements.

1.3.8 Recommendations for Advanced Practice Nurse Roles

There have been attempts to develop a universal standard for advanced practice nursing roles; however, doing so is challenging due to the geographical variations that influence these roles, such as policy development, legislation, regulation and healthcare demands. Chang et al. (2011) identify that a contextually appropriate framework for APNs should be the goal of healthcare organisations. Bryant-Lukosius and DiCenso (2004) provide a useful participatory, evidence-informed, patient-centred process for advanced nursing practice role development, implementation and evaluation (the PEPPA framework). This framework aims to overcome barriers to role implementation through knowledge and understanding of the roles and environments and outlines nine steps to assess, prepare, introduce and evaluate advanced nursing practice roles. A universal framework such as PEPPA can be modified to incorporate contextual variations.

1.4 Conclusion

Healthcare demands will continue to rise due to the ageing population and global epidemic of chronic disease. To respond to the changing health needs of the population, the demand for nursing will likely require a range of generic and specialist skills (Holloway et al. 2009). There continues to be support for nurses advancing their practice beyond initial registration (Dowling et al. 2013) and a growing demand for advanced practice nursing roles (Bryant-Lukosius and DiCenso 2004).

This is due to the need for expert nurses working at an advanced level of practice (Kleinpell et al. 2014). APNs can add value, increase access to healthcare and strengthen the workforce (Woo et al. 2017).

The emergence of advanced nursing practice worldwide and the introduction of APN roles such as the clinical nurse specialist and nurse practitioner have resulted in robust discussions attempting to identify the distinguishing characteristics of these new roles and levels of nursing practice (ICN 2020). There is abundant literature on advancing nursing practice, much of which highlights the ongoing confusion regarding the definitions and terminologies used. Despite the plethora of literature, the debate continues on clarifying advancing nursing practice and APN roles. Calkin (1984) stated almost 40 years ago that there was a lack of a simple definition for advanced practice nursing, and only in 2020 did the ICN provided guidelines for advanced practice nursing to unlock this stalemate.

There has been debate on the key issues related to advanced nursing practice, such as minimum education requirements and levels of practice; however, it is recognised that geographical variations must be considered, so a universal template may not be appropriate. The guidelines published by the ICN (2020) provide standards for advanced nursing practice, offering a universal guide for countries to consider. This will take time and involve an investment in the nursing profession with regard to developing nurses to a higher level of skills and knowledge and an advanced level of practice and autonomy. APN roles elevate the level of care provided to patients and can improve patient outcomes. They also provides opportunities for career progression for nurses. One of the valuable APN roles that contributes is the clinical nurse specialist role, which is the focus of Chapter 2.

References

American Academy of Nurse Practitioners. (2019). Discussion paper: scope of practice for nurse practitioners. https://www.aanp.org/advocacy/advocacy-resource/position-statements/scope-of-practice-for-nurse-practitioners (accessed 16 September 2022).

American Association of Colleges of Nursing. (2004). Position statement on the practice doctorate in nursing.

Apold, S. (2008). The doctor of nursing practice: looking back, moving forward. *Journal for Nurse Practitioners* 42: 101–107.

Arslanian-Engoren, C. (2019). Conceptualizations of advanced practice nursing. In: *Hamric and Hanson's Advanced Practice Nursing: An Integrative Approach*, 6e (ed. M.F. Tracy and E.T. O'Grady), 25–61. Missouri: Elsevier, Chapter 2.

Barton, T.D. (2012). The development of advanced nursing roles. *Nursing Times* 108 (24): 18–20.

Benner, P. (1984). *From Novice to Expert: Excellence and Power in Clinical Nursing Pratice*. Menlo Part, CA: Addison-Wesley Publishing.

Bryant-Lukosius, D. and DiCenso, A. (2004). A framework for the introduction and evaluation of advanced practice nursing roles. *Journal of Advanced Nursing* 48 (5): 530–540.

Calkin, J.D. (1984). A model for advanced nursing practice. *Journal of Nursing Administration* 14: 24–30.

Callaghan, L. (2008). Advanced nursing practice: an idea whose time has come. *Journal of Clinical Nursing* 17: 205–213.

Canadian Nurses Association. (2010). Canadian nurse practitioner core competency framework. https://www.cno.org/globalassets/for/rnec/pdf/competencyframework_en.pdf (accessed 16 September 2022).

Carney, M. (2016). Regulation of advanced nurse practice: its existence and regulatory dimensions from an international perspective. *Journal of Nursing Management* 24: 105–114.

Castledine, G. (2001). Can we standardize titles and levels of nursing? *British Journal of Nursing* 10 (13): 891.

Chang, A.M., Gardner, G.E., Duffield, C., and Ramis, M.A. (2011). Advanced practice nursing role development: factor analysis of a modified role delineation tool. *Journal of Advanced Nursing* 68 (6): 1368–1379.

Daly, W.M. and Carnwell, R. (2003). Nursing roles and levels of practice: a framework for differentiating between elementary, specialist and advancing nursing practice. *Journal of Clinical Nursing* 12: 158–167.

Delamaire, M. and Lafortune, G. (2010). Nurses in advanced roles: a description and evaluation of experience in 12 developed countries. OECD Health Working Papers, no. 54. https://doi.org/10.1787/5kmbrcfms5g7-en.

Department of Health. (2010). Advanced level nursing: a position statement. https://www.gov.uk/government/publications/advanced-level-nursing-a-position-statement (accessed 16 September 2022).

Department of Health, Social Services and Public Safety (2016). *Advanced Nursing Practice Framework*. Northern Ireland: DHSSPS.

Dowling, M., Beauchesne, M., Farrelly, F., and Murphy, K. (2013). Advanced practice nursing: a concept analysis. *International Journal of Nursing Practice* 19: 131–140.

East, L., Knowles, K., Pettman, M., and Fisher, L. (2015). Advanced level nursing in England: organisation challenges and opportunities. *Journal of Nursing Management* 23: 1011–1019.

Gardner, G., Chang, A., and Duffield, C. (2009). Making nursing work: breaking through the role confusion of advanced practice nursing. *Journal of Advanced Nursing* 57 (4): 382–391.

Glasper, A. and Carpenter, D. (2019). Celebrating 100 years of nurse regulation. *British Journal of Nursing* 28 (22): 1490–1491.

Hamric, A.B. and Tracy, M.G. (2019). A definition of advanced practice nursing. In: *Hamric and Hanson's Advanced Practice Nursing: An Integrative Approach*, 6e (ed. M.F. Tracy and E.T. O'Grady), 202–251. Missouri: Elsevier.

Heale, R. and Buckley, C. (2015). An international perspective of advanced practice nursing regulation. *International Nursing Review* 62: 421–429.

Holloway, K., Baker, J., and Lumby, J. (2009). Specialist nursing framework for New Zealand: a missing link in workforce planning. *Policy Politics and Nursing Practice* 10 (4): 269–275.

Htay, M. and Whitehead, D. (2021). The effectiveness of the role of advanced nurse practitioners compared to physician led or usual care: a systematic review. *International Journal of Nursing Studies* 3: 1–22.

International Council of Nurses (ICN). (2008). The scope of practice, standards and competencies of the advanced practice nurse. Monograph, ICN Regulation Series.

International Council of Nurses (ICN) (2020). *Guidelines on Advanced Practice Nursing*. Geneva: ICN.

Jamieson, L. (2002). Confusion prevails in defining 'advanced' nursing practice. *Collegian* 9 (4): 29–33.

Jokiniemi, K., Korhonen, K., Karkkainen, A. et al. (2021). Clinical nurse specialist role implementation structures, processes and outcomes: participatory action research. *Journal of Clinical Nursing* 30: 2222–2233.

Kapu, A.N., Sicoutris, C., Broyhill, B.S. et al. (2017). Measuring outcomes in advanced practice nursing: practice-specific quality metrics. In: *Outcome Assessment in Advanced Practice Nursing*, 4e (ed. R.M. Kleinpell). New York: Springer Publishing Company.

Kerr, H., Donovan, M., and McSorley, O. (2021). Evaluation of the role of the clinical nurse specialist in cancer care: an integrative literature review. *European Journal of Cancer Care* 30 (3): 1–13.

Ketefian, S., Redman, R.W., Hanucharurnkul, S. et al. (2001). The development of advanced practice roles: implications in the international nursing community. *International Nursing Review* 48: 153–163.

Kleinpell, R., Scanlon, A., Hibbert, D. et al. (2014). Addressing issues impacting advanced nursing practice worldwide. *The Online Journal of Issues in Nursing* 19 (2): 5.

Leary, A. and MacLaine, K. (2019). The evolution of advanced nursing practice: past, present and future. *Nursing Times* 115 (11): 18–19.

MacDonald, J.A., Herbert, R., and Thibeault, C. (2006). Advanced practice nursing: unification through a common identity. *Journal of Professional Nursing* 22 (3): 172–179.

National Council of State Bodies of Nursing (2020). A global profile of nursing regulation, education, and practice. *The Journal of Nursing Regulation* 10: 1–116.

Nursing and Midwifery Council (2020–2025). *Strategy 2020–2025: Consultation of Draft Strategic Themes*. London: NMC.

Oulton, J.A. and Cardwell, P. (2016). Nurses. In: *International Encyclopaedia of Public Health*, 2e (ed. W.C. Cockerham). USA: Elsevier.

Por, J. (2008). A critical engagement with the concept of advanced nursing practice. *Journal of Nursing Management* 16: 84–90.

Pulcini, J., Jelic, M., Gul, R., and Yuen Loke, A. (2010). An international survey on advanced practice nurse education, practice and regulation. *Journal of Nursing Scholarship* 42 (1): 31–39.

Registered Nurses Association of British Columbia (2001). RNABC policy statement advanced nursing practice. *Nursing BC* 33 (5): 10–12.

Royal College of Nursing (2018). *Advanced Level Nursing Practice: Introduction.* London: Royal College of Nursing.

Sheer, B. and Wong, F.K.Y. (2008). The development of advanced nursing practice globally. *Journal of Nursing Scholarship* 40 (3): 204–211.

Stasa, H., Cashin, A., Buckley, T., and Donoghue, J. (2014). Advancing advanced practice – clarifying the conceptual confusion. *Nurse Education Today* 34: 356–361.

Stievano, A., Caruso, R., Pittella, F. et al. (2019). Shaping nursing profession regulation through history – a systematic review. *International Nursing Review* 66: 17–29.

Wilson, K. (2005). The evolution of the role of nurses: the history of nurse practitioners in pediatric oncology. *Journal of Pediatric Oncology Nursing* 22 (5): 250–253.

Woo, B.F.Y., Lee, J.X.Y., and Tam, W.W.S. (2017). The impact of the advanced practice nursing role of quality of care, clinical outcomes, patient satisfaction, and cost in the emergency and critical care settings: a systematic review. *Human Resources for Health* 15 (63): 1–22.

World Health Organisation (2020). *State of the World's Nursing 2020: Investing in Education, Jobs and Leadership.* Geneva: WHO.

2

Emergence and Evolvement of the Clinical Nurse Specialist Role in Cancer Care

Helen Kerr

Abstract

This chapter focuses on the emergence and evolvement of the clinical nurse specialist role. It commences by setting the context of how this role emerged as one of the advanced practice nurse roles outlined in Chapter 1. The components of the clinical nurse specialist role will be provided, highlighting geographical variations. There will be a discussion of recommendations with regards to educational requirements. Outcomes associated with this role will be outlined. Content will be highlighted related to the components of the role in cancer nursing, which provides the foundation for subsequent chapters.

2.1 Introduction

This chapter will focus on the emergence and evolvement of the clinical nurse specialist (CNS) role and the importance of establishing an identity and professional standards. The components of the role from a policy and practice perspective will be outlined, highlighting global variations. The components of the role will be discussed and outcomes associated with the role identified, along with a brief overview of recommendations for future developments of the role.

2.2 Advanced Nursing Practice

Chapter 1 focused on the development of advanced nursing practice and advanced practice nurse (APN) roles, but a brief overview will be provided here to set the context for the emergence of the CNS role. From nursing's inception as a profession, it has been continually evaluated in response to health, societal and person-centred care challenges (International Council of Nurses [ICN] 2020). One aspect of the evaluation is the growing global interest in extending nursing practice beyond the level of initial registration (East et al. 2015). Advanced nursing practice is 'an umbrella term describing an advanced level of clinical nursing practice that maximizes the use of graduate educational preparation, in-depth nursing knowledge and expertise in meeting the health needs of individuals, families, groups, communities and populations' (Canadian Nurses Association 2010, p. 14, cited in Oulton and Caldwell 2017). One component of advanced nursing practice is the evolvement of APN roles. 'An Advanced Practice Nurse is one who has acquired, through additional education, the expert knowledge base, complex decision-making skills and clinical competencies for expanded nursing practice, the characteristics of which are shaped by the context in which they are credentialed to practice' (ICN 2008, cited in ICN 2020, p. 9).

APN titles vary in countries around the globe (Delamaire and Lafortune 2010). One study identified 52 APN roles in 26 countries (Heale and Buckley 2015), with an increasing number of these roles being highlighted (Maier et al. 2017). Some of the APN role titles include the CNS, advanced nurse practitioner, nurse practitioner (NP), higher level practitioner, nurse consultant, specialist practitioner, nurse therapist and physician's assistant (Daly and Carnwell 2003). Dowling et al. (2013) state that the two most common advanced practice roles are the CNS and NP, the former being the focus of this chapter.

2.3 Historical Context

The CNS role is said to date back to the 1940s (LaSala et al. 2007; Lewandowski and Adamle 2009) and was motivated by the growth of hospitals in the 1940s, advances in medical specialists (ICN 2020) and an identified need for speciality practices (Lusk et al. 2019). The CNS role subsequently developed in the second half of the twentieth century (Ketefian et al. 2001), with the psychiatric CNS, nurse anaesthetists and nurse midwives leading the way (Lusk et al. 2019; ICN 2020).

The CNS role was introduced at various time points in different countries. In the USA, the CNS role was introduced in the 1960s (Jokiniemi et al. 2021), and in Canada, the CNS role first emerged in the 1970s (ICN 2020). In the UK, the specialist nurse was reported to be developed in the 1970s (Castledine 2002).

From its inception in the mid-twentieth century, the CNS role has continued to develop in response to population healthcare needs and environments (ICN 2020) and is now well integrated into healthcare services (Cannaby et al. 2020). Whilst the CNS role was originally introduced in hospitals (Delamaire and LaFortune 2010), it has evolved to provide specialised care for patients with complex and chronic conditions in outpatients, emergency departments, home and community settings and long-term care settings (Kilpatrick et al. 2013; Bryant-Lukosius and Wong 2019). The CNS role is now recognised internationally (Kaasalaimen et al. 2010) and embedded in healthcare services in many European countries, Asia, Canada and the USA, with other countries beginning to develop the role (Fulton 2018). Lewandowski and Adamle (2009) state that the evolvement of the CNS role has been one of the most important developments in nursing and is argued to be one of the successes of modern healthcare (Smy et al. 2011). There is increasing enthusiasm for advanced practice nurse roles such as the CNS (ICN 2020), and CNSs are now recognising their own value to the nursing workforce (Bamford and Gibson 2000).

2.4   Specialists vs. Generalists

APN roles can be categorised as either generalists or specialists. Advanced-level practitioners who are generalists provide care to patients at any age with a range of healthcare needs (Royal College of Nursing [RCN] 2018). One example of an APN role that is considered more generalist is the NP (Barton 2012). NPs are generalist nurses who, after additional education at a minimum of a master's degree, are autonomous clinicians who diagnose and treat conditions (ICN 2020).

'Specialisation involves the development of expanded knowledge and skills in a selected area' in nursing (Hamric and Tracy 2019, p. 206). The term *specialist* in nursing can be traced back to the turn of the twentieth century (Doody and Bailey 2011; Lusk et al. 2019), with the beginnings of specialism associated with Florence Nightingale early in the 1900s when she taught women how to deliver care to wounded soldiers during the Crimean War (Lewandowski and Adamle 2009). Specialisation is, therefore, not a modern phenomenon, as it was recognised that patient groups and settings require practitioners with specialised knowledge and skills (Oulton and Caldwell 2017). Kaasalaimen et al. (2010) state that the term *specialist* was initially used to describe what is now known as the CNS.

Generalised preparation is considered to provide the foundation of a specialist role in nursing (Oulton and Caldwell 2017), and nurses can then progress from a generalist nurse to a specialist nurse through appropriate programmes of education. However, there is a difference between a nurse working in a specialty and a specialist nurse (ICN 2020). Although nurses who practice in various specialties may consider themselves to be specialised nurses, the designated CNS has an advanced-level clinical specialty focus (ICN 2020). As a result, the CNS has additional in-depth knowledge and critical thinking and decision-making skills that provide the foundation for an advanced level of practice and decision-making (ICN 2020).

2.5   Definition of a CNS

CNSs have advanced knowledge of a specific practice area (Doody and Bailey 2011), so their strength is in providing complex specialised care (ICN 2020). Back in 1986, Anderson and Hicks offered a simple definition of a CNS as an 'expert clinical practitioner in a specialised area of nursing' (1986, p. 36). More recently, the Canadian Nurses Association (2021) state that a CNS is a registered nurse with advanced nursing knowledge and skills who makes complex decisions and has expertise in a clinical nursing specialty. The ICN (2020) recently provided a definition of a CNS as 'an Advanced Practice Nurse who provides expert clinical advice and care based on established diagnoses in specialised clinical fields of practice along with a systems approach in practicing as a member of the healthcare team' (p. 6). In its regional guide for the development of specialised nursing practice, the World Health Organization Eastern Mediterranean Regional Office (WHO-EMRO) provides the following definition: 'A specialist nurse holds a current license as a generalist nurse, and has successfully completed an education programme that meets the prescribed standard for specialist nursing practice. The specialist nurse is authorised to function within a defined scope of practice in a specified field of nursing' (2018, p. 7, cited in ICN 2020). These definitions highlight that the CNS has advanced knowledge and skills and specialises in an area of nursing.

2.5.1   Role Blurring

There have been challenges in determining the definitive characteristics of the CNS role and the distinctions with other APN roles, particularly the NP. To provide clarity, the ICN (2020) have published information identifying both the similarities and differences between the CNS and NP. Some of the similarities relate to a recommendation that both roles have a master's degree as a minimum educational qualification, have a generalised nursing qualification, and are recognised through a system of credentialing. Both are also autonomous and accountable to an advanced level. Differences highlighted relate to the CNS having an identified specialty, where the NP is considered more generalist; the CNS provides direct and indirect care to patients with an established diagnosis, whereas the NP provides direct clinical care to patients with undiagnosed conditions in addition to providing ongoing care to those with an established diagnosis; the CNS frequently shares clinical responsibility with other healthcare professionals, and the NP assumes full clinical responsibility for the management of their patient population; the CNS may or may not have some level of prescribing, with the NP commonly having prescribing authority; and the CNS evaluates patient outcomes to identify and influence system clinical improvements, in comparison to the NP, who frequently has the authority to refer and admit patients (ICN 2020). Although there are variations, the CNS is reported to be more commonly based in a hospital or healthcare institution, whereas the NP is more commonly based in primary care (Delamaire and Lafortune 2010), although there are geographical variations.

A recent national study comparing CNSs and NPs in Canada demonstrated that while there are many common features, the main differences between the CNS and NP are related to the CNS having a greater involvement in nonclinical (indirect) activities related to the support of systems, education, publications and professional leadership and research (Bryant-Lukosius et al. 2010). Involvement in direct clinical care was high for both the CNS and NP, but differences in scope of practice were reflected in greater NP involvement in diagnosing, prescribing and treating various conditions or illnesses. Similar to these findings, additional studies highlight that NPs engage in direct care activities to a greater extent than CNSs (Donald et al. 2010; Carryer et al. 2018); however, there may be variations across the globe.

2.6 Components of the Clinical Nurse Specialist Role

Back in 2000, Bamford and Gibson stated that elucidating the components of the CNS role continues to be an area of debate (Bamford and Gibson 2000); however, over the past two decades, clarity has been provided. Broadly, it is accepted that the CNS is an expert clinician in a specialty that may be defined by population, disease or type of problem (ICN 2020). The strength of the CNS role is in providing complex specialty care (ICN 2020).

The role of the CNS is considered to be multifaceted (Bamford and Gibson 2000). The Canadian Nurses Association (2016) state there are four components of the CNS role, relating to clinical care, system leadership, advancements of nursing practice and evaluation and research. Bamford and Gibson (2000) suggest similar components, which align to the clinical component: researcher, educator and consultant. Schreiber et al. (2005) identified multiple components to the CNS role, including direct care, coordination of care, education, policy and programme development, administration, leadership, research and consultation. A review of the literature with papers representing 10 countries identified three substantive areas related to the CNS role, including managing the care of complex and/or vulnerable populations, educating and supporting interdisciplinary staff and facilitating innovation and change within healthcare systems (Lewandowski and Adamle 2009). Donald et al. (2010) outline the CNS's primary responsibilities, including clinical practice, consultation, education, research and leadership. RCN (2010) found five components to the CNS role; these included the clinical component, accounting for 67% of the role; administration, accounting for 21%; educational accounting, 6%; research accounting, 4%; and consultation, 2%.

In the cancer healthcare environment, an integrative literature review identified four components to the CNS role: providing psychological support, information provision, symptom management and service coordination (Kerr et al. 2021). Additional components not identified in the papers in this literature review were suggested by these authors to be invisible components of the role, such as involvement in research activities.

Although there are variations in the role of the CNS (Doody and Bailey 2011), the components of the role can be categorised into direct and indirect care, with some possible overlap in these categories. Direct care relates to the clinical and/or practitioner component and involves interaction and care of patients, families and groups (ICN 2020). Indirect care is provided through education, consultation and collaboration with the multidisciplinary team, facilitating change and innovation in healthcare systems (Lewandowski and Adamle 2009), leadership in the use of research and evidence, directing programmes of care and evaluating patient outcomes (ICN 2020).

2.6.1 Direct Patient Care

First and foremost, the CNS is a clinician who provides direct care in a specialist area of nursing (ICN 2020). The CNS role provides an advanced level of clinical practice that requires expert knowledge, skills and competencies (Kilpatrick et al. 2013) and critical thinking and decision-making skills (ICN 2020). The scope of practice reflects a sophisticated core body of practical, theoretical and empirical nursing and healthcare knowledge. The role may involve health promotion, risk reduction, management of symptoms and functional problems, and it may include diagnosis and treatment of disease. However, an interesting finding by Bryant-Lukosius et al. (2010) stated that the CNS role has limited involvement in direct patient care, with the exception of cancer and palliative care contexts. Norton et al. (2012) reported that 62% of the CNS's time is spent in clinical practice activities; whilst Leary et al. (2008) found that 48% of the CNS's time was on clinical activities, with the remaining time on indirect activities such as administration, education and research activities, again highlighting a variability.

2.6.2 Indirect Care

Indirect care is also a component of the CNS role. Holloway et al. (2009) suggest that the CNS has a role in clinical leadership (leadership is the focus of Chapter 10 of this book). Kilpatrick et al. (2013) also highlight that the CNS has knowledge, skills and competencies related to leadership. One of the roles the CNS often occupies is that of a key worker (Cannaby et al. 2020). The key worker role requires leadership skills and overlaps with direct clinical care. CNSs also have a crucial role in the functioning of multidisciplinary teams (LaSala et al. 2007; Vidall et al. 2011; ICN 2020), advocating for patients in team meetings and contributing to recommendations for patient care.

An additional component of the CNS role is involvement in educating patients, carers, and staff, which relates to direct and indirect care. CNSs are considered leaders in advancing nursing practice through their teaching role and ensuring that nursing practice is evidence-based (ICN 2020). Bryant-Lukosius and Martin-Misener (2016) state that the CNS role has responsibilities for nonclinical work, which includes education, highlighting the importance of this component in supporting colleagues in their care of patients and their families.

The CNS role also involves leading and supporting nurses to provide evidence-based care and translate research evidence into practice, and may involve conducting research. This component of the role is further explored in Chapter 7. CNSs have expert knowledge, skills and competencies related to a range of components, including being a researcher (Kilpatrick et al. 2013). However, the research component can be the most challenging to implement (Bamford and Gibson 2000) and can be overlooked (Doody and Bailey 2011). As previously outlined, Kerr et al. (2021) suggested that research involvement is an invisible component of the CNS role in cancer services.

Despite these attempts to clarify the components of the CNS role, the RCN (2010) stated that this is the least well understood or articulated of all the APN roles. Nurses and healthcare professionals are also reported to lack an understanding of the CNS role (Lewandowski and Adamle 2009). This may be because CNSs are a diverse group (Glen and Waddington 1998) with wide variations related to the role (Bamford and Gibson 2000).

The CNS role has evolved, but challenges are reported with regards to fulfilling all of the components. Barriers include time constraints and a lack of resources (North West Cancer Alliances and Health Education England 2021). Kilpatrick et al. (2013) also report a lack of time as a barrier to the role, in addition to multiple job expectations and a lack of administrative support.

2.7 Professional Standards

A professional standard defines the boundaries and essential elements of practice and connects the CNS to the expected quality and competence for the role or level of practice by describing the required components of care. The CNS is responsible for meeting the standard or defined competencies for advanced practice (ICN 2020). In the context of the UK, the professional standards have been delineated by the Nursing and Midwifery Council (NMC), the UK nursing and midwifery professional body (NMC 2001). A specialist practitioner holds an NMC-recordable qualification with skills and attributes involving exercising higher levels of judgement, discretion and decision-making in clinical care in four domains (NMC 2001): clinical practice, care and programme management, clinical practice development and clinical practice leadership. There is no national framework for specialist nursing practice (Holloway et al. 2009), so there is no one-size-fits-all, and there are geographical variations. A framework cannot be prescriptive; rather, each country must consider the contextual variations affecting nursing and healthcare (Hancock 2004). However, ICN (2020) state that recognition to practice as a CNS requires submission of evidence to an authoritative credentialing body on completion of a master's or doctoral degree programme from an accredited school or department of nursing. Continuing authority to practice also depends on the renewal of the generalist nursing licence and all appropriate professional regulations for CNS practice in the relevant country.

2.8 Education Requirements

ICN (2020) outline the progression pathway from a generalist nurse to a specialist nurse, which is suggested to include a master's degree programme. There is a broad consensus that to fulfil the role of CNS, a master's level qualification is required (ICN 2020; Martin-Misener et al. 2010), with some suggestions that a doctoral qualification may be required in the future (ICN 2020). Completion of a minimum of a master's degree provides enhanced professional credibility as well as clinical credibility for nurses who progress and distinguish themselves as CNSs (ICN 2020). It is further recommended that the programme of study should be specific to the role of the CNS from an accredited school/university or department of nursing (ICN 2020). However, despite attempts to provide guidance on educational requirements for the CNS role, there are variations across the globe (Delamaire and Lafortune 2010), with an acknowledgement that for some countries, the requirement of a master's degree may be aspirational as they aim for this standard (ICN 2020). It is also reported that the qualification required for a CNS may vary at the employer's discretion (Carryer et al. 2018). Kilpatrick et al. (2013) reported results from a survey indicating that 65% of CNSs held a master's level qualification in Canada. In New Zealand, 42.7% of CNSs reported in a national survey that they had a master's degree (Carryer et al. 2018); and in the UK, it is reported that most CNS are not educated to the master's level (Cannaby et al. 2020).

2.8.1 Impact of a Master's Qualification

Canadian studies have demonstrated that self-identified CNSs who had completed a master's degree were more likely to implement all domains of advanced nursing practice than those who were not prepared at the master's level (Schreiber et al. 2005; Kilpatrick et al. 2013). ICN (2020) state that the rationale for the recommended master's level qualification is that it will further assure quality of care for diverse populations and contribute to delivering optimum safe healthcare by enhancing academic rigour, scientific reasoning and critical thinking. It will also contribute to teaching and supporting other nurses and healthcare professionals in complex clinical situations. The educational programme prepares the CNS to use and integrate research into clinical practice, regardless of setting or patient population. It also enhances professional and clinical credibility (ICN 2020). This aligns with research completed by Kerr et al. (2022), which reported that the specialist practice qualification recommended for nurses with a 'specialist' title in their role in the context of Northern Ireland enhanced nurses' professional credibility.

2.9 Outcomes of the Clinical Nurse Specialist Role

The CNS is reported to contribute to improvements in outcomes. LaSala et al. (2007) stated that the CNS contributed to improvements in the quality of life for patients with links between practice and evidence-based outcomes. Quality of life improvements are also reported by Begley et al. (2012), in addition to improved service user satisfaction related to their physical care, emotional support and practice advice. Kilpatrick et al. (2013) also reported that CNSs perceived that they influenced patient satisfaction, comfort level, quality of life and patient and family knowledge. A systematic literature review indicated that telephone contact by specialist nurses had positive results regarding communication with patients (Cook et al. 2015).

Further improvements in outcomes relate to a reduction in medication errors with the involvement of CNSs in hospital wards and operating rooms (Flanders and Clark 2010). Service user satisfaction with physical care, emotional support or practical advice was reported to be high for CNSs in a study in Ireland (Begley et al. 2012). Reduced resource usage and greater cost-effectiveness related to the role of the CNS in an outpatient setting have also been reported (Kilpatrick et al. 2014).

Bryant et al. (2015a) report on a wide range of positive outcomes associated with the CNS role. CNS care delayed time to and reduced hospitalisation, improved treatment adherence and patient satisfaction, and reduced cost and length of re-hospitalised stays for individuals with heart failure. For elderly patients and caregivers, CNS care improved caregiver depression and reduced re-hospitalisation, in addition to re-hospitalisation length of stay and costs. For high-risk pregnant women and very-low-birth-weight infants, CNS care improved infant immunisation rates and maternal satisfaction with care and reduced maternity and infant length of hospital stay and costs

(Bryant et al. 2015a). The Canadian Centre for Advanced Practice Nursing Research (CCAPNR) (2012) reported a range of positive outcomes related to the CNS role, including improved access to care for patients; reduced mortality for individuals with acute or chronic conditions; improved quality of life; lower complication rates; improved physical, functional and psychological well-being; reduced hospital admission and visits to the emergency department; and shortened hospital lengths of stay.

2.9.1 Outcomes Associated with the Clinical Nurse Specialist in Cancer Services

In the context of cancer care, Alessy et al. (2021) state that the CNS has a crucial role in improving patients' experiences across the care pathway related to better experiences, involvement in treatment decisions, care coordination and being cared for with more respect and dignity. Bryant-Lukosius et al. (2015b) reported a range of positive outcomes with the involvement of a CNS for individuals with breast cancer and colorectal cancer across the cancer trajectory. These included CNS-led care being an appropriate model of care provided by physicians for newly diagnosed patients undergoing surgery and radiation therapy. It was also reported that the addition of the CNS may improve psychological well-being and survival for individuals with a new diagnosis of cancer who are post-surgery or receiving radiotherapy or chemotherapy (Bryant et al. 2015b). In an integrative literature review, Kerr et al. (2021) reported positive outcomes of the CNS role in cancer care related to psychological outcomes for patients, improved patient satisfaction, improvements in patient knowledge, and enhanced clinical outcomes, particularly in relation to symptom management and service delivery outcomes such as increased access to services. The CNS role in cancer care was also reported to contribute to cost-effectiveness (Kerr et al. 2021).

There is increasing evidence of the positive outcomes related to the role of the CNS; however, Jokiniemi et al. (2021) state that the CNS role's effects could be further increased by optimising CNS competence. This could be partly achieved by nurses being more proactive in articulating the added contributions of CNSs (Bryant-Lukosius and Martin-Misener 2016), challenging the view that the CNS role is an unaffordable luxury (Vidall et al. 2011). Vidall et al. (2011) also suggest that the benefits of the CNS role are not always realised, and the role is sometimes viewed as an unaffordable luxury. There are challenges to demonstrating the effectiveness of the CNS role due to the multifaceted nature of the position. This has led to challenges in understanding the CNS role's impact on clinical outcomes (Chan and Cartwright 2014). Despite this ambiguity, there is growing evidence of the impact of the CNS role; however, securing evidence to demonstrate the effectiveness of the CNS role remains crucial (Vidall et al. 2011).

2.10   Specialist Practice in Cancer Care

The number of CNSs in cancer care is increasing (National Cancer Action Team 2011). CNSs in cancer care are key contacts for patients, providing support and addressing questions (North West Cancer Alliances and Health Education England 2021). They often occupy a key worker role, a recommendation from the National Institute for Clinical Excellence (NICE 2004) and the focus of Chapter 5 in this book. The RCN developed a Career Pathway and Education Framework for Cancer Nursing in 2017 (RCN 2017); it was updated in 2022 to guide nurses on the knowledge and skills for cancer nursing. The European Oncology Nursing Society (EONS) have published a Cancer Nursing Curriculum with eight modules outlining the knowledge and skills for post-registration nurses to acquire if working in the cancer setting.

2.11   Future Direction of the CNS

From an international perspective, the ICN (2020) recommend continuing to promote clarity of the CNS practice to identify how these nurses contribute to the delivery of healthcare services and guide the development of educational curricula specific to the CNS. From a European perspective, the European Specialist Nurses Organisation (ESNO 2015) recommend the development of competencies for the CNS to clarify the position and practice of the role. The identification of consistent qualifications will enable the CNS to move easily within the member states of Europe.

The ICN (2020) have recently published guidance on the components of the CNS role in an attempt to provide continuity, suggesting minimum standards and enabling the movement of nurses to work in other countries. To develop an understanding of the CNS role, the ICN (2020) have suggested a requirement for title protection, a minimum master's degree and an identifiable scope of practice as part of a credentialing process. Chapter 16 of this book is dedicated to the future direction of the CNS in cancer services, providing insights into how this role can continue to respond to health and population needs.

2.12   Conclusion

This chapter has broadly outlined the evolvement of the CNS role, identifying contextual variations across the globe. The CNS role has developed over time, becoming more flexible and responsive to population healthcare needs and environments. The fundamental strength of the CNS role is in providing complex specialty care while improving the quality of healthcare delivery through a systems approach. The multifaceted CNS profile, in addition to direct patient care in a clinical specialty, also includes indirect components such as education, research and support of other nurses and the members of the multidisciplinary team. The role provides leadership to specialty practice programme development and facilitates change and innovation in healthcare systems (Lewandowski and Adamle 2009). The components of the CNS role identified in this chapter will be the focus of subsequent chapters in this book, with an exploration that provides insights into how the role can develop.

References

Alessy, S.A., Luchtenborg, M., Rawlinson, J. et al. (2021). Being assigned a clinical nurse specialist is associated with better experiences of cancer care: English population-based study using the linked National Cancer Patient Experience Survey and cancer registration dataset. *European Journal of Cancer Care* 30: 1–11.

Anderson, B. and Hicks, S. (1986). The clinical nurse specialist: role, overview and future prospects. *The Australian Nurses Journal* 15: 36–38.

Bamford, O. and Gibson, F. (2000). The clinical nurse specialist: perceptions of practising CNSs of their role and development needs. *Journal of Clinical Nursing* 9: 282–292.

Barton, T.D. (2012). The development of advanced nursing roles. *Nursing Times* 108 (24): 18–20.

Begley, C., Elliott, N., Lalor, J. et al. (2012). Differences between clinical specialist and advanced practitioner clinical practice, leadership and research roles, responsibilities, and perceived outcomes (the SCAPE study). *Journal of Advanced Nursing* 69 (6): 1323–1337.

Bryant-Lukois, D., Carter, C., Kilpatrick, K. et al. (2010). The clinical nurse specialist role in Canada. *Journal of Evaluation of Clinical Practice* 21: 140–166.

Bryant-Lukosius, D. and Martin-Misener, R. (2016). *ICN Policy Brief Advanced Practice Nursing: An Essential Component of Country Level Human Resources for Health*. Geneva: ICN.

Bryant-Lukosius, D. and Wong, F.K.Y. (2019). International development of advanced practice nursing. In: *Advanced Practice Nursing: An Integrative Approach*, 6e (ed. M.F. Tracy and E.T. O'Grady), 129–141. St. Louis, Missouri: Elsevier.

Bryant-Lukosius, D., Carter, N., Reid, K. et al. (2015a). The clinical effectiveness and cost-effectiveness of Clinical Nurse Specialist-led hospital to home transitional care: a systematic review. *Journal of Evaluation of Clinical Practice* 21: 763–781.

Bryant-Lukosius, D., Cosby, R., Bakker, D., et al. (2015b). Practice guideline on the effective use of advanced practice nurses in the delivery of adult cancer services in Ontario. Cancer Care Ontario. https://www.cancercareontario.ca/en/guidelines-advice/types-of-cancer/2166 (accessed 31 July 2022).

Canadian Centre for Advanced Practice Nursing Research (CCAPNR). (2012). The clinical nurse specialist: getting a good return on healthcare investment. McMaster University, Hamilton, ON. https://fhs.mcmaster.ca/ccapnr/documents/onp_project/CNS_Brief_final.pdf (accessed 04 January 2022).

Canadian Nurses Association. (2010). Canadian nurse practitioner core competency framework. https://www.cno.org/globalassets/for/rnec/pdf/competencyframework_en.pdf (accessed 25 January 2022).

Canadian Nurses Association. (2016). Clinical nurse specialist. https://hl-prod-ca-oc-download.s3-ca-central-1.amazonaws.com/CNA/2f975e7e-4a40-45ca-863c-5ebf0a13 8d5e/UploadedImages/documents/Clinical_Nurse_Specialist_position_statement. pdf (accessed 04 January 2022).

Canadian Nurses Association. (2021). Advanced practice nursing. https://www. cna-aiic.ca/en/nursing/advanced-nursing-practice (accessed 31 July 2022).

Cannaby, A., Carter, V., Rolland, P. et al. (2020). The scope and variance of clinical nurse specialist job descriptions. *British Journal of Nursing* 29 (11): 606–611.

Carryer, J., Wilkinson, J., Towers, A., and Gardner, G. (2018). Delineating advanced practice nursing in New Zealand: a national survey. *International Nursing Review* 65 (1): 24–32.

Castledine, G. (2002). The development of the role of the clinical nurse specialist in the UK. *British Journal of Nursing* 11 (7): 11–24.

Chan, G.K. and Cartwright, C.C. (2014). The clinical nurse specialist. In: *Advanced Practice Nursing: An Integrative Approach*, 5e (ed. A.B. Hamric, C.M. Hanson, M.F. Tracy, and E.T. O'Grady), 359–395. St. Louis: Elsevier Saunders.

Cook, O., McIntyre, M., and Recoche, K. (2015). Exploration of the role of specialist nurses in the care of women with gynaecological cancer: a systematic review. *Journal of Clinical Nursing* 24 (5–6): 683–695.

Daly, W.M. and Carnwell, R. (2003). Nursing roles and levels of practice: a framework for differentiating between elementary, specialist and advancing nursing practice. *Journal of Clinical Nursing* 12 (2): 158–167.

Delamaire, M. and Lafortune, G. (2010). 'Nurses in advanced roles: A Description and Evaluation of Experience in 12 developed Countries.' *OECD Health Working Papers,* 54, ORVF Publishing.

Donald, F., Bryant-Lukosius, D., Martin-Misener, R. et al. (2010). Clinical nurse specialists and nurse practitioners: title confusion and lack of role clarity. *Nursing Leadership* 23 (Special Issue): 189–210.

Doody, W. and Bailey, M.E. (2011). The development of clinical nurse specialist roles in Ireland. *British Journal of Nursing* 20 (14): 868–872.

Dowling, M., Beauchesne, M., Farrelly, F., and Murphy, K. (2013). Advanced practice nursing: a concept analysis. *International Journal of Nursing Practice* 19: 131–140.

East, L., Knowles, K., Pettman, M., and Fisher, L. (2015). Advanced level nursing in England: organisation challenges and opportunities. *Journal of Nursing Management* 23: 1011–1019.

European Specialist Nurses Organizations (ESNO). (2015). Competences of the clinical nurse specialist (CNS): common plinth of competences for the common training framework of each specialty. Version 1, 17–10. https://esgena.org/assets/downloads/pdfs/general/esgena_esno_statement_competences.pdf (accessed 3 July 2022).

Flanders, S. and Clark, A.P. (2010). Interruptions and medication errors. *Clinical Nurse Specialist* 24: 281–285.

Fulton, J.S. (2018). Clinical nurse specialists international. https://www.nursingcenter.com/journalarticle?Article_ID=4805470&Journal_ID=54033&Issue_ID=4805459 (accessed 18 November 2021).

Glen, S. and Waddington, K. (1998). Role transition from staff nurse to clinical nurse specialist: a case study. *Journal of Clinical Nursing* 7: 283–290.

Hamric, A.B. and Tracy, M.F. (2019, 2017). A definition of advanced practice nursing. In: *Hamric and Hanson's Advanced Practice Nursing*, 6e (ed. M.F. Tracy and E.T. O'Grady), 61–79. Missouri: Elsevier.

Hancock, C. (2004). Unity with diversity: ICN's framework of competencies. *Journal of Advanced Nursing* 47 (2): 119.

Heale, R. and Buckley, C. (2015). An international perspective of advanced practice nursing regulation. *International Nursing Review* 62: 421–429.

Holloway, K., Baker, J., and Lumby, J. (2009). Specialist nursing framework for New Zealand: a missing link in workforce planning. *Policy Politics and Nursing Practice* 10 (4): 269–275.

International Council of Nurses (ICN). (2008). The scope of practice, standards and competencies of the advanced practice nurse. Monograph, ICN Regulation Series.

International Council of Nurses (ICN) (2020). *Guidelines on Advanced Practice Nursing*. Geneva: ICN.

Jokiniemi, K., Pietila, A., and Mikkonen, S. (2021). Construct validity of clinical nurse specialist core competency scale: an exploratory factor analysis. *Journal of Clinical Nursing* 30: 1863–1873.

Kaasalaimen, S., Martin-Misener, R., Kilpatrick, K. et al. (2010). A historical overview of the development of advanced practice nursing roles in Canada. *Canadian Journal of Nursing Leadership* 23: 35–61.

Kerr, H., Donovan, M., and McSorley, O. (2021). Evaluation of the role of the clinical nurse specialist in cancer care: an integrative literature review. *European Journal of Cancer Care* 30 (3): 1–13.

Kerr, H., McSorley, O., and Donovan, M. (2022). Registered nurses' perspectives of the impact of a post-registration qualification on patient care and clinical practice in cancer care: a qualitative study. *Journal of Cancer Education* https://doi. org/10.1007/s13187-022-02205-4.

Ketefian, S., Reman, R.W., Hanucharurnkul, S. et al. (2001). The development of advanced practice roles: implications in the international nursing community. *International Nursing Review* 148: 152–163.

Kilpatrick, K., DiCenso, A., Bryant-Lukosius, D. et al. (2013). Practice patterns and perceived impact of clinical nurse specialist roles in Canada: result of a national survey. *International Journal of Nursing Studies* 50: 1525–1538.

Kilpatrick, K., Kaasaaomem, S., Donald, F. et al. (2014). The effectiveness and cost effectiveness of clinical nurse specialists in outpatient roles: a systematic review. *Journal of Evaluation in Clinical Practice* 20: 1106–1123.

LaSala, C.A., Connors, P.M., Pedro, J.T., and Phipps, M. (2007). The role of the clinical nurse specialist in promoting evidence-based practice and effecting positive patient outcomes. *The Journal of Continuing Education in Nursing* 38 (6): 262–270.

Leary, A., Crouch, H., Lezard, A. et al. (2008). Dimensions of clinical nurse specialist work in the UK. *Nursing Standard* 23 (15–17): 40–44.

Lewandowski, W.S. and Adamle, K. (2009). Substantive areas of clinical nurse specialist practice: a comprehensive review of the literature. *Clinical Nurse Specialist* 23: 73–90.

Lusk, B., Cockerham, A.Z., and Keeling, A.W. (2019). Highlights from the history of advanced practice nursing in the United States. In: *Hamric and Hanson's Advanced Practice Nursing: An Integrative Approach*, 6e (ed. M.F. Tracy and E.T. O'Grady), 40–108. Missouri: Elsevier, Chapter one.

Maier, C., Aiken, L., and Busse, R. (2017). Nurses in advanced roles in primary care: policy levers for implementation. OECD Health Working Paper, no. 98.

Martin-Misener, R., Bryant-Lukosius, D., Harbman, P. et al. (2010). Education of advanced practice nurses in Canada. *Canadian Journal of Nursing Leadership* 23 (Special Issue): 61–84.

National Cancer Action Team (2011). *Clinical Nurse Specialists in Cancer Care; Provision, Proportion and Performance*. England: NHS.

National Institute for Clinical Excellence (2004). *Improving Supportive and Palliative Care for Adults with Cancer*. London: NICE.

North West Cancer Alliances and Health Education England. (2021). Developing a cancer CNS capabilities framework in the north west: research briefing. Skills for Health. https://skillsforhealth.org.uk/wp-content/uploads/2021/10/Cancer-Framework-Research-Briefing.pdf (accessed 31 July 2022).

Norton, C., Sigsworth, J., Heywood, S., and Oke, S. (2012). An investigation into the activities of clinical nurse specialists. *Nursing Standard* 26 (30): 42–50.

Nursing and Midwifery Council. (2001). Standards for specialist education and practice.

Oulton, J.A. and Caldwell, P. (2017). Nurses. *International Encyclopedia of Public Health* 5: 264–270.

Royal College of Nursing (2010). Clinical nurse specialist: adding value to care.

Royal College of Nursing (2017). Career pathway and education framework for cancer nursing.

Royal College of Nursing (2018). Advanced level nursing practice. Section 1: the registered nurse working at an advanced level of practice.

Schreiber, R., MacDonald, M., Pauly, B. et al. (2005). Singing in different keys: enactment of advanced nursing practice in British Columbia. *Canadian Journal of Nursing Leadership, Online Exclusive* 18: 1–17.

Smy, J., Young, A., Barlow, H., et al. (2011). Making clinical nurse specialists make more of an impact. www.hsj.co.uk/best-practice/making-clinical-nurse-specialists-make-more-of-an-impact/5026053.article (accessed 31 July 2022).

Vidall, C., Barlow, H., Crowe, M. et al. (2011). Clinical nurse specialists: essential resource for an effective NHS. *British Journal of Nursing* 20 (17): S23–S27.

World Health Organisation-Eastern Mediterranean Region (WHO-EMRO). (2018). Regional guide for the development of nursing specialist practice.

3

Patient Perspective

Johanna McMullan

Abstract

Person-centred care is highly valued in cancer nursing. Furthermore, this approach is increasingly considered an imperative aspect of cancer nursing care, with positive outcomes reported by individuals with a cancer diagnosis, if employed. To support nurses to be empathic with individuals diagnosed with cancer, this chapter provides a personal experience of a cancer diagnosis. The chapter is written by a registered nurse who shares their story from the unusual perspective of being both a healthcare professional and a patient, providing insights into their perspectives of whether they experienced person-centred care. It is hoped this will challenge all clinical nurse specialists to reflect on the care they provide to ensure that it is individualised and holistic.

Dedication
From a 'Lyttle' seed a beautiful and vibrant sunflower grew
        In loving memory of Kerri McCracken, 7 June 1975 – 7 August 2022

I am a 47-year-old senior lecturer in education in the School of Nursing and Midwifery, Queen's University Belfast, Northern Ireland, and a proud registrant with the Nursing and Midwifery Council (NMC) with a background in emergency nursing. Therefore, I regard – or, should I say, regarded – myself as having knowledge, empathy and sympathy for those on a cancer journey. I am also a daughter, sister, auntie, friend, wife, mother and cancer survivor.

An integrative literature review by Kerr et al. (2021) found the clinical nurse specialist (CNS) role in cancer care as an essential, valuable and cost-effective member of the multidisciplinary team from the perspective of individuals with cancer, carers, clinical colleagues and the CNS, with positive outcomes reported

The Role of the Clinical Nurse Specialist in Cancer Care, First Edition. Edited by Helen Kerr.
© 2024 John Wiley & Sons Ltd. Published 2024 by John Wiley & Sons Ltd.
Companion website: www.wiley.com/go/kerr

associated with their contribution to care delivery. One of the strengths of this integrative literature review relates to the inclusion of a range of perspectives, providing a triangulation of perceptions related to the CNS role in cancer care. It would be remiss then to offer this book relating to this role without hearing from various perspectives. This is where I come in. In this chapter, I hope to give some insight into my cancer journey and the interactions with my nurse colleagues in their role as CNSs and discuss exactly how these reported positive outcomes are experienced in real life, from the perspective of the real-life person under the wig. My name is Jo.

I was 43 years old and on holiday with friends when, while applying suntan lotion, I felt the lump. Right breast, near the skin, pea-sized, round, mobile and hard. As a nurse, I had enough awareness to acknowledge that this warranted attention but also enough insight to know that it was probably nothing, like the great majority of breast lumps. I did not feel panic or fear. How many times had I said in my career as a nurse, 'Don't worry, it's probably nothing'? However, as many of my new friends I have met along the way who have also been diagnosed with cancer have reiterated, that unmistakable little voice in the back of my head was saying, 'But what if it is?' This voice was louder at night or when I thought of my children. Interestingly, the more people I talked to about my lump, and the more I heard 'Don't worry, it's probably nothing' or 'Don't panic', the more irritating, dismissive and patronising it sounded, until I wanted to scream! I was not panicking; I just wanted them to acknowledge how I was feeling.

My friend and I went to a private evening clinic that same week for several reasons. It would be more than two weeks until I could see a general practitioner (GP)/primary physician and a further three weeks for an appointment at a local breast clinic (which, frankly, is cruel). I also knew this surgeon, and I have three sons and work full time, so I did not want to take the time off – it was all an inconvenience. My friend came with me to the appointment so I could tell my children I was out shopping; no need to worry them. The surgeon examined me, told me not to worry, and suggested I 'pop down and get an ultrasound'. There, the pathologist told me not to worry, despite the fact that she had moved the probe to my underarm lymph nodes and recommended a biopsy. My friend told me not to worry even though all the other women at the clinic had come out of the room, turned left and been told their results would be in the post, but I had to go back to the waiting room. I even told myself not to panic as I watched the pathologist knock on the surgeon's door and then fetch the nurse. I was then told what I already knew: it was cancer and needed treatment – but 'Don't worry'. I was furnished with the obligatory leaflets, including one on palliative services, and it all began.

Very recently, a good friend of mine was telephoned to attend an appointment following an investigation, having been in remission for two years. She was told that she had been squeezed in at the end of clinic the next day and to bring a friend with her. I accompanied her to, as she put it, 'hear the obvious'. As the CNS led us past several empty rooms, my friend commented to me, 'Oh look, it's the bad newsroom with the nice settee, like the first time'. She was quite correct: she had lung and bone metastasis but was told not to worry.

I hope this highlights my first and most important insight into cancer services. Despite having a malignancy, individuals with cancer have not lost their sight or hearing – we are still rational human beings and can sense when something may be wrong. Second, it is, I am sure, the most uncomfortable and emotionally costly part of a CNS's role to be part of breaking bad news; but thinking you have done so in a reassuring manner by saying 'not to worry' can be close to patronising. We have a right to worry as you would.

There have been various studies related to the impact of the CNS role in cancer care. A study by Beaver et al. (2010, p. 2823) found that 'continuity of care by the same breast care nurse and the trusting relationship developed was reported to improve the experience of service delivery for individuals with breast cancer'. Conversely, in a mixed-methods study, the dimension of care that received the lowest score rating from individuals with breast cancer related to emotional support (Droog et al. 2014). Furthermore, individuals with cancer and their carers reported improvements in their overall satisfaction with services because of the contribution of the CNS (Beaver et al. 2009; Hardie and Leary 2010; Borland et al. 2014; Droog et al. 2014; Visser et al. 2015). Hardie and Leary (2010) reported improvements in the experiences of treatment for individuals with breast cancer, increasing from 38% pre-introduction of the breast care CNS service to 56% after the introduction of a CNS service.

My personal experience reflects this mixed evidence. I attended my local National Health Service (NHS) breast clinic the following week, where I met my first CNS: a breast care nurse. I find it hard to articulate why she was so fantastic. She greeted me by name, she did not call out my name while looking at a file, she had no pity in her eyes, and she did not hold my hand or deliberately make eye contact. She introduced herself and, with sincerity, told me it was nice to meet me but offered no apology for it being under 'dreadful circumstances' (another frequently used, annoying line). Her first question was, 'What can I do for you?' Hooray! No checklist, speech or well-rehearsed passing on of compulsory information. What could she do for *me*. Person-centred care at last. I explained that I was a nurse, that I knew it was malignant and that I needed surgery and after that, I supposed, maybe chemotherapy, radiotherapy, etc. She nodded but skilfully left an appropriate pause, so I continued: I was not scared, I was furious that it had happened, it was unfair, my poor boys, how would I tell my mum, what about work? The floodgates had opened. She just listened – and when I finished, I thanked her. It was exactly what I needed. On reflection, much of what I divulged to her, I had not even acknowledged to myself and certainly had not processed. To be clear, she did not suggest these fears to me or hint at them in any way; she simply created a comfortable environment that allowed me to speak and think without feeling the need to teach or give information.

Every curriculum in higher education for nursing teaches communication, and I am sure every nurse registrant, if asked, would be able to quote active listening as an essential component of effective communication. There are full texts about listening in healthcare, such as McKenna et al. (2020, p. 379), who state that 'listening serves to build trusting, caring, and therapeutic relationships'. There is no doubt of the importance and worth of listening, yet very few of the healthcare professionals I met along the way did. A plethora of research details the barriers to communication (Chan et al. 2018). In my personal experience, the biggest barrier was that open and honest communication was not regarded as worthwhile. Most of my interactions with healthcare professionals was to provide me with information; interestingly, I already knew most of it due to my profession, but no one thought to ask. A few times I said I was a nurse, which was always acknowledged with a smile; then the interaction continued at the same pace and level as before, with utter determination that I was to receive this information. But that first breast care nurse I encountered approached the situation from my perspective. Who was I? What did I know? What did I want to know? Effortlessly yet skilfully, she acquired all this information by saying nothing but truly listening.

Over the next 20 minutes, this CNS addressed everything I had said without saying 'Don't worry' once. Her care was invaluable to me; I felt valued, safe, and respected and that she was talking with Jo, not to a 'breast cancer patient'. Sadly, this fantastic nurse was not my assigned breast care nurse; she had kindly stepped in as I was 'out of sync' with the system because I had my first appointment privately. It was her day in the clinic, so she just thought she would say hello for half an hour, but I can say with sincerity that I will remember her forever with gratitude. She was the embodiment of what Griffiths et al. (2013, p. 42) reported: 'that individuals with a range of cancers felt the CNS saw their cancer in the context of the person's whole life, rather than just a set of symptoms', thus highlighting the holistic and supportive approach of the CNS role.

Every story has twists and turns, highs and lows, and this chapter should be 'warts and all' to be authentic. I do not wish to complain or in any way reprimand anyone I met on my journey. I only wish to highlight the difference with another CNS I encountered who did their job but – sadly, from my patient perspective – failed to achieve what other CNSs I encountered achieved effortlessly. They all were present when they ought to have been, but sometimes it felt that they were not fully present. Sometimes information was passed on but in a rather scripted way, which gave me the feeling that it was a chore, a job done. For example, when I received my results from surgery, a CNS was present in the room, presumably to be supportive, answer questions and so forth. As the surgeon told me the margins were clear, that it was oestrogen and progesterone positive but unfortunately also HER2 positive, I was distracted by the fact that the CNS was scrolling through her phone; she only spoke to say 'but you'll get a wig' when the surgeon said I would probably need chemotherapy, and even then she failed to lift her eyes from the screen. She was physically present but not in the moment as the surgeon was. When I left the room, I had to have blood samples taken, and the CNS started to explain how to get there. I thanked her but said I knew the way as I often worked in this hospital as a bank nurse. I was told she had to walk patients out, and along the way she felt it necessary to tell me that much younger women had been diagnosed with cancer than I, that she had lots of 'palliative patients' in her care, and that overall, I was very fortunate to have a 'good (!) cancer' that was easily treatable and nothing to worry about. I felt slightly ashamed and that I should pull myself together and remember there were indeed others much worse off than me. On reflection, however, I feel anger. I was not crying; I had attended this appointment on my own and knew it was high stakes. Were my margins clear? Was there lymph node involvement? I was prepared for chemotherapy and radiotherapy, so I was delighted with my results and was smiling and very relieved. It was a blow to be HER2 positive, but Herceptin was available, so overall it was good news. Perhaps this approach had been tried and tested, but it was not suitable. I am quite sure this nurse did not mean to be uncaring and rather was attempting to make me feel better – but she didn't. This encounter ended with her giving me her card and telling me to get in touch if I wanted to – not 'feel free to do so anytime', only if I wanted to. I will draw a line under this paragraph by saying I never felt I wanted to get in touch with this individual again, despite reaching out to many others along the way.

Next was peripherally inserted central catheter (PICC) insertion. To my surprise, it was inserted by a CNS, demonstrating what Cannaby et al. (2020, p. 608) describe as 'the vast scope of practice of CNSs'. It was done with great skill, in terms of clinical competence, and a fantastic explanation was delivered at a level appropriate to my previous knowledge, along with personable conversation. This CNS and I met again on a tour of the chemotherapy unit, where she made me feel welcome and, remembering I was a nurse, skilfully asked what I knew already and what I did not know.

The first three rounds of chemotherapy came and went, the dressing on the PICC was changed by district nurses, and blood was taken from the PICC line. I wished there was a PICC clinic, as hanging about the house all day waiting for a district nurse to call was frustrating. I understood that district nurses have many calls, but this made me feel like an invalid one day a week; the other six days, I was living life completely normally. One evening, after this weekly ritual, I found it difficult to sleep; I was on edge and thought it was probably due to cabin fever and not enough exercise or fresh air. By the small hours of the morning, I was sweating yet cold and took my temperature: it was 39 °C. I telephoned the 24-hour chemotherapy helpline and, unsurprisingly, was sent to the emergency department, where the receptionists, triage nurse and duty doctor all swung into action. I was isolated, given antibiotics and swiftly admitted under oncology. My National Early Warning Score (NEWS) was satisfactory. The following morning, more blood was taken, and all was well except that my PICC seemed to be blocked and attempts made to rectify this problem failed. By mid-morning, I felt on edge again: looking back, I had that classic feeling of impending doom (Sheehan 2021). At this point, an experienced CNS arrived who I can say at the very least saved unnecessary tests, possibly an admission to a high dependency unit (HDU), and countless cost to the NHS, but also quite possibly saved my life. The International Council of Nurses (2020) state that the role of the CNS should involve a combination of direct and indirect care. Kerr et al. (2021) found that direct care involves care to patients and families, which may include the diagnosis and treatment of disease, whilst indirect care involves the implementation of improvements in the healthcare delivery system. Direct care is borne out in the findings of this literature review identified through the components of the CNS role in providing psychological support, information and education and the clinical component of the role. Indirect care is also discernible in the findings related to the coordination of services and the advocacy role. This CNS certainly displayed all these aspects of the role.

The CNS introduced herself and looked quickly through my notes. She chatted while looking at my observations and asked how I was feeling at that moment – the first person who had asked rather than examining a chart. I admitted to her that I was not feeling great, and as she took my blood pressure again, she said she had a hunch it was my PICC line and that she would like to remove it. The PICC had been great, saving countless cannulas and needle insertions, but I did not hesitate to agree. Her manner conveyed knowledge, concern and experience, and I trusted her 100% straight away. Out of curiosity, I asked why she had this 'hunch', and she was not sure; it was the dressing change and blood being taken the day before, the PICC line being blocked on admission, and an acknowledgement that if I did not feel well, then I was not well, despite what the chart said.

The CNS removed the PICC line, sent its tip to the laboratory, inserted another peripheral cannula and commenced intravenous fluids. The junior oncologist was sure I was getting better, but this CNS insisted that my observations were to be taken half-hourly for the next few hours and assured me she would follow up with laboratory work. Unfortunately, she was right: rigours, vomiting and the classic signs of sepsis kicked in quickly. My blood pressure at one point was 76/33, and I was heading for the HDU. I cannot remember the next 24 hours, but it transpired that I had a gram-negative bacillus in my PICC line. With two intravenous doses of the specific antibiotic, I fortunately bounced back very quickly. When I say 'bounced back', over the next three days I moved classically through the hierarchy of needs from unconscious, to weak, to eating a little, to wanting my make-up bag and feeling caged. This CNS was with me every step of the way, from prescribing and administering anti-emetics and holding the emesis bowl, to comforting me when I was scared and embarrassed, to suggesting I could be part of a clinical trial whereby patients move to oral antibiotics and self-care sooner. I was able to go home much more quickly than anticipated, yet she continued to monitor and support me when I got home. Her knowledge and involvement in research were apparent but perhaps only obvious to me with my insight into this area.

Interestingly, Kerr et al. (2021) also found that an additional component of indirect care outlined by the International Council of Nurses (2020), which applies to all CNS roles, relates to contribution to research. The apparent absence of the research component of the CNS role is likely to be because it is a hidden element that is not immediately visible to patients, carers and other healthcare professionals but could be embedded in their role. This is evidenced in two studies, with research being identified by the CNS as a component of their role (Ream et al. 2009; Kim 2011); however, research was not identified by other participant groups. In the development of the CNS role in cancer care, it remains imperative that job descriptions include a contribution to the design, implementation and evaluation of research in the clinical environment. This CNS was the leader of this team and even after discharge was curious to know how I had found the whole experience and asked if I could suggest any improvements; this reflects findings from Farrell et al. (2011) and Henry (2015) identifying that additional components of the CNS role could include a leadership role and contributions to service development. During this time, I was cared for by a great many people on the multidisciplinary team; however, this CNS was what Cook et al. (2019, p. 10) describe as 'the glue of the team' by using her advanced skills to 'accurately assess the patient, with appropriate timely referrals being made to other relevant services' (Cook et al. 2019).

Unfortunately, I have two very good friends who were also diagnosed with breast cancer around the time I was. I asked them their thoughts and experiences regarding CNSs. One said the following:

> I was totally lost. I do not even know the difference between an oncologist and a surgeon. I kept getting appointments, one day to prepare for surgery, next for chemotherapy. There was a great deal of overlap, and I often thought the left hand was unaware of what the right hand was doing. The only person who seemed to have an overall picture of my situation was my CNS. At one stage I got two different appointments for the same day, and when I telephoned the CNS, it turned out I did not need either appointment, as one was a routine mammogram, but I had already had an MRI two weeks before, and the other was to have a sample of blood taken, which I already had.

The other friend had similar thoughts, saying

> I soon realised there was no point trying to contact the various departments when I had a question. It was endless being transferred from pillar to post. My breast care nurse (CNS) was always able to answer my questions or, if not, she was able to navigate the various departments with ease and always got back to me when she had found out the answer. This was usually because of overlaps in appointments or waiting for another which had not materialised.

It is easy to see why then there is a 'growing body of evidence to suggest that CNSs provide value for money in terms of patient safety, quality of service and efficiency' (Leary 2011, p. 49), yet 'nurse specialists struggle to demonstrate this to executive boards that want to see a return on their investment'.

What struck me the most after being in the care of the CNS was how equal and respectful the relationship was, how I was at the centre of the care, and how present she was, which is why I believe she was open and quite correct in her 'hunch'. I remember first hearing as a student nurse in the 1990s about Benner and Tanner (1987) work on how expert nurses use intuition, and I confess it sounded like mystical nonsense. My background is emergency department nursing, and I still do shifts at the local department some 26 years later. I have always believed my ontological perspective is that of a scientist. Everything can be explained, and I am certainly more comfortable in the world of x leads to y treated with z. However, as I get older and perhaps wiser, or maybe just gain yet another year of experience, I am fascinated by how one can teach the Manchester triage system, but hunches are real. If I override what the book tells me, am I truly an expert? It's like those 3D pictures: if you defocus your eyes from the pixels and stand back, can you see the whole picture?

Currently, with my life experience and working experience, I can appreciate that behind the obvious issues is a cause, and in the centre of this is a person. Today I am not as interested in ED traumas as recurrent falls or recurring admissions for pain relief. I find myself more and more listening to that inner voice and saying to younger colleagues, 'trust me' – but I have nothing to substantiate this other than a 'hunch'. I could recount several stories about witnessing, over the years, several experienced ED nurses just knowing, without being able to articulate, when someone was unwell. I remember clearly being a new nurse registrant, working in St. Georges Hospital, London, and observing a man being triaged with back pain and a possible urinary tract infection. I was being supervised and selected the category using the Manchester triage system based on his observations. My supervisor suggested I check the blood pressure in both arms, and they were equal. For a while, I thought she was being rather curious or even a little patronising. Nevertheless, she selected a higher category in the Manchester triage system, and he did in fact have an aortic aneurysm dissection. I was shocked and later asked how she knew, what I had done wrong, what I had missed – but she kindly reassured me by saying that I would soon develop my 'sixth sense'.

I am not claiming to be an expert or writing to gain praise, but later a young footballer presented with shortness of breath. His NEWS was zero, but he said he felt uneasy because he could not catch his breath after running in the second half of the match. I gently suggested that perhaps a young, fit athlete could have very different baseline observations than those of a generic NEWS scoring system and that if he was reporting feeling unwell, he knew himself better than we did. When his X-ray revealed a spontaneous pneumothorax, I was asked how I knew. Perhaps it was 'pattern or similarity recognition', as discussed by Benner and Tanner (1987), or maybe it was that 'sense of salience' whereby one is aware that not all events are of equal importance or relevance. I would say I have reached the proficient level of practice, but I am still in awe of experts such as a good friend of mine who is a nurse and who, while collecting a relative from the waiting room, 'spotted an ectopic pregnancy' waiting to be triaged and brought her straight through. Her explanation of how she knew was 'by the way she was sitting ... just a hunch'. This intuitive judgement cannot be taught, perhaps can never truly be captured, but must never be devalued. It is of course pertinent to all areas of expertise and all areas of nursing. What I experienced was a CNS being open, using a person-centred approach; but sadly, this was lacking in some other CNSs. It may or may not depend on length of time as a nurse registrant or in a particular work role, or courses attended, but it was very apparent in this CNS's attitude and demeanour.

Radiotherapy, 18 cycles of Herceptin, mammograms, and hair regrowth followed. I returned to work. I suppose one's journey never ends; but as I get further from these events, like a view in my car's rear-view mirror, the significance or trauma gets smaller and fainter. However, as a nurse involved in education, my curiosity prevails. What did I learn? What can I pass on in teaching nursing students? Therefore, I was more than happy to write this chapter; I am and remain a cancer survivor, nurse and teacher. Perhaps the only good that could come out of this experience is to offer my insight from these combined perspectives. Recently, in my work environment, we have embarked on a new undergraduate nursing curriculum, including a module on professionalism and another on care and communication. Interestingly, this curriculum was being developed just as I was returning to work. I heard several colleagues remarking on whether it was necessary to have such modules, as these skills should be inherent in those wishing to pursue a career in nursing. I agree that this may be the case in an ideal world.

I teach and willingly talk with students about diagnosis, treatments and even personal experiences about side effects such as constipation and hair loss, without any negative emotion. However, one class focuses on the 'Hello, my name is' campaign, and it never fails to open old wounds. This campaign is now led by the husband of a patient who lost her life to cancer and articulates how few healthcare professionals introduce themselves. I would go further: for a healthcare professional not to introduce themselves is not bad practice – it is demeaning, dismissive and, frankly, rude. It conveys that the person entering your room is in authority and in control of the situation. This campaign started in 2013, and by 2018, when I was receiving treatment, the message seemed to have reached healthcare professionals; but unfortunately, at times I got the impression that the point had been missed. Although many healthcare professionals introduced themselves, their introduction was devoid of emotion or even eye contact, a tick box exercise. It was obvious that they were doing it because they ough to. Depressingly often, 'My name is' whoever 'and I'm going to do such and such, OK?' is said with zero sincerity, challenging the view of gaining meaningful consent.

I am discussing this in this context because it beautifully demonstrates the difference between the CNSs I encountered. I can remember the names of two of the three I have discussed; I only know the name of the third because it was on the paperwork. For two of the CNSs, their introduction was natural and instinctive, which, on reflection, mirrored their entire practice. Again, NMC registrants, students and lecturers in the world of nursing discuss values-based practice, quoting 'The Code: Professional Standards of Practice and Behaviour' for nurses and midwives (NMC 2018), 'Standards of Conduct, Performance and Ethics' (HCPC 2012); 'Compassion in Practice' (Department of Health and Social Care 2012); and the NHS Constitution (Department of Health and Social Care 2015) that underpin it. Mohr et al. (2001, p. 35) state quite simply, 'values express who and what we are'.

This book is about cancer CNSs. On reflection of all my encounters with CNSs, it strikes me that some has lost sight of 'nursing', trying to be a specialist, and had moved toward a medical model. If one imagines a scoring system of 1–10 in terms of a skill or knowledge, such as prescribing, or tasks such as insertion of PICC lines, some are focused on the 7, 8, 9 and 10 out of 10 and have forgotten or perhaps discarded 1–6. However, from a cancer patient's perspective, the CNSs who are exceptional, achieving 10/10 for excellence in nursing, excel in what is often irritatingly referred to as 'the basics' rather than the fundamental aspects of nursing – values-based, person-centred care. By doing so, the therapeutic relationship established through mutual respect and trust certainly benefited me on my journey. To me, they were very special nurses who happen to look after individuals with cancer like me, and my name is Jo.

References

Beaver, K., Tysver-Robinson, D., Campbell, M. et al. (2009). Comparing hospital and telephone follow-up after treatment for breast cancer: randomised equivalence trial. *British Medical Journal* 338: 1–9.

Beaver, K., Williamson, S., and Chalmers, K. (2010). Telephone follow-up after treatment for breast cancer: views and experiences of patients with specialist breast care nurses. *Journal of Clinical Nursing* 19: 2916–2924.

Benner, P. and Tanner, C. (1987). How expert nurses use intuition. *AJN The American Journal of Nursing* 87 (1): 23–34.

Borland, R., Glackin, M., and Jordan, J. (2014). How does involvement of a hospice nurse specialist impact on the experience on informal caring in palliative care? Perspectives of middle-aged partners bereaved through cancer. *European Journal of Cancer Care* 23 (5): 701–711.

Cannaby, A.M., Carter, V., Rolland, P. et al. (2020). The scope and variance of clinical nurse specialist job descriptions. *British Journal of Nursing* 29 (11): 606–611.

Chan, E.A., Wong, F., Cheung, M.Y., and Lam, W. (2018). Patients' perceptions of their experiences with nurse-patient communication in oncology settings: a focused ethnographic study. *PLoS One* 13 (6): e0199183.

Cook, O., McIntyre, M., Recoche, K., and Lee, S. (2019). Our nurse is the glue for our team – multidisciplinary team members' experiences and perceptions of the gynaecological oncology specialist nurse role. *European Journal of Oncology Nursing* 41: 7–15.

Department of Health and Social Care. (2012). Compassion in practice.

Department of Health and Social Care. (2015). The handbook to the NHS Constitution for England.

Droog, E., Armstrong, C., and MacCurtain, S. (2014). Supporting patients during their breast cancer journey: the informational role of clinical nurse specialists. *Cancer Nursing* 37 (6): 429–435.

Farrell, C., Molassiotis, A., Beaver, K., and Heaven, C. (2011). Exploring the scope of oncology specialist nurses' practice in the UK. *European Journal of Oncology Nursing* 15: 160–166.

Griffiths, P., Simon, M., Richardson, A., and Corner, J. (2013). Is a larger specialist nurse workforce in cancer care associated with better patient experience? Cross-sectional study. *Journal of Health Services Research & Policy* 18 (1_suppl): 39–46.

Hardie, H. and Leary, A. (2010). Value to patients of a breast cancer clinical nurse specialist. *Nursing Standard* 42: 24–34.

Health and Care Professions Council. (2012). Standards of conduct, performance and ethics.

Henry, R. (2015). The role of the cancer specialist nurse. *Nursing in Practice* 24.

International Council of Nurses. (2020). Guidelines of advanced practice nursing.

Kerr, H., Donovan, M., and McSorley, O. (2021). Evaluation of the role of the clinical nurse specialist in cancer care: an integrative literature review. *European Journal of Cancer Care* 30 (3): 1–13.

Kim, M.Y. (2011). Effects of oncology clinical nurse specialists' interventions on nursing-sensitive outcomes in South Korea. *Clinical Journal of Oncology Nursing* 15 (5): E66–E74.

Leary, A. (2011). How nurse specialists can demonstrate their worth. *Gastrointestinal Nursing* 9 (6): 46–49.

McKenna, L., Brown, T., Oliaro, L. et al. (2020). Listening in health care. In: *The Handbook of Listening* (ed. D.L. Worthington and G.D. Bodie), 373–383. Wiley.

Mohr, W.K., Deatrick, J., Richmond, T., and Mahon, M.M. (2001). A reflection on values in turbulent times. *Nursing Outlook* 49 (1): 30–36.

Nursing and Midwifery Council. (2018). The code. Professional standards of practice and behaviour for nurses, midwives and nursing associates.

Ream, E., Wilson-Barrnett, J., Faithfull, S. et al. (2009). Working patterns and perceived contribution of prostate cancer clinical nurse specialists: a mixed method investigation. *International Journal of Nursing Studies* 46: 1345–1354. https://doi.org/10.1016/j.ijnurstu.2009.03.006.

Sheehan, J.L. (2021). The patient with anxiety. In: *Inpatient Psychiatric Nursing: Clinical Strategies and Practical Interventions* (ed. J.L. Sheehan, C. Alexandre, M.H. Hohenhaus, and J.M. Matthew), 23. Springer Publishing Company.

Visser, A., Bos, W.C., Prins, J.B. et al. (2015). Breast self-examination education for BRCA mutation carriers by clinical nurse specialists. *Clinical Nurse Specialist* 29 (3): E1–E7.

4

Carer's Perspective

Trevor Wightman

Abstract

This chapter focuses on the role of a carer for an individual diagnosed with cancer. Trevor outlines his role in caring for his wife, Carol, until she sadly died in 2017. He openly shares his feelings along the journey from diagnosis to treatment to end of life, identifying how the title 'carer' involved major life changes. Trevor identifies the contribution of the clinical nurse specialist over key points in the three-year period when valuable support and advice were provided above what was 'required'.

Before I start, I would like to introduce myself. My name is Trevor, and a short time ago, I marked my 67th birthday. I am a retired civil servant but prior to that trained as an electrician and spent some time in the Merchant Navy. I also dabbled in self-employment. I have a grown-up family and was married twice, most recently to the lady who is the main focus of this chapter: Carol. In 2014, I officially became a 'carer' for Carol, and continued until 2017.

Being asked to contribute to this book has given me a wonderful opportunity for some self-reflection. From the outset, I would like to say that anything I share should not be interpreted as criticism of any individual or healthcare unit. With the passage of time, some memories may have faded, but the care, empathy and respect shown to my wife and me were faultless. Therefore, I have decided to anonymise this piece to protect the identity of the professional staff who cared for Carol and me.

In modern parlance, this is where I imagine I should explain my 'journey'. I struggle with that description, as any journey I have undertaken has involved at least some element of planning and structure, and I could not have anticipated being a carer. This role throws you into the deep end. I appreciate that this is my opinion, and others may disagree; however, it is how I feel as I reflect on my personal caring experience.

The Role of the Clinical Nurse Specialist in Cancer Care, First Edition. Edited by Helen Kerr.
© 2024 John Wiley & Sons Ltd. Published 2024 by John Wiley & Sons Ltd.
Companion website: www.wiley.com/go/kerr

In April 2014, following major abdominal surgery, my wife Carol was diagnosed with metastatic cancer with an unknown primary tumour. She was advised that, although it not entirely certain, the primary cancer was in all likelihood located in her bowel. At this stage, Carol was 52 years of age. As anyone who has received this news will be aware, the words being spoken feel like you have been run over by a bus. After the initial shock, there is time spent waiting for the surgery to heal. Then, finally, it is the day of the initial oncology appointment to discuss the next stage of treatment. In many ways, this is where the story truly starts regarding my role as a carer.

There is no preparation possible for what you are about to experience as a carer. This was the first time I was introduced to a clinical nurse specialist (CNS), who was also present in this initial meeting. For the purposes of this chapter, I will use Karen as a pseudonym for the CNS. I may have been advised in this meeting that Karen's title was CNS, but the reality for me was that she was a 'nurse' who worked closely with the oncologists. At this meeting, Carol was advised that a course of nine chemotherapy treatments would be available, and these would commence a few weeks later. The treatments involved Carol attending the oncology outpatient clinic at the local hospital every two weeks, with the chemotherapy administered intravenously over a three-hour period. Carol was advised that there were possible side effects. These included, but were not limited to, nausea, vomiting, headaches, fluctuating temperature and insomnia. As the chemotherapy treatment cycles progressed, I became aware of the varied roles the CNS was responsible for, and my admiration grew with regards to the value of their role to me as a carer. It would be difficult to list the many times I came to rely on Karen, so for the purposes of this chapter, I will provide a few examples to outline my experience of the valuable role of the CNS.

From the initial consultation with the oncologist, let me say that I completely understand that the full focus of the professional staff is on the service user. This is perfectly sensible and correct, but in the flurry of information, most of which I was attempting to process and analyse, I felt almost invisible. All questions were directed to Carol, and clearly there was a protocol relating to the chemotherapy treatment plan that had to be discussed. Once this was completed and the oncologist outlined the treatment to be followed in the coming months, Carol accepted the invitation to go with Karen to be orientated to the treatment area where she would receive the chemotherapy and be introduced to staff who would be involved in administering the chemotherapy. I was taken to another room, and a short time later, Karen returned. I vividly remember the first question Karen asked me directly: 'Will you be Carol's carer?' This totally threw me off guard; I explained that I was Carol's husband, only to be informed that they were aware of this but still needed to establish who would be Carol's 'primary carer'. At this time, I realised that a 'role' had been created for me and that this was clearly a vital part of the protocol and what Carol needed. To this day, I still struggle with the concept of being a 'carer', as to me, it was a labour of love.

Having established in this meeting with Karen that I would indeed be the primary carer, we then moved on to the practicalities of the caring 'role'. I had very little experience dealing with the medical profession prior to this, but within a short time I became aware of just how much input I would have into the 'care package' for Carol. This included details of contact numbers of healthcare professional staff that might be useful as the treatments progressed, cancer charities and counselling services. Karen delivered this information in a clear manner. I know Karen was working through a 'checklist', but she demonstrated clear empathy and acknowledged how difficult this was for a layperson to absorb. I honestly cannot remember how long this initial meeting lasted, but I do remember leaving it laden with literature and a checklist of things I needed to put in place. This included emergency phone numbers and simple advice pages. Oh! I almost forgot; I was advised to make sure I bought a good thermometer. My initial thought was, 'Why do I need that?' When I asked Karen, she advised that while it would hopefully never be needed, it was vital to have a thermometer available at home. As it transpired, virtually everything I was given or advised to get was needed over the next three years. Not surprisingly, Karen was proven to be correct.

In hindsight, this initial encounter set the tone for all future visits to the hospital unit on treatment days when chemotherapy was being administered. At the time, I did not fully grasp the enormity of what a 'carer' was responsible for. Certain aspects of my conversations with Karen remain with me today. These conversations did not all happen in one or two treatment visits to the hospital but over a couple of years. Perhaps the most enlightening conversation related to being told that I was the eyes and ears of the treatment team. It was mentioned that they would only see Carol every two to three weeks when she attended hospital for chemotherapy treatment, while I would be with her 24/7. For this reason, it was vitally important that I inform staff on treatment days how I believed Carol was coping with her treatment. Karen was also the first person to explain that as a 'carer', I would be responsible for overseeing the drug regime at home between chemotherapy treatments. I was advised that I was also responsible for ensuring that Carol's diet remained healthy and that she took exercise when able, and for making mental notes on the side effects of the chemotherapy and how it was affecting Carol both physically and mentally. In addition, I was responsible for monitoring Carol's temperature and was advised at what stage I needed to seek advice from the hospital unit. As one of Carol's treatments involved coming home attached to a chemotherapy infusion via a peripherally inserted central catheter (PICC) line, I was also trained to use the spill kit I was issued and told what course of action I needed to take should a spill occur. All of this was explained to me with great care by Karen.

I believe that early in the first treatment cycle, Karen was very astute and identified that Carol was an 'I don't want to make a fuss' type of person. This meant Carol might communicate that she was coping better than she was in reality. In making this observation, Karen again demonstrated her knowledge and insight into what makes people 'tick'. On the second or third clinic visit, Karen asked me to join her for a cup of tea while Carol had her chemotherapy treatment. When we were alone, she said the time had come for me to be completely honest about how Carol was coping. I was fully aware that when at home, Carol struggled with all the side effects of chemotherapy, but on entering the treatment unit, she would paint a smile on her face; when asked, she would simply say 'I am fine'. On reflection, this is probably when the trust between Karen and myself really grew. Karen put me at ease by explaining that she fully understood my loyalty to Carol and that telling it 'as it was' might feel like I was betraying her confidence. She explained that by Carol 'holding back' in not sharing the reality of her chemo- therapy experiences, she was not helping the oncologist determine the correct drug doses required. Up until that point, I was unaware they could modify the various drugs and amounts to suit the individual patient. This caused a crisis of conscience for me, but Karen provided a convincing case to share the reality of how Carol was coping – so much so that I agreed to be the eyes and ears I had originally been asked to be and to be honest in sharing how Carol was coping.

Over repeated chemotherapy cycles, this is how it continued. Carol in her pre- chemotherapy consultation would not create 'a fuss', and then Karen would make me a tea and find out exactly how Carol was coping. Very quickly, we both knew this could not continue, so Karen suggested she speak to Carol and me together. Again, I have nothing but respect for her ability to 'read' people. It transpired that Carol knew I was 'telling tales' on how she was keeping; but once Karen explained why and what could be done to make life easier, Carol clearly understood the need to be honest in reporting how the treatment was impacting her. From this point on, Carol was able to be totally honest with Karen about how she was coping. This was completely down to Karen recognising the right time and approach to help Carol share her experience of chemotherapy.

Another example of the valuable role of the CNS was an occasion when Karen went 'the extra mile'. I think it was at the beginning of Carol's third chemotherapy treatment cycle, and she was really struggling to cope with the side effects, to the extent that I telephoned the chemotherapy unit for advice. I spoke to Karen, who asked me to take Carol's temperature every 30 minutes and share exactly how Carol was feeling. She also arranged for the district/community nurse to attend and take blood samples and have these urgently processed through the laboratory. After several hours, Karen telephoned again and asked that Carol attend the hos- pital for a blood transfusion. As this was a new experience for me as a carer, I was unaware of what was going on behind the scenes regarding blood results and organising a blood transfusion. What I can say, however, is that Karen kept me fully informed and was a key contact person over this challenging time. When we arrived at the hospital, everything had been arranged, and Carol was seen by healthcare professionals immediately. After she was discharged from hospital, Karen telephoned me to see how everything had gone and check on how Carol was feeling.

My involvement with Karen continued through three separate chemotherapy treatment cycles. The week Carol passed away, she was due to start a fourth chemotherapy treatment. On admission to hospital, after being advised that no further treatment could be offered, Carol asked me to inform the chemotherapy unit that she would not need the slot for treatment and to allocate it to someone else. When I went to the unit, it was Karen I spoke to. She comforted me and offered to help in any way she could. A few hours later, she arrived on the ward where Carol had been admitted with a few of the unit nurses to visit Carol and me. To me, this was over and above any requirement as a 'professional' nurse. This was someone showing compassion and respect, and it will stay with me forever.

I suppose, like many people, I felt that once my involvement with the chemotherapy unit was over, it would be a case of out of sight, out of mind. To disprove this, about six months after Carol died, I met Karen and her family out shopping in the local town. On most occasions, I imagine there might have been a polite hello and a parting of the ways. Not this time. Karen suggested we go for a coffee, and she arranged to meet her family later. We went to a local cafe and had coffee and a chat. She did not rush and seemed totally at ease talking to me about Carol and how I had been coping. This was another example to me of someone going way beyond what was expected.

A final example is more recent. In 2017, a few months before Carol died, we became involved, through a small charity, with a local university in developing a website providing help and advice to carers of those with cancer: www.cancercaringcoping.com. I am still involved today in helping keep the content of this site current. As a result of this involvement, in 2020, I was asked to speak at an oncology conference at the same local university in Northern Ireland to outline the 'carer' role. While waiting for the conference to commence, I was sitting at a table when Karen and some of the chemotherapy unit nurses attended. Karen told me they had been invited to the conference, but on seeing my name down as one of the speakers, they decided to attend and offer me support. Amazing!

What do I believe a CNS to be, and what attributes do I think necessary for the role? At its most basic level, the core skills are likely to be identical to what leads anyone into the nursing profession. These include excellent communication skills, care and compassion, courage, competence and an ability to empathise. The CNS to me is someone who has taken these skills to a higher level. They have the ability to communicate complicated medical procedures in a language that is easy for patients and carers to understand. Karen brought and supported me along the 'journey', and every step of the way was explained fully with regards to what would happen. She demonstrated her knowledge, compassion and empathy, and nothing was ever too much trouble.

In relation to what attributes I believe a CNS should possess, in addition to knowledge, the ability to clearly demonstrate empathy is massive. CNSs are dealing with people during a horrific time, and being able to adapt their approach to each individual patient and/or carer is paramount. I am aware that this is a current 'buzzword', but person-centred care is crucial. I have only dealt with the role of the CNS in relation to oncology, as this is the area I encountered. I know the role of the carer is much wider than my experience, but perhaps my views are similar to other carers.

Finally, although the CNS has been anonymised in this chapter, I want to say a heartfelt 'thank you' to Karen for making what was a long and arduous journey easier. I will never forget you or your kindness to both myself and Carol.

5

Key Worker Role

Karen Armstrong and Helen Kerr

Abstract

Each individual with a diagnosis of cancer should be allocated a key worker to improve continuity and coordination of care. The key worker role is often an important component of clinical nurse specialists in cancer services, who are ideally placed to fulfil this role. The role may be operationalised using different titles, such as key worker in the United Kingdom, professional cancer navigator in Canada and the United States of America and cancer care coordinator in Australia. Irrespective of the title, key workers are known to positively impact patient care through the delivery of information, provision of emotional and supportive care and coordination of services. Identifying the appropriate professional to be a patient's named key worker is often driven by the cancer multidisciplinary team, and challenges remain regarding consistency of provision and effectively communicating this to patients. Care should be taken to avoid over-reliance on the key worker role within the multidisciplinary team and to ensure ongoing patient empowerment.

5.1 Introduction

The term *key worker* has been used frequently in the media during the COVID-19 global pandemic. In a broad sense, *key worker* is used to define an essential employee working in the public or private sector in a profession considered essential to society (Betterteam 2021). A key worker in healthcare, particularly the oncology setting, is a 'person who, with the patients' consent and agreement, takes a key role in coordinating the patient's care and promoting continuity, ensuring the patient knows who to access for information and advice' (National Institute for Health and Care Excellence (NICE) 2004, p. 42). This chapter will explore the concept of a key worker in cancer services and consider whether the cancer clinical nurse specialist (CNS) is often best placed to be a patient's named key worker. It will consider the advanced nursing skills required to successfully navigate the role and how these intertwine to impact direct and indirect patient care. Drawing on the first author's experience, the chapter will provide an overview of the key worker role in practice and discuss how challenges may be effectively managed. The chapter will conclude with a clinical example of challenges in practice and how the first author addressed these to change routine practice.

The first author is currently working as a band 6 gynaecological oncology CNS in the Northern Ireland Cancer Centre, Belfast, providing direct patient care for individuals with a diagnosis of gynaecology cancer. This is a unique role, as the author works across both gynaecology oncology surgical services and gynaecology clinical oncology services. The author has held this post from its creation in 2017, having previously worked in an inpatient gynaecology and breast surgical oncology ward for three years. The second author is a senior lecturer at the School of Nursing and Midwifery, Queen's University Belfast, with a clinical nursing background in cancer and palliative care.

5.2   The Key Worker

The 'key worker' concept was introduced within Cancer Peer Review measures and supported by NICE guidelines to improve the continuity and coordination of care for patients with cancer (NICE 2004; NHS England 2010; Ling et al. 2013). NICE (2016) guidelines advocate that each individual with a diagnosis of cancer should be allocated a key worker. The key worker should be a core member of the multidisciplinary team (Belfast Health and Social Care Trust (BHSCT) 2019) and may be a community nurse, allied health professional, nurse specialist or social worker (NICE 2004).

The idea that the key worker role is a 'role' rather than a job title allows professionals with the appropriate knowledge, experience and skills to fulfil this role. This means being a key worker is an aspect of the healthcare professional's role. The key worker is an individual designated to provide advice, information and emotional support; coordinate care; and help the individual navigate services. There are a number of drivers to be considered in deciding who is best placed to be a patient's named key worker, such as the context, patient needs and skills/ knowledge required to support patients and their families.

In the cancer setting, multidisciplinary teams (MDT)s are required to identify a named key worker (NICE 2004). Although there is no national guidance on how the key worker role should be implemented, most cancer services in the United Kingdom (UK) have an agreed key worker policy that sits within or alongside the MDT operational policy. These policies are likely to have been developed in response to Cancer Peer Review measures as outlined by the NICE guidelines (NICE 2004). These policies often advocate that the key worker allocation should be reviewed at key points in the patient's cancer journey and in doing so may transfer to another named professional, depending on the patient's personal circumstances or clinical condition: for example, at diagnosis, commencement of treatment, completion of treatment, disease recurrence and the point of recognised incurability (Welsh Government 2014; BHSCT 2019). However, the transfer of a key worker should be made with caution, with changes kept to a minimum and appropriately documented and communicated to patients and the wider MDT to ensure continuity of care (BHSCT 2019).

The key worker policy outlines skills required to fulfil the key worker role, and many document as essential criteria advanced communication, advocacy skills and the appropriate knowledge or ability to source relevant information to meet the needs of the patient (Welsh Government 2014; Macmillan Cancer Support 2015; BHSCT 2019). These are areas where the cancer CNS is known to make key contributions to cancer care (NHS England 2010), which supports the ethos that the CNS have been long since recognised as ideally placed to assume the role of key worker for patients with cancer (NICE 2004; NHS England 2010; MacmillanCancer Support 2015; Department of Health Northern Ireland 2022). Furthermore, data from the Northern Ireland (NI) Cancer Patient Experience Study (Department of Health Northern Ireland 2018) demonstrated that the support of a CNS is the single most important factor in a patient's experience of care. This sentiment was also supported in a recent literature review that included 14 worldwide studies and identified the oncology CNS role as one that contributes to improving patient outcomes and enhancing cancer care (Kerr et al. 2021).

A key worker policy recognises that a patient should have a named key worker identified within the MDT; as previously outlined, this may change during the course of the patient's care pathway depending on the patient's personal circumstances or clinical condition (BHSCT 2019; Barnett 2014). Patients from a small in-depth UK survey highlighted that they would prefer their named key worker to remain the same throughout their pathway, irrespective of changing treatment modalities (Ling et al. 2013). Within its evaluation of the contribution of the oncology CNS, Macmillan Cancer Support also advocate that the CNS should act as a key worker across the whole care pathway (NCAT 2010).

Whilst there is clear guidance for quality assurance through peer review (NHS England 2011), this may not always occur (Department of Health Northern Ireland 2010; Ling et al. 2013). For example, the MDT may identify and document the CNS as the patient's key worker; however, the patient may not be informed that the CNS present at their diagnosis is their key worker. This widespread lack of patient awareness is further highlighted in patient experience surveys (Department of Health Northern Ireland 2010; Quality Health 2018), where, confusingly, reference is made to CNSs rather than to key workers. The interchangeable and inconsistent use of terminology has the potential to confuse patients and reduce continuity and coordination of care (Ling et al. 2013). Furthermore, staff from a number of studies disliked the term *key worker* as a replacement for their own specialist roles (Ling et al. 2013; Martins et al. 2016).

Despite roles being operationalised using different titles – for example, *key worker* in the UK (Ling et al. 2013), *professional cancer navigator* in Canada and the USA (Martins et al. 2016) and *cancer care coordinator* in Australia (Freijser et al. 2015), the roles share three core characteristics. These relate to the provision of information, provision of emotional and supportive care, and coordination of services (Martins et al. 2016), and each will be explored further.

5.2.1 Provision of Information

Abrahamson et al. (2010) advocate that meeting the individual's information needs, as identified by them, leads to patient empowerment and an increase in patient participation in their own care. With improvements in digital technologies and the introduction of social media, there is also the emergence of an 'e-patient' (De Bronkart 2015; Richards et al. 2015). This brings a change in the flow and accessibility of knowledge. Patients now have access to information that may have previously been reserved for those in the medical profession. Combining the key worker's training and clinical experience with the patient's new knowledge, life experience, needs and priorities can help improve overall care, increase patient autonomy and encourage shared responsibility (De Bronkart 2015; Richards et al. 2015).

Despite this, some apprehension remains within the medical profession regarding the credibility and reliability of online information and the value of patients 'googling' their conditions (De Bronkart 2015). Online support groups, which may not be governed by a recognised body, may also be criticised in that they lack regulation and offer individual opinion-based advice, which may not be factual or helpful to patients. This further highlights the need for the key worker to assess patient information requirements and provide verbal and written information concerning their diagnosis, investigations, treatment options, living with cancer and signposting to local support services (BHSCT 2019).

5.2.2 Provision of Emotional and Supportive Care

Patients with a diagnosis of cancer often experience multifactorial distress that can encompass psychological, social and spiritual elements, which may result in patients being frightened and vulnerable and, often, unable to understand the full implications of the treatment they are being offered (Buckley et al. 2018).

The cancer CNS or other key worker can provide supportive care, appropriate information and individualised care planning for the patient and their carers/relatives, as well as acting as an advocate for the patient within the wider multiprofessional team (Dempsey et al. 2016).

Providing direct care by way of psychological support to patients and their loved ones is recognised within the NI Cancer Patient Survey (Department of Health Northern Ireland 2018) as instrumental in improving the patient's journey. A primary aim of the CNS key worker role is to offer holistic, whole-patient care whereby patients feel supported and know whom to contact with their queries and concerns (NICE 2004). Several tools and interventions have been developed over the years to move away from acute, episodic care to a holistic, personalised approach that is well coordinated and integrated. One such example is the Macmillan Cancer Support Recovery Package, now further developed and named Personal Care and Support Planning (PCSP) (Macmillan Cancer Support 2021). PCSP facilitates patient support conversations and holistic needs assessments (HNA). Although this can be utilised by any professional, it is often the CNS, as the patient's key worker, who offers and completes the HNA and/or PCSP with patients at key points of their care pathway. These supportive conversations and completion of the HNA not only help to build rapport between the CNS and the patient but also allow the patient to take an active and empowered role in the way their care is planned and delivered. They offer opportunities for information giving, patient teaching and interventions tailored around the things that matter most to the patient and in the context of their life and family situation (Macmillan Cancer Support 2021). In addition, they facilitate proactive management of care, which is thought to result in better patient outcomes in terms of survival, quality of life and decisions at end of life (Leary et al. 2014). In practice, support conversations may also be informal and reactive, recognising that most interactions between the CNS and patient are an opportunity to ensure that patients feel supported and empowered.

5.2.3 Coordination of Services

The advanced nursing skills of the CNS – and, as defined by NICE (2004), the skills required of a key worker – offer effective communication and coordination of patient care and ensure that patient information needs are met (NICE 2004; Buckley et al. 2018). Working collaboratively with other professionals, the CNS is often the patient's advocate within the MDT and regularly imparts details regarding patient fitness, awareness of their disease and patient choice (Dempsey et al. 2016; Buckley et al. 2018). Recognising that in practice, the rigid hierarchy or power and influence within healthcare organisations may create barriers to effective communication within MDTs further highlights the need to identify and understand the CNS key worker role and their contribution to the efficacy of the

MDT (Wilcocks 2018). In fact, Wilcocks (2018) outlines that teams with higher efficacy demonstrate shared leadership in which all MDT members are nurtured and supported and feel empowered to contribute.

Earlier in the chapter, it was acknowledged that as a named key worker, the CNS often coordinates patient care through the complex and multifaceted oncology system. The CNS, as the patient's key worker, advocates for the patient within the MDT, often requesting that appointments and scans are as timely as possible whilst also referring to wider community services such as health physiotherapy. Evidence shows that patient outcomes are better when nurses lead care coordination (Forbes 2014; Martins et al. 2016).

Direct access to a CNS, as the patient's key worker, has proven beneficial in minimising or preventing admissions; however, accessibility to services varies geographically and according to cancer type (Leary et al. 2014). Challenges such as size and nature of caseload, organisational structure and allocation of resources have been suggested as reasons for inconsistency in CNS service provision (NHS England 2013; Leary et al. 2014). In a lung cancer audit (Healthcare Quality Improvement Partnership 2012), patients with a known CNS, in comparison to those who did not have a CNS, were more likely to receive treatment (60% versus 30%). It is thought that patient performance status and survival may be improved with CNS interventions; this, together with enhanced information giving, facilitated better-informed decision-making and thus patients who were more likely to proceed with treatment (Leary et al. 2014).

The NICE (2004) advocate that a named key worker should be accessible and available. This is likely to vary according to the individual fulfilling the role, and clear communication should be given both verbally and in writing to patients regarding key worker availability. In the context of the CNS, the role is usually not usually available over a 24-hour period and also over 7 days, but this may be a consideration for future developments of the role.

5.3 Key Worker/Clinical Nurse Specialist Impact on Direct and Indirect Patient Care

Many components specified within the remit of the key worker role are considered to already be integral elements of the CNS role (Ling et al. 2013); thus there is value in briefly considering the impact of the CNS on patient care as a whole. The International Council of Nursing (ICN) (2020) advocate that the CNS role impacts and influences both direct and indirect patient care: the former through holistic psychological patient support, coordination and continuity of care, information giving, patient teaching and clinical management; and the latter through cost savings, implementing improvements and translating research evidence into clinical practice to improve clinical and fiscal outcomes (ICN 2020; Kerr et al. 2021).

Elements with a direct impact on patient care were explored earlier in this chapter under the headings of provision of information, provision of emotional support and coordination of care. The indirect impact of the CNS key worker role on patient care may be found in cost savings from the introduction of nurse-led services such as review clinics. These are well-established worldwide and are often run by nurses with specialist knowledge in their field, such as CNSs. Multiple studies have shown that nurse-led services afford health trusts considerable monetary cost savings compared to consultant-led clinics, with no detriment to patient care (Henry 2015; Latter et al. 2019). Nurse-led care is the focus of Chapter 11 of this book.

Often, nurse-led services are timelier and thus help reduce patient waiting times for review. In the UK, documents such as 'Transforming Your Care' (Department of Health Northern Ireland 2010) look at risk-stratified follow-up pathways. These include patient-directed aftercare and are driven by nurse-led services, usually managed by the CNS as the patient's key worker. Certain disease sites such as breast, prostate, and gynaecology oncology services have embraced patient-directed aftercare; this is now embedded in the follow-up pathway, relieving pressure on both nurse-led and consultant-led review clinics whilst supporting patients with piece of mind via a rapid-access clinic (nurse-led), should the patient have concerns (NHS England 2016).

The CNS role has developed over time, becoming more flexible and responsive to the population's healthcare needs and environments (ICN 2020). The fundamental strength of the CNS role is in providing complex speciality care while improving the quality of healthcare delivery through a systems approach (ICN 2020). In the UK, the development of the CNS role has included many aspects of care that were traditionally in the domain of the medical profession and have underpinned many key changes in the NHS, such as shortened (or avoidance of) hospital stays, personalised care planning and rapid-access diagnostics (Henry 2015). CNSs are also in the driving seat of the ongoing initiative to address the lifelong needs of cancer survivors (Torjesen 2010), taking the concept of continuity of care beyond the confines of ongoing clinical management (Vidall et al. 2011). In its 2010 report, the Royal College of Nursing (RCN) describe specialist nurses as adding value to care and providing an optimal return on investment in relation to income generation, patient safety, efficiency, cost savings and improvements in patient care and experience (Royal College of Nursing 2010).

5.4 Challenges in Practice

The Cancer Strategy for Northern Ireland (Department of Health Northern Ireland 2022) highlight that despite the positive associations related to key worker support through a CNS, not all patients have access to a CNS. For many, support is limited to only some elements of their pathway rather than following the individual patient throughout their cancer journey (Department of Health Northern Ireland 2022). As a key worker, the CNS provides a unique set of services at all system outcome levels and is an essential part of the healthcare team (Mohr and Coke 2018). It is important that employers model workloads and allocation of resources efficiently, as doing so contributes to service delivery (White and Goodchild 2019). In the UK, CNS need has been calculated on the national dataset of new diagnoses/incidences (White and Goodchild 2019). However, this negates to include the ongoing caseload of patients who continue to use CNS services.

Furthermore, it is reported that for some disease sites, such as ovarian and lung cancer, patients access CNS key worker services but are then diagnosed as benign, which is not reflected in the CNS workload (Healthcare Quality Improvement Partnership 2012; Leary et al. 2014). This has led to a chronic shortage in CNS provision over the years as incidences of new cancer diagnosis rise and patients continue to live longer with cancer (McConnell et al. 2016).

In the context of NI, there had been a drive for CNS provision to be brought in line with mainland UK levels. Following a workforce planning review and collaboration with charity groups, funding was made available for 60 new CNS posts across the province in 2016 (Department of Health Northern Ireland 2016). This work is ongoing, and phase two of the CNS expansion plan continues with the recognition of incidence, prevalence, complexity and benchmarking of CNS provision against that of England and Wales (Department of Health Northern Ireland 2022).

Before the COVID-19 worldwide pandemic, there were ongoing investigations to estimate the gap in the provision of specialist cancer nurses (White and Goodchild 2019). With the further redeployment of CNS provision due to COVID-19, the development of newer roles and stretched resources, there is a risk of the cancer CNS role – and, by association, the key worker role – being eroded and devalued (Skills for Health 2021).

The non-tangible impact of the CNS key worker role on patient care is hard to define and quantify; thus there is a need to continue to develop robust data on clinical outcomes, a task which can be difficult to do in practice (Royal College of Nursing 2009). The CNS role is often critiqued for struggling to demonstrate their worth and not having clearly defined evidence of the impact of their activity on patient outcomes (Latter et al. 2019). A larger study of lung cancer in the UK identified that caseload size and nature is a determinant of workload in terms of time available for the CNS to provide holistic complex cancer care to the optimum best practice standard (Leary et al. 2014). In a study of the complexity of metastatic breast care work by CNS key workers, patient-initiated contacts such as telephone calls are recognised as 'hidden appointments' and should be formally identified and recorded to evidence workload and fed into clinical outcomes data, which should in turn drive CNS workforce provision (Leary et al. 2014).

The complex, multifaceted role of the CNS and lack of understanding within the wider MDT often result in duplication of work with other disciplines and confusion for patients as to who their key worker is and who best to direct their concern to (Cook et al. 2019). Education and effective communication of the role of the cancer CNS to non-CNS colleagues, in addition to clear pathways for the maintenance of the descriptor *key worker* in the eyes of the patient, will guide support and ensure that misunderstandings do not negatively affect the delivery of care and patient support (Vidall et al. 2011). An appreciation of the skills of other members of the MDT is important, in order to not overlook what other nurses, disciplines and specialities can offer the patient (Cook et al. 2019). For example, whilst undertaking radiotherapy, patients may be best placed to seek guidance from the radiotherapy nursing team or specialist radiographers rather than their oncology CNS key worker. Again, this raises the question of whether the key worker role should transfer to other specialities or disciplines within the patient treatment pathway.

5.5 'First Impressions Count'

The diverse nature of tumour-specific sites and varied treatment modalities can impact how and when patients are first introduced to their CNS key worker. Macmillan Cancer Support advocate that patients should be referred to a CNS (key worker) at first diagnosis, but they recognise that not all areas of cancer have a CNS (Macmillan Cancer Support 2021). For cancers with multiple treatment modalities, there may be several CNSs with specialist knowledge and skills pertaining to each sphere of the treatment pathway. For example, gynaecology malignancies may first be managed with surgery and then referred for adjuvant chemotherapy +/− radiotherapy +/− brachytherapy. In the first author's experience, the gynaecology oncology surgical CNS has specialist knowledge of all five gynaecology cancers and their surgical management. As per Northern Ireland Cancer Network (NICaN) guidelines (BHSCT 2019), patients are introduced to or given contact details of their surgical CNS as their key worker at their first diagnosis appointment. This relationship ends when the patient is referred via the MDT to the appropriate clinical oncology or medical oncology team for onward treatment. The CNS connected to these teams then aims to see the patient and introduce themselves as a key worker at their first appointment to discuss treatment. A study of gynaecology oncology CNSs in Australia highlighted that the CNS, as the patient's central contact within the team, was responsible for the smooth transition of care between departments and episodes of care (Cook et al. 2019). Research from multiple patient surveys has shown that early input from an oncology CNS improves the patient experience (NCAT 2010; Department of Health Northern Ireland 2018).

In a further study by Regan et al. (2012), the specialist nurses interviewed identified their key worker role as 'everything to everyone'. This raises concern about the possibility of patients and MDT members becoming over-dependent on the CNS in the role of key worker. An overreliance could contribute to disempowering individuals, with team members completing tasks that patients may be able to do for themselves (Regan et al. 2012; Cook et al. 2019). In essence, the CNS key worker role should be part of the system rather than the system itself.

5.6 Example of Change in Practice

It has already been highlighted that there is debate as to whether a patient should be given a named cancer key worker who remains constant throughout their cancer journey or if the key worker should change as the patient progresses through the various stages of their cancer pathway. As outlined earlier in the chapter, Ling et al. (2013) completed a small study with patients and staff and identified that staff felt the key worker role should transfer to other members of the care team, while patients expressed a desire to have the same key worker. This highlights the importance of continuity for the patient in this relationship. Dempsey et al. (2016) suggest that the CNS may pass the key worker role on to another relevant professional when the patient is on a particular part of the pathway, as this may be in the patient's best interests and provide the best support at that particular point of their journey. By contrast, a large study commissioned by Macmillan Cancer Support states that patients benefited positively by having a single named CNS in charge of their care (Macmillan Cancer Support 2015).

Empowering patients with knowledge facilitates them in making informed choices as to who is best to contact for support when they need it. Indeed, we identified earlier that a core element of the key worker role is to ensure that patients have appropriate information and to support their understanding of it. The regional gynaecology oncology centre in NI delivers both chemotherapy and radiotherapy to patients by the same team and in the same treatment centre. As such, patients come into contact with clinical specialist site radiographers (CSSRs) and specialist nurses, including CNSs, at the same time during their pathway. Initially, patients were given two separate contact cards for the CSSR and CNS as their points of contact. Patients reported either that they were unsure which to contact and so contacted both the CSSR and CNS, resulting in possible duplication of work, or that they felt overwhelmed and contacted neither, resulting in an unsatisfactory patient outcome. To address this concern, the team in NI innovatively explored collaborative approaches of working to enhance communication and improve patient pathways across multiple treatment modalities. A key worker information leaflet was created for patients and highlights not only how a key worker can support patients but, more helpfully, whom patients should contact and when. This new information leaflet is given to patients at their first treatment consultation by the CSSR/CNS or medical team, with an emphasis placed on the joint supportive roles available throughout the treatment and follow-up pathway. It is hoped that the joined approach with one information leaflet rather than two separate contact cards provides clarity to patients and gives them confidence that they have contacted the right person to support their needs at that time.

5.7 Conclusion

The cancer key worker role is complex and multifaceted and recognised as vital to improving clinical outcomes for patients with cancer. Much of the key worker role mirrors the CNS role and hence offers strong support that the CNS is ideally placed to fulfil the role of patient key worker. CNSs are often best placed to impact and influence direct and indirect patient care through holistic psychological patient support, coordination and continuity of care, information giving, and patient teaching and clinical management whilst generating cost savings, implementing improvements and translating research evidence into clinical practice to improve clinical and fiscal outcomes. Further work needs to be undertaken to clarify the key worker site-specific role requirements and consistent use of terminology within the wider clinical team to avoid overlap of services. This should then be clearly documented and cascaded to patients to provide clear direction of the support available. Care should be taken to avoid over-reliance on the CNS key worker role by the MDT. The development of robust methods to evidence CNS key worker activity to feed into clinical outcomes data should contribute to driving CNS workforce provision and help meet the NICE (2004) recommendation that each individual with a diagnosis of cancer be allocated a key worker.

References

Abrahamson, K., Durham, M., and Fox, R. (2010). Managing the unmet psychosocial and information needs of the patient with cancer. *Patient Intelligence* 2: 45–52.

Barnett, L. (2014). Cancer services – 'key worker' policy. Doncaster and Bassetlaw Hospitals NHS Foundation Trust, England.

Belfast Health and Social Care Trust (2019). *Operational Policy for Belfast Trust Specialist Gynae-Oncology Multidisciplinary Team*. Belfast: BHSCT.

Betterteam. (2021). What is a key worker in the U.K.? https://www.betterteam.com/uk/what-is-a-key-worker (accessed 3 April 2022).

Buckley, L., Robertson, S., Wilson, T. et al. (2018). The role of the specialist nurse in gynaecological cancer. *Current Oncology Reports* 20: https://link.springer.com/article/10.1007/s11912-018-0734-6 (accessed 22 September 2022).

Cook, O., McIntyre, M., Recoche, K., and Lee, S. (2019). Our nurse is the glue for our team–multidisciplinary team members' experiences and perceptions of the gynaecological oncology specialist nurse role. *European Journal of Oncology Nursing* 41: 7–15.

De Bronkart, D. (2015). From patient centred to people powered: autonomy on the rise. *British Medical Journal* 350: 1–3.

Dempsey, L., Orr, S., Lane, S., and Scott, A. (2016). The clinical nurse specialist's role in head and neck cancer care: United Kingdom National Multidisciplinary Guidelines. *The Journal of Laryngology and Otology* 130 (suppl2): S212–S215.

Department of Health Northern Ireland. (2010). Transforming your care. https://www.health-ni.gov.uk/topics/health-policy/transforming-your-care (accessed 26 November 2021).

Department of Health Northern Ireland. (2016). Health minister announces £11.5m investment in cancer care. https://www.health-ni.gov.uk/health-minister-announces-ps115m-investment-cancer-care (accessed 28 November 2021).

Department of Health Northern Ireland (2018). *Career framework for specialist nursing roles*. Northern Ireland: DoH.

Department of Health Northern Ireland. (2022). A cancer strategy for Northern Ireland 2022–2032. https://www.health-ni.gov.uk/publications/cancer-strategy-northern-ireland-2022-2032 (accessed 12 October 2022).

Forbes, T.H. (2014). Making the case for the nurse as the leader of care coordination. *Nursing Forum* 49 (3): 167–170.

Freijser, L., Naccarella, L., McKenzie, R., and Krishnasamy, M. (2015). Cancer care coordination: building a platform for the development of care coordinator roles and ongoing evaluation. *Australian Journal of Primary Health* 21 (5): 157–163.

Healthcare Quality Improvement Partnership. (2012). National Lung Cancer Audit Report 2011. https://www.hqip.org.uk/resource/national-lung-cancer-audit-report-2011/#.YsfRrmDMLrc (accessed 7 July 2022).

Henry, R. (2015). The role of the cancer specialist nurse. Nursing in Practice. https://www.nursinginpractice.com/clinical/cancer/the-role-of-the-cancer-specialist-nurse (accessed 22 July 2022).

International Council of Nurses (2020). *Guidelines of Advanced Practice Nursing*. Geneva: ICN.

Kerr, H., Donovan, M., and McSorley, O. (2021). Evaluation of the role of the clinical nurse specialist in cancer care: an integrative literature review. *European Journal of Cancer Care* 30 (3): 1–13.

Latter, K.A., Purser, S., and Chisholm, S. (2019). Divisional review of the nurse specialist role. *Nursing Standard* 34 (5): 31–34.

Leary, A., White, J., and Yarnell, L. (2014). The work left undone. Understanding the challenge of providing holistic lung cancer nursing care in the UK. *European Journal of Oncology Nursing* 18: 23–28.

Ling, J., Smith, K.E., Brent, S., and Crosland, A. (2013). Key workers in cancer care: patient and staff attitudes and wider implications for role development in cancer services. *European Journal of Cancer Care* 22: 691–698.

Macmillan Cancer Support. (2015). Impact briefs: cancer clinical nurse specialists. https://www.macmillan.org.uk/documents/aboutus/research/impactbriefs/clinicalnursespecialists2015new.pdf (accessed 10 November 2022).

Macmillan Cancer Support. (2021). Caught in the maze. Delivering personalised, integrated care for people with cancer. https://www.macmillan.org.uk/_images/caught-in-the-maze-report_tcm9-359697.pdf (accessed 23 June 2022).

Martins, A., Aldiss, S., and Gibson, F. (2016). Specialist nurse key worker in children's cancer care: professionals' perspectives on the core characteristics of the role. *European Journal of Oncology Nursing* 24: 70–78.

McConnell, H., White, R., and Maher, J. (2016). *Understanding Variations. Outcomes for People Diagnosed with Cancer and Implications for Service Provision.* England: Macmillan.

Mohr, L.D. and Coke, L.A. (2018). Distinguishing the clinical nurse specialist from other graduate nursing roles. *Clinical Nurse Specialist* 32 (3): 139–151.

National Institute for Health and Care Excellence. (2004). Improving supportive and palliative care for adults with cancer. https://www.nice.org.uk/guidance/csg4 (accessed 27 November 2021).

National Institute for Health and Care Excellence. (2016). Breast cancer. https://www.nice.org.uk/guidance/qs12/resources/breast-cancer-pdf-2098481951941 (accessed 3 April 2022).

NHS England. (2010). Excellence in cancer care: the contribution of the clinical nurse specialist. National Cancer Action Team.

NHS England. (2011). Quality in nursing. Clinical nurse specialists in cancer care; provision, proportion and performance. A census of the cancer specialist nurse workforce in England 2011. National Cancer Action Team. https://www.england.nhs.uk/improvement-hub/wp-content/uploads/sites/44/2017/11/Clinical-Nurse-Specialists-in-Cancer-Care_Census-of-the-Nurse-Workforce_Eng-2011.pdf (accessed 27 November 2021).

NHS England. (2013). The Alexa toolkit – Calculating optimum caseload guidance for lung cancer nurse specialists. National Cancer Action Team.

NHS England. (2016). Innovation to implementation: stratified pathways of care for people living with cancer – a 'how to guide'. https://www.england.nhs.uk/publication/innovation-to-implementation-stratified-pathways-of-care-for-people-living-with-or-beyond-cancer-a-how-to-guide (accessed 8 July 2022).

Quality Health (2018). *National Cancer Patient Experience Survey*. Derbyshire: Quality Health Limited.

Regan, M., Mills, J., and Ristevki, E. (2012). Cancer care coordinators relationships with the multidisciplinary team and patients: everything to everyone. *Australian Journal of Cancer Nursing* 13 (1): 12–19.

Richards, T., Coulter, A., and Wicks, P. (2015). Time to deliver patient centred care. *British Medical Journal* 350: 1–2.

Royal College of Nursing (2009). *Specialist Nurses Make a Difference*. London: RCN.

Royal College of Nursing (2010). *Clinical Nurse Specialists: Adding Value to Care*. London: RCN.

Skills for Health. (2021). Developing a cancer CNS capabilities framework in the north west. https://www.skillsforhealth.org.uk/wp-content/uploads/2021/12/Cancer-Framework-Research-Report-Final.pdf (accessed 28 April 2023).

Torjesen, I. (2010). A new approach to aftercare. *Health Service Journal* 120 (suppl 2–3).

Vidall, C., Barlow, H., Crow, M. et al. (2011). Clinical nurse specialists: essential resource for an effective NHS. *British Journal of Nursing (Oncology Supplement)* 20 (17): S23–S27.

Welsh Government. (2014). Principles and guidance – key workers for cancer patients. https://gov.wales/sites/default/files/publications/2019-07/principles-and-guidance-key-workers-for-cancer-patients.pdf (accessed 20 July 2022).

White, R. and Goodchild, J. (2019). *Estimating the Gap in the Provision of Specialist Cancer Nurses in England*. England: Macmillan Cancer Support.

Willcocks, S. (2018). Exploring team working and shared leadership in multi-disciplinary cancer care. *Leadership in Health Services* 31 (1): 98–109.

6

Psychological Support

Caroline McCaughey, Edel Aughey, and Susan Smyth

Abstract

This chapter examines the psychological sequelae of a cancer diagnosis for the patient and their loved ones. It focuses on three time points – diagnosis, treatment decisions and survivorship – as these have been described in the literature as phases of relevance. The chapter seeks to provide evidence-based insights into the varied psychological responses that patients may experience and strongly advocates for a personalised approach to the support and management of the patient by the clinical nurse specialist (CNS). Furthermore, it explores tools and approaches that may foster an effective therapeutic relationship between the CNS and the individual with cancer. Finally, the emotional consequences of ongoing care by the CNS are acknowledged, and the value of self-care, peer supervision and managerial support is discussed.

6.1   Introduction

This chapter is approached not as an exhaustive exploration of the vast topic of psychological care provided by the cancer clinical nurse specialist (CNS) but rather from the perspective of experiential insights gleaned from practice and the literature. These have been accrued from the viewpoints of the three authors: a practice educator/honorary senior lecturer at Queen's University Belfast, whose role involves the education of CNSs (CMcC); a nurse consultant with line management responsibility for CNSs (EA); and a haematology specialist nurse (SS). All three have extensive experience in providing care to individuals with cancer and their families.

This chapter will approach psychological support in two parts. The first part will explore the impact of a cancer experience on the individual diagnosed with cancer and their family/significant others and the psychological care that the CNS

The Role of the Clinical Nurse Specialist in Cancer Care, First Edition. Edited by Helen Kerr.
© 2024 John Wiley & Sons Ltd. Published 2024 by John Wiley & Sons Ltd.
Companion website: www.wiley.com/go/kerr

should provide in a supportive and empowering manner. The second part will focus on the inextricably linked aspect of support and self-care for the CNS so that they can effectively sustain the challenge of providing psychological care unrelentingly throughout a career in cancer nursing.

6.2   Part One: The Impact of a Cancer Diagnosis

A cancer diagnosis is a life-changing event, understandably causing acute psychological distress often characterised by shocked disbelief, anxiety, denial, anger and sadness (Matthews et al. 2019). Indeed, McDonald (2016) identifies that one-third of individuals with cancer are thought to be at high risk of a psychological disorder within the first year of diagnosis. According to Johnson et al. (2015), the adverse impact is related to the existential threat of the disease, potential psychosocial consequences on employment and family/social life, and disease- or treatment-related symptomologies such as pain, dyspnoea, nausea and altered body image. In a recent study, Muzzatti et al. (2022) recognised anxiety and depression as related (yet distinct) dimensions of psychological distress. This study reported incidence rates of 17% for anxiety and depression simultaneously, and 21% of patients had either anxiety or depression. They affirm that psychological distress is common and disturbing for all patients during the cancer trajectory and advocate for the usefulness of assessing both the intensity and prevalence of anxiety and depression using tools such as the validated Hospital Anxiety and Depression Scale (HADS). Seiler and Jenewein (2019) and Hauk et al. (2021) acknowledge that the traumatic and uncontrollable nature of the often sudden diagnosis of cancer can make individuals vulnerable to long-lasting negative psychological outcomes incorporating distress, anxiety, insomnia, fatigue, depression and reduced quality of life. Consequently, Tauber et al. (2019) identify that this may lead to the overuse of scarce healthcare services or, conversely, non-engagement behaviours with health services.

In a literature review regarding risk factors for psychological distress, Arroyo et al. (2019) reported that whilst study findings lacked consistency, commonly cited factors included younger age, lower education level, unmarried status, non-engagement in physical activity, menopausal symptoms, employment status, aggressiveness of anti-cancer therapy and presence of other comorbidities. Hardardottir et al. (2022) also identify a history of psychological morbidity as an additional risk factor for psychological distress. Although this awareness is important for the CNS, the divergent study findings emphasise the necessity of an individualised patient assessment.

Fradgley et al. (2019) outlines how the International Psycho-oncology Society (IPOS) emphasise that distress should be measured as the sixth vital sign alongside temperature, blood pressure, pulse, respiratory rate and pain and that treating distress is an essential component of high-quality care. The National Comprehensive Cancer Network (Riba et al. 2019) define distress as a multifactorial, unpleasant emotional experience that is psychological, social, spiritual and/or physical and may interfere with an individual's ability to cope with a cancer diagnosis, symptoms and treatment. Despite the prevalence of distress, particularly in the initial weeks post-diagnosis (Hardardottir et al. 2022), Molassiotis et al. (2020) uncover issues of inadequate psychosocial care, symptom control and unmet information needs. They identify the essential role of the specialist nurse in completing a holistic needs assessment (HNA), providing and coordinating supportive care, and associating this intervention with improved emotional functioning and symptoms, thus lowering service utilisation and reducing cost. Macmillan Cancer Support (2021) advocate for an HNA as a key intervention to structure conversations, identifying patient concerns and thus developing a more personalised, collaborative care and support plan. Whilst not consistently utilised in practice, Snowdon et al. (2011) suggest the distress thermometer, commonly included in an HNA, as a well-validated screening tool with a brevity that makes it ideal to incorporate into clinical practice.

The National Institute for Health and Care Excellence (NICE) (2004) postulate that psychological support can be separated into two categories (Table 6.1).

Table 6.1 Categories of psychological support.

	Level	Group	Assessment	Intervention
Recommended model of professional psychological assessment and support				
	1	All health and social care professionals	Recognition of psychological needs	Effective information-giving, compassionate communication and general psychological support
↑ Self-help and informal support ↓	2	Health and social care professionals with additional expertise	Screening for psychological distress	Psychological techniques such as problem-solving
	3	Trained and accredited professionals	Assessed for psychological distress and diagnosis of some psychopathology	Counselling and specific psychological interventions, such as anxiety management and solution-focused therapy, delivered according to an explicit theoretical framework
	4	Mental health specialists	Diagnosis of psychopathology	Specialist psychological and psychiatric interventions such as psychotherapy, including cognitive behavioural therapy (CBT)

Category one incorporates level one and level two and can be provided by healthcare professionals who have some training in assessment and frontline management of psychological problems but are not mental health practitioners. Category two incorporates levels three and four and can be provided by trained, accredited practitioners such as counsellors or mental health professionals. The CNS role sits within the definition of level two support, which incorporates professionals who are guided by holistic assessment to formally detect distress and offer interventions to enhance self-care and adjustment on a daily basis. Furthermore, they may need to offer referral to more specialised services.

Person-centred practice is advocated globally as an approach to care for all healthcare professionals and has been demonstrated to improve patient outcomes. It is 'an approach to practice established through the formation and fostering of healthful relationships between all care providers, service users and others significant to them in their lives. It is underpinned by values of respect for person, individual right to self-determination, mutual respect and understanding. It is enabled by cultures of empowerment that foster continuous approaches to practice development' (McCormack and McCance 2017, p. 3).

In order to maintain a focus on adopting a person-centred approach, the theory will be applied to a case study, which for confidentiality and anonymity purposes will be a hybrid of a number of patients who have taught the authors valuable lessons in their nursing careers to date. There will be a focus on three significant points in the patient trajectory, cited by Samuelsson et al. (2021) as phases of relevance: the point of diagnosis, treatment decision-making, and embarking on survivorship. It is recognised by Arroyo et al. (2019) and Samuelsson et al. (2021) that the cancer trajectory often follows a winding path, with overlap along the survivorship and palliative care routes. Whilst it is recognised how critical psychological support is in the palliative and end-of-life phase, the focus will remain on the three time points outlined, with the understanding that many of the evidence-based skills and strategies are transferable to any point of the patient's pathway.

6.2.1 Time Point One: Breaking Significant News

Case study: Sarah (she/her) is a 52-year-old senior laboratory technician, married to Michael (he/him), and together they have two children. Aoife is 20 years old and currently studying at university, and Matthew is 16 years old and currently at school. Sarah presented to the emergency department with a six-week history of reduced appetite, abdominal discomfort and constipation. A computed tomography (CT) scan showed an abdominal mass. Biopsies were taken, and once Sarah's symptoms were managed, she was discharged with an oncology appointment date.

Table 6.2 SPIKES framework.

S	**Set up** the interview – consider privacy, uninterrupted time, rapport building.
P	Review the patient's **perception** of the illness.
I	Get an **invitation** from the patient to deliver the news – determine how much information the patient wants, and provide a 'warning shot' that bad news is coming.
K	Give the patient **knowledge** and information.
E	Respond to the patient's **emotions.**
S	**Summarise** the treatment plan, and review all that has been discussed.

Given the potential enormity of a cancer diagnosis, Matthews et al. (2019) conducted a meta-synthesis to explore the experiences of patients and their families receiving bad news about cancer. Conclusions reported that the impact could be modulated by the quality of how the difficult news is delivered, with additional training suggested to enhance the healthcare professional's ability to deliver this news sensitively and with appropriate support. This would reflect the first author's (CMcC) experience, having been responsible for co-facilitating a two-day Wilkinson Model communications skills training course for healthcare professionals in the cancer setting (Wilkinson et al. 2008; Rutherford and McCaughey 2015). The training provides resources and tools that have been utilised by all the authors in their roles as nurses in cancer clinical practice. The first of the models is the SPIKES framework (Table 6.2) outlined by Baile and Parker (2017). This anagram is easily understandable and, importantly, can be applied to many situations throughout the cancer trajectory, including diagnosis, recurrence and transition to palliative care.

Interestingly, Blanckenburg et al. (2020) note that the SPIKES protocol was designed from a healthcare professional's perspective. To address this, they conducted a study to ascertain patients' preference for the communication of bad news, with the motivation that person-centred communication is less anxiety-provoking. Implications of their findings were that all SPIKES components were seen as highly relevant, with an emphasis on the importance of tailoring support and approaches to individual preferences whilst incorporating the six steps. Patient feedback stressed the need to explore concerns, provide an opportunity to express feelings and involve the patient in decision-making.

Case study: The first meeting with Sarah and Michael was at the haematology outpatient clinic, where the diagnosis of lymphoma was explained. Whilst the haematologist was relaying the information regarding Sarah's diagnosis, it was evident from Sarah's non-verbal cues that this was indeed a huge shock, although she did not say very much during this initial consultation. As a CNS, the final author (SS) accompanied Sarah and Michael into another room, away from the busy clinic, to gauge their reactions and offer support.

This case study highlights the use of a second tool called ICE (ideas, concerns and expectations), promoted by Finn et al. (2017) and designed to assess patients in a more holistic and individualised way. By exploring ideas, the CNS establishes the patient's thoughts, beliefs and feelings about their condition whilst eliciting specific concerns at this point in their illness. Finally, expectations facilitate an enquiry into the patient's hopes and what they would like to happen, providing insight into the degree to which they correlate with what the CNS anticipates. The authors have found this tool particularly useful in uncovering any unrealistic patient expectations, which the CNS may gently and sensitively explore. In this situation, we would utilise the 'Wish, Worry, Wonder' communication support framework (Dana-Farber Cancer Institute 2016, p. 12). 'I wish' allows the CNS to align with the patient's hopes, with the expression of 'I worry' providing an opportunity for being truthful about the situation. 'I wonder' provides a subtle insight to make an alternative recommendation or introduce a different perspective.

> Case study: These frameworks were particularly appropriate in this situation: they facilitated Sarah to verbalise her anger, which surprised Michael, who attempted to intervene with soothing words.

This highlights the often-different needs required by patients and their families, necessitating that the CNS be cognisant of the individualised person-centred approach required in their care delivery and assist all involved parties with their emotional and informational needs to reduce the psychological distress so often felt at this pertinent time (Samuelsson et al. 2021). Rodenbach et al. (2019) suggest that tensions can arise when there are conflicting perspectives between the patient and family member and advise that anticipating these emotionally charged exchanges can help the CNS deal calmly with family tensions.

Whilst imparting knowledge and information is an important step in the SPIKES framework, Korsvold et al. (2016) caution that communication can be inappropriately dominated by one-way information-giving, a position that Zimmermann and Del Piccolo (2007) concur with. These authors contend that one of the crucial challenges in communication is being attentive to patients' expressions of emotions and needs; these often indicate emotional distress of clinical significance and can be expressed with cues. Korsvold et al. (2016) identify that patients often express their emotions indirectly, using hints and cues, and there are large variations in how healthcare professionals respond. This may lead to missed opportunities for empathic opportunities. Korsvold et al. (2016) elaborate on the importance of acknowledging and validating the patient's emotions rather than simply responding with medical facts; otherwise, if a patient does not feel heard and understood, they may be less satisfied with their care, remember less information and be more reluctant to follow advice. Zimmermann and Del Piccolo (2007) clarify that cues differ from concerns, which are mostly verbalised emotions; as patients often hide emotions, healthcare professionals may only uncover them if they pay adequate attention. As well as verbal hints, cues may also be non-verbal and expressed by, for example, body posture or voice inflexion. Zimmermann and Del Piccolo (2007) found that clinicians often missed cues by interrupting, avoidance, discouraging expression of emotions, giving information or providing premature reassurance, thus alerting us to be observant for these blocking behaviours in our practice. Cues subsequently can be acknowledged and explored using clarifying, open and probing questions. Zimmermann and Del Piccolo (2007) make the salient point that cues take listeners into the patient's agenda and thus are a vital addition to the ICE framework.

Dr Kathryn Mannix, a palliative care consultant, provides challenging and enlightening insights in her book *Listen,* and we recommend this reading material to all CNSs (Mannix 2021). Dr Mannix emphasises not just listening but attentive listening to understand. Her writing resonates, as on reflection, CNSs would be likely to acknowledge that the quality of listening may be imperfect. Often, CNSs are too busy thinking of the next question to ask the patient and thus miss vital cues and information in the moment. We hope the following excerpt provides some challenge and reflection.

> When was the last time ... you felt that someone appreciated not only the words you were saying, but why the matter under discussion was important to you? ... What we are considering here is not simply being listened to, but being heard.
>
> *(Mannix 2021, p. 25)*

Dr Mannix suggests the alternative phrase 'unwelcome news' as preferable to 'bad news', as it conjures up the many times CNSs may deliver information that the patient finds undesirable, even though we may not have considered it as significant as diagnostic/prognostic news. Moreover, along with other authors (Matthews et al. 2019; Mailankody and Rao 2021), Dr Mannix emphasises the importance of truth-telling, underscoring that truth with kindness is core.

> I've been using the word tender to describe sensitive conversations for several years now.... 'Courageous/challenging/difficult conversations' all evoke a self-defence response that as the very opposite of the 'I'm here for you' mindset that these conversations require. Tenderness seemed to me to conjure the disposition most helpful for discussions that are painful to one or both parties. It acknowledges the presence of pain not as something to be overcome, but an experience to be held with sensitivity and respect.... It's not about difficulty, courage or challenge. It's simply about being intentionally, fully present.
>
> *(Mannix 2021, p. 37)*

A particular reassuring point made by Mannix (2021) is that it is understandable to feel that we do not always know what to say. She acknowledges the complexity of the situations and dilemmas patients face, and cautions us to be mindful that our task is not always to solve but sometimes simply to listen. With this approach, she proposes that words will come from the heart rather than the head and convey the authentic empathy and concern that Jeffrey (2016) rates as valuable. Like Pease (2017), Mannix dwells on the importance of silence in painful conversations to provide space to think; slowing down the pace helps to focus on what is being said.

6.2.2   Time Point Two: Treatment Decision-Making

> Case study: Returning to Sarah, following the initial consultation regarding the diagnosis of cancer and planning of further tests, the next appointment related to treatment planning. SPIKES components were also pertinent at this stage, in addition to tailoring the information to the individual to minimise psychological distress. It became clear that Sarah needed more specific information, so in partnership with the pharmacist, relevant articles were sourced that attempted to meet her need for scientific information. As Hyatt et al. (2022) explain, not all information is helpful to all patients, and it is imperative to gauge the health literacy of each individual patient. This point is echoed by Fahmer et al. (2022), who concluded that responding to a patient's individual health literacy, results in higher satisfaction with both information and care and an increase in self-efficacy. For Sarah, this type of scientific information was in a format and language she was readily acquainted with, making it an appropriate source of information for her.

In addition to understanding the information regarding the proposed treatment, patients must also be prepared to manage at home. This may include dealing with side effects, self-administering supportive medications and being aware of the Chemotherapy Helpline, if available. Hyatt et al. (2022) provide a reminder that this information can be complex, and it is essential that patients understand. Strategies such as chunk and check (Gilligan et al. 2017; Lehmann et al. 2020) and teach back (Nouri and Rudd 2015; Neville Miller et al. 2021; Shersher et al. 2021) are invaluable at this stage.

Delivering information in small units and assessing understanding systematically is a straightforward method of tailoring information for the patient whilst simultaneously reducing their psychological distress and maximising their recall (Lehmann et al. 2020). The strategy of *chunk and check* allows optimisation of what can be limited time in a busy clinical area and simultaneously prevents overloading patients with information they are unable to manage at this time (Lehmann et al. 2020). Using this strategy assists in keeping the dialogue person-centred and tailored towards the patient's needs.

Teach back allows the patient to repeat back their understanding of information or relevant instructions and can allow the CNS to assess knowledge, elicit recall and correct any errors or misconceptions (Shersher et al. 2021). Neville Miller et al. (2021) take this further and propose that as a strategy, teach back enhances patient self-efficacy.

> Case study: After the meeting, a telephone call was arranged between the specialist nurse and Sarah to follow up on what had been discussed and to ascertain if she had any further questions about any of the material she had been given.

Herrmann et al. (2018) proposed that treatment consultations can be overwhelming for patients and that two separate shorter consultations can be more beneficial and ease the psychological burden felt by patients at this important time. Understandably, with clinics at capacity, this may seem an impossible proposition. However, allowing a break for the patient to take a cup of tea and then reconvening may be sufficient, or, alternatively, arranging a follow-up telephone call. This may not be necessary for every patient; the salient point is tailoring information to avoid the mechanical information-giving that Prip et al. (2022) allude to in their study, concluding that the CNS role is pivotal in turning what can potentially be a unilateral flow of information, into the empathic, collaborative encounter and active engagement valued by individuals with cancer (McDonald 2016).

Interestingly, despite the increased availability of alternative sources of information for many patients today, Rutten et al. (2016) found that talking with their CNS remained a key resource for individuals with cancer. The importance of information being given within a trusted, established relationship is a repeated concept throughout much of the literature associated with providing psychological support for patients with cancer (Atherton et al. 2018; Matthews et al. 2019; Prip et al. 2022).

6.2.3   Time Point Three: Survivorship and Resilience

Whilst the early phase of the cancer experience undeniably has a profound psychological impact, which can have long-lasting outcomes, many patients with cancer can manifest remarkable resilience, as overcoming adversity provides an opportunity for personal growth (Seiler and Jenewein 2019; Tamura et al. 2021). However, each person has their own individual valid response. Tamura et al.'s systematic literature review (Tamura et al. 2021) recognises that there are trends related to psychological morbidity, including individual personality traits, cancer type (particularly metastatic disease) and treatment stage. These can influence the incidence of anxiety, depression and resilience, which they define as the ability to adapt to difficult situations. According to Tamura et al. (2021), highly invasive/intensive treatments and long-term physical symptoms as a result of the disease and/or treatment can threaten mental health. Moreover, they identify a trend of lower resilience in females and those who live alone, have a lower level of education or are from an ethnic minority.

Both Seiler and Jenewein (2019) and Tamura et al. (2021) concur that resilience may be modifiable to promote successful adaption to cancer. Factors they identify as facilitative include the ability of the individual to make meaning of their situation. King et al. (2015) report that cancer specialist nurses have the capacity to help patients reframe the experience of illness more positively, enabling better adaption and coping skills. Patients who feel a degree of hope and optimism, anticipate survival, have social support and draw on spirituality are also identified as more resilient (Seiler and Jenewein 2019).

For the CNS, Seiler and Jenewein (2019) identify the positive influence of a meaningful relationship with healthcare providers, with both social and professional support enabling a sense of being valued and subsequently reducing stress. The CNS, who often fosters a long-term patient relationship, is in an invaluable position to encourage adaptation as the patient's life circumstances change over time. Indeed, Tamura et al. (2021) contend that maintaining mental health, which is inextricably linked with good physical symptom management (Costa et al. 2016), is an important role in cancer nursing and can promote completion of treatment and improved quality of life. Whilst Tamura et al.'s (2021) recommendations of psychotherapy and pharmacotherapy to promote resilience may be outside of the skill set of many CNSs, the role of the CNS in co-coordinating referrals will play an invaluable part.

Thus, for some patients, the CNS may contribute to what Tamura et al. (2021) refer to as *post-traumatic growth*, defined as subjective, positive psychological changes and new insights that arise following a major life crisis, whereby life becomes richer and more meaningful. However, each patient's perspective is highly subjective. Costa et al. (2016) identify that the time after treatment completion can be a difficult transition, which is also recognised by Burney (2019) as a time when feelings of abandonment may be experienced as healthcare contact is less frequent.

Case study: An aspect of the CNS role is to provide an HNA after the completion of treatment. This can provide an opportunity to identify any areas of concern for Sarah. The feeling of abandonment was something Sarah anticipated, so reiterating that she had the CNS's contact number provided reassurance.

Atherton et al. (2018) talk of a secure base, again affirming the value of the continued relationship and contact between the CNS and patient that is invaluable, as advocated by Lim et al. (2022).

6.2.4 Fear of Recurrence

Tauber et al.'s (2019) systematic review and meta-analysis elucidate that despite improved treatment and prognoses, many survivors of cancer live with high levels of uncertainty and fear of cancer recurrence (FCR). These fears can pervade the disease trajectory from completion of active treatment into survivorship and are reported by patients as a common unmet need among survivors of cancer. Of note, low levels of FCR may encourage positive health behaviours and alert patients to early signs of recurrence; however, persistent, excessive fear can be very debilitating and conversely result in avoidance behaviours. Tauber et al. (2019) advocate that cognitive therapies can be efficacious but reassuringly note that FCR tends to stabilise over time.

> Case study: The fear of cancer recurrence for Sarah was very real and identified during the HNA appointment. With her consent, Sarah was referred to a Macmillan Cancer Support survivorship course that helps patients deal with these very issues. It aims to assist them in managing those fears and returning to some form of normalcy, which has particular significance for families (Kuswanto et al. 2018).

Kuswanto et al. (2018) report that parents, particularly mothers, may have an increased risk of stress responses and FCR. Interventions they advocate to minimise stress responses in parents include tangible, practical support such as management of treatment side effects, guiding parents on how to talk to their children and facilitating the maintenance of family routines to promote normalcy. Schiena et al. (2019) additionally promote the provision of relevant information and utilising a warm, family-centred and flexible approach, which the CNS could be influential in offering. Indeed, Kuswanto et al. (2018) note that emotional disruption is exacerbated if the mother feels objectified as a 'patient' by healthcare providers, bringing into sharp focus the advantage of personalisation and collaboration. We suggest asking each patient throughout their journey the question promoted by Macmillan: 'What matters (or what's important) to you?'

> Case study: Currently, Sarah still attends clinic appointments every three months for what she terms 'check-ins'. She has stated that whilst, on the one hand, she dreads the blood tests or scan results, she acknowledges the need for the appointments to continue and that the ever-present support from her CNS helps her to feel like a person and not just a patient with cancer.

6.3 Part Two: Self-Care and the Clinical Nurse Specialist

Much has been written about nursing being a stressful profession, specifically within cancer services, with challenges around uncertain disease trajectories, sudden deterioration and end-of-life care (Potter et al. 2010; Button et al. 2017; Wells-English et al. 2019). The provision of psychological support is a pivotal role of the CNS, as evidenced throughout this chapter in the patient case study; however, this may have implications for the CNS in relation to their mental and physical wellbeing. It may also have implications for the nursing profession, with stress experienced perhaps contributing to challenges with recruitment and retention within this speciality (Toh et al. 2012). This highlights the need for a proactive approach to self-care.

Concepts such as compassion fatigue (Figley 2002) and burnout (Maslach et al. 2001) have been described as the cost of caring and have been documented in the literature over many years. *Compassion fatigue* (CF), introduced by Figley (2002), is described as the emotional cost of caring: the negative consequence of absorbing the suffering of others, which over time can lead to a loss of empathy or even negative feelings towards a patient, leading to sub-standardisation of care (Jenkins and Warren 2012). *Burnout*, conceptualised by Maslach et al. (2001), encompasses three dimensions – emotional exhaustion, depersonalisation and reduced personal accomplishment – and is measured by the Maslach Burnout Inventory (MBI) tool (Maslach et al. 2001). It leads to feelings of apathy and frustration and is associated with low morale, absenteeism and high staff turnover (Toh et al. 2012; Jones et al. 2013).

The level of meaningful engagement by the CNS with individuals with cancer and their families requires a significant and empathic investment by the CNS. Jeffrey (2016) states that empathy is a process in which one person imaginatively enters the experience of another but, critically, without losing awareness of its difference from one's own. Jeffrey proposes that it is necessary to distinguish between our own and another's perspective. Otherwise, we can make assumptions that they feel as we do, so not only do we fail to understand their experience, but we also assume that we do, which leads to false assumptions and places the CNS at risk of personal distress that may lead to burnout.

Jeffrey (2016) also explores how to empathise without becoming overwhelmed and concludes that detachment is not beneficial, as empathy is critical to learn more of the patient's perspective and facilitate them to participate more fully in decision-making. Indeed, Jeffrey (2016) presents evidence that health professions with higher empathy have greater job satisfaction and less burnout and engender a trusting patient relationship. Thus, he concludes that empathy can be fostered and can motivate health professions to help but must be differentiated from sympathy, which is characterised by pity and a self-orientated perspective that risks health professions feeling overwhelmed.

Mannix (2021) agrees that empathy is a more sophisticated emotional response than sympathy, which identifies with suffering and recognises that either there may be no way to fix it or the solutions must come from the patient's viewpoint rather than that of the CNS. In contrast, sympathy generally aims to make it better. Mannix (2021) argues that even the suggestion that the persons suffering can be 'fixed' is demeaning. Instead of focusing on doing something – an approach nurses are often comfortable with – empathy offers to be with someone in their suffering, checking and being aware of their perspective.

However, Jeffrey (2016) cautions that sharing the emotions and feelings of another can lead to distress, particularly if we over-identify with the individual's situation, which can distort one's understanding and threaten the therapeutic process. Also of note, professionals may distance themselves from patients, avoiding emotion and focusing on medical facts as a protective mechanism. To prevent these maladaptive protective mechanisms, the CNS can develop certain skills to ensure that they can continue to provide meaningful person-centred care for individuals with cancer and their families without detriment to their own health and wellbeing. This is particularly significant as an empathetic presence is associated with positive patient outcomes (McDonald 2016; Matthews et al. 2019; Hauk et al. 2021), highlighting the importance of the organisation investing in nurturing those skills required to foster that empathic relationship.

Wilkinson et al. (2008) and McDonald (2016) assert that communication skills training and re-training of the so-called soft skills are not always valued, yet conveying empathy is embedded in what a CNS says and how they say it. This places much significance on the CNS's ability to communicate effectively, especially given that Wilkinson et al. (2008) and McDonald (2016) concur that poor communication negatively affects not just the patient experience but also the wellbeing of the healthcare professional. These studies demonstrate the importance of building confidence and increasing knowledge for cancer nurses, especially related to communication skills and areas of psychosocial care. This very point was identified in the newly published 'A Cancer Strategy for Northern Ireland 2022–2032' (Department of Health Northern Ireland 2022), demonstrating its relevance to the cancer workforce.

The importance of educating staff regarding communication is a pervading theme within cancer nursing, with all advocating for continuing education (Peterson et al. 2010; Leung et al. 2011; Philips and Volker 2020). In Northern Ireland, advanced communication skills training using the Dr Susie Wilkinson Model (Wilkinson et al. 1999) is delivered, which involves video-recorded role-play situations with facilitated discussion, providing valuable learning opportunities in a safe environment. This two-day course has been positively evaluated in Northern Ireland by senior multidisciplinary team members, with 93.5% of participants (N = 66, over 11 advanced communication skills courses) stating they would definitely recommend it to a colleague (Rutherford and McCaughey 2015). Furthermore, Emold et al. (2011) reported that nurses who were confident with their communication skills also felt fulfilled in their jobs. Additionally, they found significant associations between communication skills, self-efficacy and burnout. Higher levels of emotional exhaustion were associated with lower self-efficacy in specific topics, such as communicating unwelcome news or helping a patient deal with uncertainty, leading Emold et al. (2011) to suggest that self-perception of communication abilities impacted levels of burnout and stress felt by cancer nurses.

An additional skill that requires nurturing and is cited as being of utmost relevance to both the patient and CNS in terms of coping is resilience. 'Resilience: The Power Within', a paper published by Grafton et al. (2010), aimed to advance understanding of resilience as an innate resource with potential and relevance in managing workplace stress for cancer nurses. Resilience, the ability to cope with or recover from the impact of stress and turn it into a positive learning experience (Richardson 2002; Jackson et al. 2007), is claimed in the literature to assist nurses to better manage the impact of stress and lead to sustained wellbeing (Hodges et al. 2005). Therefore, it is incumbent on organisations to support and develop resilience amongst CNS staff to ensure that workplace stress is managed and CNSs have space to flourish and grow in a positive environment that values their role and contribution to patient care. Wittenberg-Lyles et al. (2013) found that regular peer clinical support groups facilitated learning and increased the level of support amongst staff in the oncology/haematology care setting. These support groups were positively evaluated, although securing time away from the clinical area was a major impediment and required senior management commitment. *This mirrors the experience of the final author (SS) as a CNS, as regular meetings facilitate the sharing of knowledge, expression of emotions and debriefing.* These moments of protected time foster resilience, allowing CNSs to continue to provide exceptional care to patients and their families.

From an organisational perspective, facilitating this protected time is one way of providing a nurturing work environment or culture. Wu et al. (2016) cited that supportive work environments effectively decreased compassion fatigue and burnout. This study also noted a cohesive team approach to mitigate burnout and compassion fatigue. Given the evidence from this study, proposing a multi-professional approach to clinical supervision may assist with team dynamics and engender positive working relationships within the oncology team (Wu et al. 2016).

Gribben and Semple (2021) studied a sample of 78 haemato-oncology nurses from the island of Ireland to determine the prevalence and predictors of burnout and work-life balance. They found that levels of burnout were high amongst the nurses studied and suggested organisations had a responsibility to teach approaches to stress management, self-care and how to foster resilience within their workforce. Furthermore, they found that where work-life balance was better, nurses were much less likely to experience burnout. In the final author's experience, the value of regular one-to-one meetings where work-life balance and job plans can be reviewed cannot be underestimated. In addition, annual appraisals provide a means of offering the CNS dedicated time to talk to their manager to share concerns, aspirations or wishes, thus fostering a sense of the value of the CNS role.

However, the responsibility to develop skills such as empathy, communication and resilience does not lie solely at the feet of the organisation; the CNS must also take ownership of their psychological wellbeing. Health and Social Care Trusts throughout Northern Ireland offer free or subsidised classes/initiatives for staff, encompassing many options for wellbeing and stress management. These include mindfulness, music, yoga, Pilates and physical exercise classes to appeal to the preferences of as many professionals as possible. Acrimon-Pagès et al. (2019) propose that unless self-help is encouraged, the oncology workforce will continue to experience burnout and/or compassion fatigue, resulting in a high turnover of staff (Toh et al. 2012). 'One can think of self-care, then, as a form of insulation against stress' (Sherman 2004, p. 52). Self-help interventions such as mindfulness, yoga and exercise are all reported to decrease burnout and stress and foster compassion for oneself and others; additionally, they increase resilience and teach emotional regulation (Ceravolo and Raines 2019; Green and Kinchen 2021; Hilcove et al. 2021).

Furthermore, flexible working policies to promote work-life balance exist in all the Health and Social Care Trusts in Northern Ireland. Similar to the flexibility valued by patients to minimise interruptions to family life, these policies may offer an opportunity for the CNS to discuss family-friendly arrangements, which are feasible within the confines of service provision, and thus promote a better work-life balance. Crelin and Quinn (2010) also highlight the efficacy of a counselling service for oncology staff and patients; this opportunity is an option in each of the authors' workplaces.

6.4 Conclusion

It is evident that patients and their loved ones will present with variable emotional responses at different stages of their cancer trajectory. Whilst a diagnosis of a malignancy is indisputably highly distressing, with the passage of time, many patients manifest remarkable resilience to overcome the adversity, which may even provide an opportunity for personal post-traumatic growth. An effective relationship and communication with a CNS can be pivotal and has the potential to not only improve the patient and family experience but also increase job satisfaction for the CNS. In order to retain the resilience needed for this demanding role, the CNS needs to feel valued through organisational support, such as protected time for supervision, the opportunity for appraisal and educational investment. By empowering the CNS with self-care skills and communication tools, the resilience of both the patient and the CNS may be maximised.

The thread that has run through this entire chapter is that of empathic, personalised, family and person-centred care to promote psychological health. It is striking that these patient-care values reflect the approach that is also required to foster and support the CNSs who are journeying alongside them.

References

Acrimon-Pagès, E., Torres-Puig-Gros, J., Fernández-Ortega, P., and Canela-Soler, J. (2019). Emotional impact and compassion fatigue in oncology nurses: results of a multicentre study. *European Journal of Oncology Nursing* 43: 1–6.

Arroyo, O.M., Vaillo, Y.A., Lopez, P.M., and Garrido, M.J.G. (2019). Emotional distress and unmet supportive care needs in survivors of breast cancer beyond the end of primary treatment. *Supportive Care in Cancer* 27: 1049–1057.

Atherton, K., Young, B., Kalakonda, N., and Salmon, P. (2018). Perspectives of patients with haematological cancer on how clinicians meet their information needs: "managing" information versus "giving" it. *Psycho-Oncology* 27: 1719–1726.

Baile, W.F. and Parker, P.A. (2017, 2017). Breaking bad news (chapter 12). In: *Oxford Textbook of Communication in Oncology and Palliative Care*, 2e (ed. D. Kissane, B. Bultz, P. Butow, et al.). Oxford: Oxford University Press.

Blanckenburg, P., Hofman, M., Riel, W. et al. (2020). Assessing patients' preferences for breaking bad news according to the SPIKES-protocol: the MABBAN scale. *Patient Education and Counseling* 103: 1623–1629.

Burney, S. (2019). Psychological issues in cancer survivorship. *Climacteric* 22 (6): 584–588.

Button, E., Chan, R.J., Chamber, S. et al. (2017). A systematic review of prognostic factors at the end of life for people with a haematological malignancy. *BMC Cancer* 17 (213): 1–15.

Ceravolo, D. and Raines, D.A. (2019). The impact of a mindfulness intervention for nurse managers. *Journal of Holistic Nursing* 37 (1): 47–53.

Costa, D., Mercieca-Bebber, R., Rutherford, C. et al. (2016). The impact of cancer on psychological and social outcomes. *Australian Psychologist* 51 (2): 89–99.

Crelin, R. and Quinn, S. (2010). The benefits of hospital-based counselling for patients and staff. *Cancer Nursing Practice* 9 (9): 28–30.

Dana-Farber Cancer Institute. (2016). Serious illness care program reference guide for clinicians. https://divisionsbc.ca/sites/default/files/Divisions/Powell%20River/ClinicianReferenceGuide.pdf (accessed 22 September 2022).

Department of Health Northern Ireland. (2022). A cancer strategy for Northern Ireland 2022–2032. https://www.health-ni.gov.uk/publications/cancer-strategy-northern-ireland-2022-2032 (accessed 12 October 2022).

Emold, C., Schneider, N., Meller, I., and Yagil, Y. (2011). Communication skills, working environment and burnout among oncology nurses. *European Journal of Oncology Nurses* 15 (4): 358–363.

Fahmer, N., Faller, H., Engehausen, D. et al. (2022). Patients' challenges, competencies, and perceived support in dealing with information needs – a qualitative analysis in patients with breast and gynecological cancer. *Patient Education and Counseling* 105: 2382–2390.

Figley, C.R. (2002). Compassion fatigue: psychotherapists' chronic lack of self care. *JCLP/In Session: Psychotherapy in Practice* 58 (11): 1433–1444.

Finn, A., King, E., and Wilkinson, S. (2017). The implementation of advanced communication skills training for senior healthcare professionals in Northern Ireland: the challenges and rewards. In: *Oxford Textbook of Communication in Oncology and Palliative Care*, 2e (ed. D. Kissane, B. Bultz, P. Butow, et al.). Oxford: Oxford University Press.

Fradgley, E.A., Bultz, B.D., Kelly, B.J. et al. (2019). Progress toward integrating distress as the sixth vital sign: a global snapshot of triumphs and tribulations in precision supportive care. *Journal of Psychosocial Oncology Research and Practice* 1 (1): e2.

Gilligan, T., Coyle, N., Frankel, R.M. et al. (2017). Patient-clinician communication: American Society of Clinical Oncology Consensus Guideline. *Journal of Clinical Oncology* 31: 3618–3632.

Grafton, E., Gillespie, B., and Henderson, S. (2010). Resilience: the power within. *Oncology Nursing Forum* 37 (6): 698–705.

Green, A.A. and Kinchen, E.V. (2021). The effects of mindfulness meditation on stress and burnout in nurses. *Journal of Holistic Nursing* 39 (4): 356–368.

Gribben, L. and Semple, C. (2021). Prevalence and predictors of burnout and work-life balance within the haematology cancer nursing workforce. *European Journal of Oncology Nursing* 52: 1–16.

Hardardottir, H., Aspelund, T., Zhu, J. et al. (2022). Optimal communication associated with lower risk of acute traumatic stress after lung cancer diagnosis. *Supportive Care in Cancer* 30: 259–269.

Hauk, H., Bernhard, J., McConnell, M., and Wohlfarth, B. (2021). Breaking bad news to cancer patients in times of COVID-19. *Supportive Care in Cancer* 29: 4195–4198.

Herrmann, A., Sanson-Fisher, R., Hall, A. et al. (2018). A discrete choice experiment to assess cancer patients' preferences for when and how to make treatment decisions. *Supportive Care in Cancer* 26: 1215–1220.

Hilcove, K., Marceau, C., Thekdi, P. et al. (2021). Holistic nursing in practice: mindfulness-based yoga as an intervention to manage stress and burnout. *Journal of Holistic Nursing* 39 (1): 29–42.

Hodges, H.F., Keeley, A.C., and Grier, E.C. (2005). Professional resilience, practice longevity, and Parse's theory for baccalaureate education. *Journal of Nursing Education* 44: 538–554.

Hyatt, A., Shelly, A., Cox, R. et al. (2022). How can we improve information for people affected by cancer? A national survey exploring gaps in current information provision, and challenges with accessing cancer information online. *Patient Education and Counseling* 105: 2763–2770.

Jackson, D., Firtko, A., and Edenborough, M. (2007). Personal resilience as a strategy for surviving and thriving in the face of workplace adversity: a literature review. *Journal of Advanced Nursing* 60: 1–9.

Jeffrey, D. (2016). Empathy, sympathy and compassion in healthcare: is there a problem? Is there a difference? Does it matter? *Journal of the Royal Society of Medicine* 109 (2): 446–452.

Jenkins, B. and Warren, N.A. (2012). Concept analysis, compassionate fatigue and effect upon critical care nurses. *Critical Care Nursing Quarterly* 35 (4): 388–395.

Johnson, A., Rees, J., Delduca, C., and Criddle, R. (2015). *Psychological Support. Sharing Good Practice. Winter 2015.* UK: Macmillan Cancer Support.

Jones, M.C., Wells, M., Gao, C. et al. (2013). Work stress and wellbeing in oncology settings: a multidisciplinary study of health care professionals. *Psycho-Oncology* 22: 46–53.

King, A., Evans, M., Moore, T. et al. (2015). Prostate cancer and supportive care: a systematic review and qualitative synthesis of men's experiences and unmet needs. *European Journal of Cancer Care* 24: 618–634.

Korsvold, L., Mellblom, A., Lie, H. et al. (2016). Patient-provider communication about the emotional cues and concerns of adolescent and young adult patients and their family members when receiving a diagnosis of cancer. *Patient Education and Counseling* 99: 1576–1583.

Kuswanto, C., Stafford, L., Sharp, J., and Schofield, P. (2018). Psychological distress, role and identity changes in mothers following a diagnosis of cancer: a systematic review. *Psycho-Oncology* 27: 2700–2708.

Lehmann, V., Labrie, N.H.M., van Weert, J.C.M. et al. (2020). Tailoring the amount of treatment information to cancer patients' and survivors' preferences: effects on patient-reported outcomes. *Patient Education and Counseling* 103: 514–520.

Leung, D., Esplen, M.J., Peter, E. et al. (2011). How haematological cancer nurses experience the threat of patients' mortality. *Journal of Advanced Nursing* 68 (10): 2175–2183.

Lim, C.Y.S., Laidsaar-Powell, R.C., Young, J.M. et al. (2022). The long haul: lived experiences of survivors following different treatments for advanced colorectal cancer: a qualitative study. *European Journal of Oncology Nursing* 58: 1–15.

Macmillan Cancer Support. (2021). Caught in the maze. Delivering personalised, integrated care for people with cancer. https://www.macmillan.org.uk/_images/caught-in-the-maze-report_tcm9-359697.pdf.

Mailankody, S. and Rao, S.R. (2021). PENS approach for breaking bad news – a short and sweet way! *Supportive Care in Cancer* 29: 1157–1159.

Mannix, K. (2021). *Listen. How to Find the Words for Tender Conversations.* Dublin: Harper Collins.

Maslach, C., Schaufeli, W.B., and Leiter, M.P. (2001). Job burnout. *Annual Review of Psychology* 52: 397–422.

Matthews, T., Baken, D., Ross, K. et al. (2019). The experiences of patients and their family members when receiving bad news about cancer: a qualitative meta-synthesis. *Psycho-Oncology* 28: 2286–2294.

McCormack, B. and McCance, T. (2017). *Person-Centred Practice in Nursing and Health Care: Theory and Practice*, 2e. West Sussex: Wiley Blackwell.

McDonald, A. (2016). *A Long and Winding Road. Improving Communication with Patients in the NHS*. UK: Marie Curie.

Molassiotis, A., Liu, X.L., and Kwok, S.W. (2020). Impact of advanced nursing practice through nurse-led clinics in the care of cancer patients: a scoping review. *European Journal of Cancer Care* 30e: 1–17.

Muzzatti, B., Agostinelli, G., Bomben, F. et al. (2022). Intensity and prevalence of psychological distress in cancer inpatients: cross-sectional study using new case-finding criteria for the hospital anxiety and depression scale. *Frontiers in Psychology* 13: 1–7.

National Institute for Health and Care Excellence. (2004). Improving supportive and palliative care for adults with cancer. https://www.nice.org.uk/guidance/csg4.

Neville Miller, A., Zraick, R., Atmakuri, S. et al. (2021). Characteristics of teach-back as practiced in a university health center, and its association with patient understanding, self-efficacy, and satisfaction. *Patient Education and Counseling* 104: 2700–2705.

Nouri, S.S. and Rudd, R.E. (2015). Health literacy in the "oral exchange": an important element of patient-provider communication. *Patient Education and Counseling* 98: 565–571.

Pease, N. (2017). Palliative medicine: communication to promote life near the end of life. In: *Oxford Textbook of Communication in Oncology and Palliative Care*, 2e (ed. D. Kissane, B. Bultz, P. Butow, et al.). Oxford: Oxford University Press.

Peterson, J., Johnson, M., Halvorson, B. et al. (2010). Where do nurses go for help? A qualitative study of coping with death and dying. *International Journal of Palliative Nursing* 16 (9): 432–437.

Philips, C.S. and Volker, D.L. (2020). Riding the roller coaster. *Cancer Nursing* 43 (5): E283–E289.

Potter, P., Deshields, T., Divanbeigi, J. et al. (2010). Compassion fatigue and burnout: prevalence among oncology nurses. *Clinical Journal of Oncology Nursing* 14 (5): E56–E62.

Prip, A., Pii, K.H., Nielsen, D.L., and Jarden, M. (2022). Patients' experience of communication during their course of treatment in an oncology outpatient department. *Cancer Nursing* 43 (1): E187–E195.

Riba, M., Donovan, K., Andeerson, B. et al. (2019). Distress management version 3. *Journal of the National Comprehensive Cancer Network* 17 (10): 1229–1249.

Richardson, C.E. (2002). The metatheory of resilience and resiliency. *Journal of Clinical Psychology* 58: 307–321.

Rodenbach, R.A., Norton, S.A., Wittink, M.N. et al. (2019). When chemotherapy fails: emotionally charged experiences faced by family caregivers of patients with advanced cancer. *Patient Education and Counseling* 102: 909–915.

Rutherford, L. and McCaughey, C. (2015). Evaluation of the two day versus the three day advanced communication skills training in Northern Ireland using the Susie Wilkinson Model. Unpublished internal report by the Northern Ireland Regional Advanced Communication Skills Training Facilitators Group.

Rutten, L.J.F., Agunwamba, A.A., Wilson, P. et al. (2016). Cancer-related information seeking among cancer survivors: trends over a decade (2003–2013). *Journal of Cancer Education* 31: 348–357.

Samuelsson, M., Wennick, A., Jakobsson, J., and Bengtsson, M. (2021). Models of support to family members during the trajectory of cancer: a scoping review. *Journal of Clinical Nursing* 30: 3072–3098.

Schiena, E., Hocking, A., Joubert, L. et al. (2019). An exploratory needs analysis of parents diagnosed with cancer. *Australian Social Work* 72 (3): 325–335.

Seiler, A. and Jenewein, J. (2019). Resilience in cancer patients. *Frontiers in Psychiatry* 10: 1–35.

Sherman, D.W. (2004). Nurses' stress and burnout: how to care for yourself when caring for patients and their families experiencing life-threatening illness. *American Journal of Nursing* 104 (5): 48–56.

Shersher, V., Haines, T.P., Sturgiss, L. et al. (2021). Definitions and use of teach-back method in healthcare consultations with patients: a systematic review and thematic synthesis. *Patient Education and Counseling* 104: 118–129.

Snowdon, A., White, C.A., Christie, Z. et al. (2011). The clinical utility of the distress thermometer. *British Journal of Nursing* 20 (4): 220–227.

Tamura, S., Suzuki, K., Ito, Y., and Fukawa, A. (2021). Factors related to the resilience and mental health of adult cancer patients: a systematic review. *Supportive Care in Cancer* 29: 3471–3486.

Tauber, N., O'Toole, M., Dinkel, A. et al. (2019). Effect of psychological intervention on fear of cancer recurrence. A systematic review and meta-analysis. *Journal of Clinical Oncology* 37 (31): 2899–2915.

Toh, S.G., Ang, E., and Devi, K.M. (2012). Systematic review on the relationship between the nursing shortage and job satisfaction, stress and burnout levels among nurses in oncology/haematology settings. *International Journal of Evidence-Based Healthcare* 10 (2): 126–141.

Wells-English, D., Giese, J., and Price, J. (2019). Compassion fatigue and satisfaction. *Clinical Journal of Oncology Nursing* 23 (5): 487–493.

Wilkinson, S., Bailey, K., Aldridge, J., and Roberts, A. (1999). A longitudinal evaluation of a communications skills programme. *Palliative Medicine* 13 (4): 341–348.

Wilkinson, S., Perry, R., Blanchard, K., and Linsell, L. (2008). Effectiveness of a three-day communication skills course in changing nurses' communications skills with cancer/palliative care patients: a randomised controlled trial. *Palliative Medicine* 22: 365–375.

Wittenberg-Lyles, E., Goldsmith, J., and Reno, J. (2013). Perceived benefits and challenges of an oncology nurse support group. *Clinical Journal of Oncology Nursing* 18 (4): E71–E76.

Wu, S., Singh-Carlson, S., Odell, A. et al. (2016). Compassion fatigue, burnout, and compassion satisfaction among oncology nurses in the United States and Canada. *Oncology Nurse Forum* 43 (4): E161–E169.

Zimmermann, C. and Del Piccolo, L. (2007). Cues and concerns by patients in medical consultations: a literature review. *Psychological Bulletin* 133 (3): 438–463.

7

Integrating Research and Evidence-Based Practice

Adrina O'Donnell, Ruth Boyd, and Clare McVeigh

Abstract

Evidence-based practice (EBP) is the integration of current evidence with clinical expertise and patient preferences. Whilst barriers exist in its implementation in the clinical setting, the clinical nurse specialist (CNS) has a pivotal role in the delivery of EBP in cancer care. Clinical examples are provided in this chapter to illustrate this. Inherent in the CNS role is engagement in research. One component of research relates to cancer clinical trials (CCTs), which are vital for the development of innovation in cancer treatment and care. Working with the research team, the CNS has a valuable role in supporting individuals with decision-making regarding participation and navigating CCTs.

7.1 Introduction

This chapter will explore the important role of research in informing evidence-based practice (EBP) among clinical nurse specialists (CNS)s working in the cancer setting. The concepts of EBP and research will be outlined, with a particular emphasis on the integral relationship between them. EBP will be defined and its importance highlighted in the healthcare setting. The specific need for CNSs to deliver EBP when caring for people with cancer and their families will be emphasised. The chapter will provide clinical examples of implementing EBP in the cancer setting, acknowledging the barriers to optimal EBP delivery. Additionally, the important role of cancer clinical trials (CCT) and the integration of research will be discussed to enhance the CNS's knowledge of this crucial aspect of EBP.

The first author, Adrina O'Donnell, is a Macmillan Gynae-Oncology CNS specialising in ovarian cancer and is based at a regional cancer centre in Northern

The Role of the Clinical Nurse Specialist in Cancer Care, First Edition. Edited by Helen Kerr.
© 2024 John Wiley & Sons Ltd. Published 2024 by John Wiley & Sons Ltd.
Companion website: www.wiley.com/go/kerr

Ireland; she has a background in gynae-oncology and CCTs spanning over 25 years. Ruth Boyd is a Cancer Research UK senior research nurse based at a regional cancer centre in Northern Ireland and has over 25 years of experience in CCTs. Dr Clare McVeigh is a lecturer at the School of Nursing and Midwifery, Queen's University, Belfast, and a registered nurse with over 15 years of experience in oncology and palliative care.

7.2 Evidence-Based Practice

EBP is a crucial underpinning to the provision of care in any healthcare setting. It is firmly embedded in the healthcare curriculum and underpins the delivery of effective patient care, contributing to optimal patient outcomes. EBP evolved as a concept from Florence Nightingale in the nineteenth century, with its foundations further recognised in medicine in the 1970s and subsequently in nursing in the 1990s (Mackey and Bassendowski 2017). David Sackett, a medical professor, McMaster University, Canada, is regarded as a leading pioneer in evidence-based medicine; the approach emphasises the importance of combining research evidence with clinical skills and patient values and preferences (Smith and Rennie 2014).

Within nursing specifically, the delivery of evidence-based care – often referred to as evidence-based nursing (EBN) – based on the most recent clinical research contributes to the delivery of safe and optimal person-centred care (Kerr and Rainey 2021). Similar to evidence-based medicine, EBP has been defined as the integration of three components: the most up-to-date evidence and the clinician's own expertise, also incorporating the individualised needs and values of the patient (Hoffman et al. 2017). The World Health Organisation (WHO) highlighted that the key to achieving optimum patient outcomes at the lowest cost is the pursuit of EBP (Jylhä et al. 2017). Profetto-McGrath et al. (2010) suggested that EBP has become the desired standard to optimise patient outcomes within all health disciplines, with Malik et al. (2015) identifying the role of nurses in consistently developing EBP outcomes. Kerr and Rainey (2021) suggest that the nursing profession should be supported to implement and integrate evidence within their clinical expertise, as this will contribute to promoting optimal patient outcomes. In the context of the UK, EBP is a key component of standards published by the professional body of nursing, the Nursing and Midwifery Council (NMC) (2018), which outlines the importance of nursing care being based on the best available evidence.

One of the three key components of EBP is integrating the most up-to-date evidence, and research makes a significant contribution. Robust research is essential for the development of scientific knowledge and best practice. Critical thinking and appraisal are central to synthesising and applying research and developing nursing knowledge. CNSs have an integral role in synthesising and integrating research in the care of individuals with cancer (Bruinooge et al. 2018).

7.3 Barriers to the Implementation of Evidence-Based Practice in the Clinical Setting

Whilst EBP is a fundamental aspect of nursing practice and the role of the CNS, implementation within the clinical setting can be challenging. An Australian study explored the knowledge, skills and attitudes of nurse educators, clinical coaches and nurse specialists towards EBP (Malik et al. 2015). The findings revealed that senior nurses had positive attitudes towards EBP but experienced major barriers such as limited time and resources and also lacked knowledge and skills in appraising and utilising EBP (Malik et al. 2015). However, these findings demonstrated that participants acknowledged these challenges and welcomed educational opportunities and protected time to further develop a more research-orientated culture.

Cooper et al. (2021) were involved in designing and implementing a novel pro-gramme for nurses and allied healthcare professionals (AHPs) to develop capacity for evidence-informed clinical practice at a UK hospital. They found that with clinical leadership support, it was feasible to employ a multi-strategy approach to educate nurses and AHPs to use research evidence in clinical practice. Caldwell et al. (2017) reported findings from a survey undertaken in a cancer centre among clinical staff to identify research awareness and attitudes towards research. Again, positive attitudes were demonstrated related to the principles of research; however, a lack of knowledge, skills, training, time and line management support were all identified as barriers. Roberts (2013) previously identified similar themes and highlighted barriers to implementing EBP such as inadequate knowledge and skills pertaining to its use, in addition to insufficient resources and a lack of line management support. Roberts (2013) emphasised that a culture of EBP must be sustained in healthcare rather than a trend that will come and go.

Addressing these challenges is crucial. An international nursing research organisation, the Joanna Briggs Institute (JBI), have developed the JBI model of evidence-based healthcare (Jordan et al. 2019). The aim is to guide professionals to achieve an evidence-based approach to clinical decision-making. The United Kingdom Oncology Nursing Society (UKONS) is a registered charity managed by cancer nurses for cancer nurses. Their mission is to inspire cancer nursing by providing support in their research, learning and development. The continual pursuit of excellence in cancer care is their underlying ethos. Furthermore, the provision of EBP in healthcare across the European region has the nursing and midwifery professions at its core (Jylhä et al. 2017).

7.4   Role of Evidence-Based Practice in Caring for Patients with Cancer and Their Carers

The multi-faceted impact of cancer is recognised globally due to its significant burden on personal and public health. From diagnosis to living and/or dying with cancer, this disease can profoundly impact patients and their informal caregivers (Santin et al. 2014). Dunniece and Slevin (2000) suggested that few things in life can surpass the trauma of receiving a cancer diagnosis, as expectations of future living can be negatively impacted by the threat of impending death. Cancer impacts not only a person's physical health but also their holistic wellbeing, alongside that of their informal caregivers (Treanor et al. 2019). Without a doubt, it can be a time fraught with complexity, turmoil and uncertainty.

The provision of high-quality holistic nursing care is imperative for all patients with a diagnosis of cancer. Central to this is providing evidence-based care, and this approach has steadily gained momentum across all health and social care disciplines from its inception. One of the key recommendations highlighted in 'A Cancer Strategy for Northern Ireland 2022–2032' (Department of Health Northern Ireland 2022) for optimal cancer care is the development of an appropriate infrastructure to deliver a robust research function, a key component of EBP. It acknowledges that participation in research improves patient outcomes across all aspects of the patient pathway. It is foundational to the delivery of care excellence and not an add-on to care delivery.

7.5   Providing Evidence-Based Care as a Clinical Nurse Specialist

The role of the CNS is diverse and multi-faceted within healthcare. Gordon et al. (2012) indicated that CNSs in the United States of America (USA) encompassed the EBP roles of expert clinician, educator, team leader and chaplain. They believed strategies they employed using EBP not only improved patient care but also decreased costs overall. It has been internationally recognised that the CNS role is ideally placed to act as a link between evidence and its implementation in practice (Profetto-McGrath et al. 2010). The European Specialist Nurses Organisations (ESNO) (2015) compiled 'Competences of the CNS', and inherent in this is their involvement in research. They suggested that this supports CNSs to evolve practice by adding to the evidence base and enhancing patient care through their involvement in research.

CNSs are pivotal members of the multidisciplinary team (MDT). They hold a valued and privileged position, accompanying the patient and their family from the point of a cancer diagnosis through treatment, into follow-up and hopefully on to living with and beyond cancer. The presence of a robust evidence base has never been more essential due to the evolving nature of the CNS role and the complexities related to holistic symptom management. This is supported by Benea (2014), who highlights the importance of research competencies as being core to CNS practice. La Salsa et al. (2007) suggest that the knowledge and expertise of the CNS are crucial to the quality of care a patient receives. They indicated their contribution to improving patient care is critical through linking professional practice with EBP and outcomes.

7.6 Clinical Application of Evidence-Based Practice by Clinical Nurse Specialists

The CNS's contribution in delivering evidence-based care is not a new phenomenon. CNS practice has been described as comprising multiple roles, including clinical expert, educator, consultant, leader, administrator and researcher (Kerr et al. 2021). CNSs make a significant contribution to oncology services, with reports of positive patient experiences (Alessy et al. 2021). Involvement in recruiting patients to a research study reflects effective partnerships between clinical practice and academia. The CNS is appropriately placed to lead on this activity and introduce the research-related concepts. This facilitates the next steps of the study and the overall study design, ensuring that the patient remains central to all activities.

It is essential that the CNS embraces and promotes research, as this will progress the evidence base for cancer treatment and care. CNSs can be involved in the conduct of research in a range of ways, which may include direct or indirect involvement. Direct involvement may include leading on research studies or participating in an aspect of a research study, such as inviting participants to consider engaging in research, data collecting, data analysis, dissemination and implementing findings. Indirect involvement may include peer-reviewing research protocols and co-authoring research papers. A systematic review of published intervention research led or facilitated by cancer nurses indicated that the majority were delivered by specialist cancer nurses (Charalambous et al. 2018), highlighting the potential role of the CNS in research. The CNSs role is valuable as a conduit between research and clinical teams by promoting research engagement with potential participants (Gettrust et al. 2016). CNS are considered agents of change, with a crucial role in supporting the adoption of research findings in practice (Kristensen et al. 2016).

Vignette
As a CNS, my ongoing collaboration with external academic partners in a University setting has resulted in the implementation of a research study (Exercise and Ovarian Cancer) involving individuals with ovarian cancer. I was directly involved in the recruitment phase of this study. When I was conducting the patients' scheduled nurse-led clinical review, if the patient met the inclusion criteria, I introduced the study and provided information if they were interested. Recruitment data was subsequently forwarded to the researcher at the university. This highlights effective, interdisciplinary engagement between clinical practice and academia in research activities. The ultimate aim of this cross-organisation engagement is that evidence is gathered related to effective nursing care.
Internal collaboration with the Cancer Trials Network within the Hospital Trust is another way in which my role as a CNS contributes to research. I work closely with Clinical Research Nursing colleagues from this Network in the delivery of bespoke research studies which recruit individuals with a diagnosis of ovarian cancer to clinical trials. These important contributions advance the body of scientific knowledge, ultimately enhancing patient outcomes for individuals with cancer.
Adrina O'Donnell, Macmillan Gynae-Oncology CNS

Despite the CNS's positive contributions to developing the evidence base for safe and effective care through research, challenges may be experienced. In the UK, Leary et al. (2008) found that research, education and consultation were the areas of practice that accounted for the least CNS time compared to clinical work and administration. In Canada, Benea (2014) reported that research remained the most challenging and underused domain of CNS practice but recognised that involvement in research teams could bring professional and career development opportunities for the oncology CNS. In the USA, 41.7% of CNSs had acted as a principal or co-investigator in research studies but reported that barriers to conducting research included getting access to the literature and lack of research mentors (Albert et al. 2016). These challenges for the CNS must be acknowledged and addressed.

7.7 Cancer Research and Clinical Trials

Advances in cancer treatment are among the factors contributing to increasing cancer survival rates (Arnold et al. 2019; Siegel et al. 2022). CCTs are a vital part of the research tapestry and translate practice-based ideas and pre-clinical laboratory evidence into approved protocols, recruiting patients to determine the safety and effectiveness of an intervention to find better approaches in cancer prevention, screening, diagnosis, treatment, surveillance, quality of life and care. There is growing evidence that a hospital's research culture and activity also correlate with lower mortality outcomes for emergency admissions (Ozdemir et al. 2015), reduced mortality and improved quality outcomes and hospital performance (Jonker and Fisher 2018), better processes of care (Boaz et al. 2015) and better outcomes for all patients with colorectal cancer (Downing et al. 2017). In the cancer treatment setting, many milestones have been achieved through trials ranging from the development of the human papilloma virus (HPV) vaccine for the prevention of cervical and other cancers to immunotherapy and chimeric antigen receptor (CAR) T-cell therapy and the use of cancer genomics in precision medicine (Danovi and Sadanand 2020; National Cancer Institute 2020).

CNSs located in cancer treatment centres are likely to encounter drug trials, which are fundamental to the drug development process, systematically evaluating the safety and efficacy of novel products or combinations through Phase I to Phase IV trials. A key objective of Phase I trials is to identify the recommended dose for the next phase. In addition, drug safety and pharmacological characteristics are evaluated. Phase II trials continue to assess toxicity and efficacy. With increasing numbers of patients participating in successive phases, Phase III trials usually involve hundreds of patients randomised to either the study treatment arm or the control arm, the current best standard of care. After a positive Phase III randomised controlled trial, a dossier of evidence is submitted to the relevant national regulatory authority for marketing approval (Hackshaw and Stuart 2020). Phase IV trials occur after a drug is licensed, assessing longer-term safety and effectiveness.

Patients have reported positive outcomes in relation to their involvement in CCTs. Results of a survey in England, UK, identified that research participants were more likely to feel informed about their care and condition, reported better interactions with staff and were almost twice as likely to have been assigned a CNS (McGrath-Lone et al. 2015). Benefits of participation reported by patients included access to the intervention itself and additional monitoring. Patients viewed participation in trials positively, and some actively chose to attend a teaching hospital to increase the opportunity to participate in a trial.

There is increasing recognition that people affected by cancer are vital members of the research team, not just on an individual participant basis but also with a wider influence across the cancer research agenda, including CCT portfolio development, research priorities, study design, recruitment strategies, patient documents and dissemination of results (Pii et al. 2019). Patients are often advocates for trial participation. Working in partnership with patients and carers is essential to enhance the quality and appropriateness of research (Brett et al. 2014).

CNSs are in an ideal position to signpost interested patients and carers to patient advocacy opportunities in research, as their insights into their unmet needs means they have a key contribution in identifying and reinforcing research priorities for patients, carers and families impacted by cancer.

7.8 Cancer Clinical Trials, Research Nurses and the Role of the Clinical Nurse Specialist

In the USA, whilst there are efforts to gain a greater understanding of attitudes and roles of oncology advanced practitioners (including CNSs) relating to CCTs, this role dimension has been largely undocumented in the last decade (Braun-Inglis et al. 2022). Time constraints may impact discussions about clinical trials; however, cancer nurses have reported barriers such as a lack of confidence in communicating clinical trials and have indicated the need for specialised training to increase confidence and knowledge to support patients through decision-making (Ulrich et al. 2012; Flocke et al. 2017). Local roles along the patient pathway will vary, but research nurses and CNSs are vital mutual resources. CCTs are conducted in a scientific, regulated and monitored manner to safeguard research quality and protect participants. This time and resource-intensive activity requires investment in clinical research infrastructure, including expanding the cancer research nurse workforce (Ness 2020; Hong et al. 2021). The research nurse and the clinical trial co-ordinator are key members of the research team, supporting both the conduct of the study at the local site and care of patients participating in clinical trials (Purdom et al. 2017). Study-specific training is required alongside knowledge of national and local research regulations, good clinical practice (GCP) (International Council for Harmonisation of Technical Requirements for Pharmaceuticals for Human Use (ICH) 2016) and the ethical standards of the Declaration of Helsinki (World Medical Association 2013).

Fisher et al. (2022) reported that the most frequent activities of the research nurse were recruitment of research participants, monitoring participants for adverse events and providing nursing leadership within the interdisciplinary team. The CNS and research nurse roles may share some similarities but are distinct and can be synergistic in providing care. A shared care model has been described (Thornton 2017), outlining the CNS having a role in discussing CCTs with the patient. Alongside improved patient experience, it is proposed that an added benefit of this teamwork approach may be improved nurse experience and shared learning, specialist knowledge, skills and experience (Lavender and Croudass 2019). The cancer CNS should be familiar with the clinical trial process in order to effectively collaborate with researchers and research nurses.

Vignette

As a CNS working with research nurses and patients on colorectal cancer clinical trials, it is important to establish clarity of nursing roles when providing care to patients. During my CNS induction, I spent some time with the Research Nurse in colorectal cancer to become more familiar with their work. I am based in a small centre, and we know colleagues well, and there is a lot of mutual respect for each other's roles. Patients on clinical trials and standard care treatments meet the same medical doctors at their visits so the CNS and research nurses can be in the same clinics, and I have found this promotes communication. Familiarity with clinical trial protocols is important, particularly to check if certain treatment interventions could be study exclusion criteria or contraindicated.

A patient I cared for was ZX (pseudonym), who was a woman in her 50s with metastatic colorectal cancer. I was her key worker during the journey through standard therapies, and I assessed her holistic needs, which included pain control and financial issues. As treatments were unfortunately no longer effective, I 'peppered' the conversation with information about early phase clinical trials. In the environment in which I work, during trial treatment, the Research Nurse is the primary nurse. I am usually more on the periphery if the patient moves to participating in a clinical trial. However, there were certain times I became more involved again in ZX care, such as urological complications and palliative radiotherapy and when the study concluded. We emphasise to patients that if they have questions, they should ask either the CNS or research nurse throughout the clinical trial; however, we share information as appropriate and have discussions on who best can support the patient. The priority is that the patient makes contact when they have a need and receive person-centred care if they have questions or concerns so staff are not territorial. My experience is that patients have had no difficulty navigating these distinct nursing roles of the research nurse and the CNS.

Allison Irwin, Macmillan CNS Colorectal Cancer, Northern Ireland

7.9 The Role of the Clinical Nurse Specialist Along the Cancer Clinical Trial Patient Pathway

Figure 7.1 illustrates the patient pathway in CCTs and highlights the elements of this process where the CNS, as the patient's key worker, has a pivotal role in patient care and collaboration with the research team. Each of the six stages is further delineated below, highlighting the potential contribution of the CNS. Knowledge of the clinical trial process can help guide, prepare and manage patient and carer

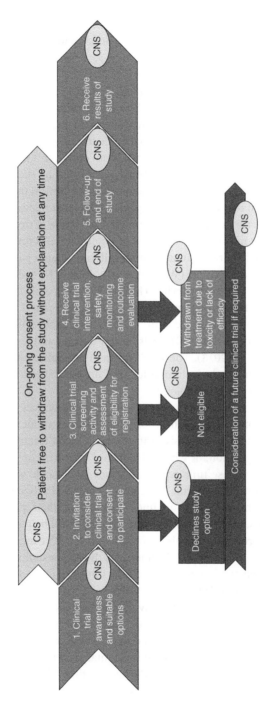

Figure 7.1 The patient clinical trial pathway and potential CNS role interface points.

expectations, providing support not just as patients enter the pathway but also as they navigate the pathway alongside the uncertainties and then move beyond the pathway.

1) Cancer clinical trial awareness and suitable options

   Public information about clinical trials is increasingly accessible; however, due to the dynamic nature of research, there is no guarantee that a suitable clinical trial will be available at a patient's treating hospital. Referral to another centre for trial participation may be an option if it is in the patient's interest. The website https://clinicaltrials.gov, hosted by the USA National Library of Medicine, is an international database of clinical trials, though for the CNS, the local research team will provide the most relevant information about the local portfolio open to recruitment. Discussion of treatment options at MDT meetings may include a review of potential CCTs for an individual. CNS patient insights are invaluable in identifying when a patient is eligible or not for trial participation (Wallace et al. 2019). CNS-led clinics are an increasing feature of cancer services (Kerr et al. 2021), and CNSs have a role in referring interested patients to the research team (Lancaster and Dumville 2019). Providing general information about clinical trials in advance can support patient CCT decision self-efficacy and reduce decisional conflict (Miller et al. 2013). The CNS can help normalise clinical trials for patients by explaining the potential for trial opportunities and introducing research concepts and terminology.

2) Invitation to consider a clinical trial and consent to participate

   CCTs usually become an option for consideration when a patient is at a significant milestone, such as diagnosis, primary or adjuvant treatment, or cancer recurrence or progression, or when all standard treatment options have been exhausted. Clearly, these time points are likely to coincide with the patient receiving bad news. The CNS role, which has established a therapeutic consistent patient relationship, with an understanding of their past experience, knowledge, hopes, fears, motivations and priorities, will help shape appropriate holistic support. The vulnerability of individuals with cancer with nothing to lose in the early phase of a CCT highlights the responsibility of healthcare professionals to ensure that patients are fully informed of study requirements and realistic outcomes (Murphy et al. 2020).

   Initial discussions with patients may need to address misconceptions about research including, where appropriate, false hope (Sawyer et al. 2021). Throughout the CCT pathway, it is vital that patients know available alternatives and understand that participation is voluntary and they are free to decline to take part or to withdraw from the CCT at any time without explanation or penalty (ICH 2016). Capacity to consent is an aspect of care that the CNS will be well placed to assess and contribute to discussion of other eligibility factors such as performance status and a patient's ability to comply with study requirements.

It is reported that over half of patients, if offered the opportunity to take part in a CCT, will agree (Moorcraft et al. 2016; Kearns et al. 2020; Unger et al. 2021). Alongside altruism, hope of medical benefit is a strong motivator for CCT participation (Harrop et al. 2016; Moorcraft et al. 2016; Sawyer et al. 2021). There may be many structural and clinical barriers to recruitment and patient burden factors such as finance, insurance and travel to academic centres (Sawyer et al. 2021; Unger et al. 2021) or treatment concerns (Manne et al. 2015; Moorcraft et al. 2016; Unger et al. 2021) beyond the CNS's control. Increased equity, diversity and inclusion are required (Oyer et al. 2022) to address under-representation in trials across under-served groups (McGrath-Lone et al. 2015; Unger et al. 2021; Oyer et al. 2022). Strategies including cultural competency training, increasing trust and a person-centred approach that promotes the feeling of being seen as an individual (Bodicoat et al. 2021) must be supported by the CNS.

Manne et al. (2015) indicates that patients with lower education and financial support may need more decisional support, a recognised role of the CNS in cancer treatment choices (Carroll 1998).

Cancer nurses see their role as patient educators and advocates in the CCTs discussion (Flocke et al. 2017). In the UK, CNSs felt they were well placed to invite patients to consider research without putting them under pressure, given the time they had with the patient and the trust and rapport developed with patients (French and Stavropoulou 2016). The value of CNS neutrality when discussing CCTs was also echoed by teenagers and young adults with bone cancer, expressing the value of an honest friend to work through concerns and simplify information (Pearce et al. 2018). Alongside a positive research culture and teamwork, specialist nurses' attitudes, skills and experience are identified as key facilitators in inviting patients to participate (French and Stavropoulou 2016), with CNS involvement in clinical trials leading to increased participation (Lancaster and Dumville 2019).

3) Clinical trial screening activity and assessment of eligibility for registration
   After consent, access to the study is still not guaranteed for the individual with cancer. Suitability for study registration is not confirmed until baseline and screening activities have been completed. If a patient is not eligible at this stage, they may be disappointed, especially when the CCT was the only active treatment option available at that time. Patients planning to take part in Phase I or II trials have reported anxiety and depression waiting for results and trial spaces and being upset if they were not eligible to take part, with feelings that this was a death sentence (Sawyer et al. 2021). CNS knowledge of the research process can support patients in managing expectations throughout the consent and screening process.

4) Receive clinical trial intervention, safety monitoring and outcome evaluation
   Compliance with the clinical trial protocol is key to patient safety and research quality. During clinical trial treatment, assessments and safety evaluations are undertaken. Patients need access to 24/7 care, as required, throughout treatment. All drug-related adverse events are recorded, and where these are serious and require admission, they will be reported to the study sponsor by the research team within 24 hours of becoming aware. Through pharmacovigilance, overall study safety is evaluated. Where the CNS becomes aware of patient experience of adverse events, timely communication with the research team is crucial and invaluable.

   The patient may also have to end their trial participation if toxicity is too severe. It is important that the patient reports their experience so this can be evaluated accurately. Participants in Phase I and II studies have reported experiencing conflict between wanting to stay on treatment and fearing that disclosing side effects may mean treatment would be withdrawn (Sawyer et al. 2021). In this setting, the CNS relationship with the patient and education and advocacy for patient safety and wellbeing can support the patient experiencing any conflict.

5) Follow-up, end of study and withdrawal at any stage
   The patient schedule and duration of trial participation depend on the length of the intervention and the endpoints being measured, such as acute toxicity, quality of life and survival. The period beyond the trial has been associated with a mix of emotions, including relief, disappointment, hope of future help, uncertainty and abandonment (Wootten et al. 2011). In the Phase I setting, it has been noted that the patient may feel lost in transition at the end of a study, and this time has led to a range of psychological and social needs (Ferrell et al. 2020). Interviews undertaken with patients withdrawn from CCTs in the USA (Ulrich et al. 2021), primarily because of disease progression (65%) or adverse effects (25%), highlighted the emotional impact of this period of transition. Patients described a sense of failure of the drug or trial or blamed the cancer. After withdrawal, while some reported regret that they had participated in the trial, 75% wished to enrol in another trial; 70% also expressed fear of death, as CCTs represented hope and a key to survival. These findings echo earlier research by Cox (1999), specific to the Phase I and II setting in the UK, with patients who had no standard care option reporting a sense of disappointment, a feeling of relief and a fear of feeling abandoned. Again, despite some negative emotions, 78% reported that they would participate in a clinical trial again (Cox 1999).

   Ulrich et al. (2021) indicated that 90% of patients withdrawn from CCTs relied on personal and professional support to cope emotionally during this time. This further endorses the potential significance of the role of the CNS at this point in the patient pathway, when it may feel as though there is no clear path forward (Ulrich et al. 2021). Wilson et al. (2007) identified that closure is important for patients at the end of trial treatment. Patients may also be experiencing ongoing adverse effects of treatment so referral or ongoing palliative care may be appropriate (Ferrell et al. 2020).

6) Receive results of the study

The impact of the study for each participant will be part of the ongoing, timely clinical communication in regard to treatment response, adverse events, follow-up and next steps. However, at the conclusion of a trial, a study patient is also entitled to be informed of the outcome and share in the benefit, which may include access to the intervention (World Medical Association 2013). Despite this ethical principle, there is not a standard format of communication at the study conclusion. Recognition of the need for transparency and publication of results has grown in momentum (Moorthy et al. 2015; Health Research Authority 2021). The vast majority of CCT participants would like to know the study results, with a preference to be informed verbally (Fernandez et al. 2009; Cox et al. 2011). Both patients and clinicians acknowledge that reporting results could, in some cases, risk a negative psychological impact (Cox et al. 2011); thus, ongoing CNS support is of further value at this time.

Participation in CCTs becomes a very significant personal journey for many individuals with cancer. This is an important arena for the CNS to develop knowledge and skills to support patients and help support their decision-making process, including whether to enter a CCT or not, and support them to navigate the clinical trial journey and beyond.

7.10 Conclusion

Cancer knows no boundaries; it has become integral in the healthcare landscape. It remains highly challenging and an ongoing health concern. In the pursuit of individualised, high-quality nursing care, a robust evidence base informed by research is critical. The three components of EBP are of equal value; the best available evidence, combined with clinical experience and patient values and preferences. It is crucial that adopting the principles of EBP in healthcare should be firmly embedded in practice. CNSs must keep this at the forefront of their agenda when delivering holistic nursing care to individuals with cancer and their families. As a cohort of professionals, ownership of this vital component of practice needs to be fully endorsed. Athanasakis (2013) advocates that research-based nursing and EBP need to be organised by nurses themselves. Therein, benefits will truly be realised, both in enhanced care delivery and in heightening critical thinking and autonomy of the nursing profession, which includes the CNS role.

References

Albert, N.M., Rice, K.L., Waldo, M.J. et al. (2016). Clinical nurse specialist roles in conducting research: changes over 3 years. *Clinical Nurse Specialist* 30 (5): 292–301.

Alessy, S.A., Luchtenborg, M., Rawlinson, J. et al. (2021). Being assigned a clinical nurse specialist is associated with better experiences of cancer care: English population-based study using the linked National Cancer Patient Experience Survey and Cancer Registration Dataset. *European Journal of Cancer Care* 30 (6): 1–11.

Arnold, M., Rutherford, M.J., Bardot, A. et al. (2019). Progress in cancer survival, mortality, and incidence in seven high-income countries 1995–2014 (ICBP SURVMARK-2): a population-based study. *Lancet Oncology* 20 (11): 1493–1505.

Athanasakis, E. (2013). Nurses research behaviour and barriers to research utilisation into clinical nursing practice: a closer look. *International Journal of Caring Sciences* 6 (1): 16–28.

Benea, A. (2014). The challenge and opportunity of research in the oncology clinical nurse specialist role. *Canadian Oncology Nursing Journal* 24 (4): 295–298.

Boaz, A., Hanney, S., Jones, T., and Soper, B. (2015). Does the engagement of clinicians and organisations in research improve healthcare performance: a three-stage review. *British Medical Journal Open* 5 (12): 1–14.

Bodicoat, D.H., Routen, A.C., Willis, A. et al. (2021). Promoting inclusion in clinical trials – a rapid review of the literature and recommendations for action. *Trials* 22: 1–11.

Braun-Inglis, C., Boehmer, L.M., Zitella, L.J. et al. (2022). Role of oncology advanced practitioners to enhance clinical research. *Journal of Advanced Practice Oncology* 13 (2): 107–119.

Brett, J., Staniszewska, S., Mockford, C. et al. (2014). Mapping the impact of patient and public involvement on health and social care research: a systematic review. *Health Expectations* 17 (5): 637–650.

Bruinooge, S.S., Todd, A.P., Vogel, W. et al. (2018). Understanding the role of advanced practice providers in oncology in the United States. *Journal of Oncology Practice* 14 (9): e518–e532.

Caldwell, B., Coltart, K., Hutchinson, C. et al. (2017). Research awareness, attitudes and barriers among clinical staff in a regional cancer centre. Part 1: a quantitative analysis. *European Journal of Cancer Care* 26: 1–12.

Carroll, S. (1998). Role of the breast care clinical nurse specialist in facilitating decision-making for treatment choice: a practice profile. *European Journal of Oncology Nursing* 2 (1): 34–42.

Charalambous, A., Wells, M., Campbell, P. et al. (2018). A scoping review of trials of interventions led or delivered by cancer nurses. *International Journal of Nursing Studies* 86: 36–43.

Cooper, S., Sanders, J., and Pashayan, N. (2021). Implementing a novel programme for nurses and allied health professionals to develop capacity for evidence-informed clinical practice. *Journal of Research in Nursing* 26 (5): 395–404.

Cox, K. (1999). Researching research: patients' experiences of participation in phase I and II anti-cancer drug trials. *European Journal of Oncology Nursing* 3 (3): 143–152.

Cox, K., Moghaddam, N., Bird, L., and Elkan, R. (2011). Feedback of trial results to participants: a survey of clinicians' and patients' attitudes and experiences. *European Journal of Oncology Nursing* 15 (2–4): 124–129.

Danovi, S. and Sadanand, S. (eds.) (2020). *'Nature Milestones.'* Cancer, pp. S1-S17.

Department of Health Northern Ireland. (2022). A cancer strategy for Northern Ireland 2022–2032. https://www.health-ni.gov.uk/publications/cancer-strategy-northern-ireland-2022-2032 (accessed 5 March 2022).

Downing, A., Morris, E.J.A., Corrigan, N. et al. (2017). High hospital research participation and improved colorectal cancer survival outcomes: a population-based study. *Gut* 66: 89–96.

Dunniece, U. and Slevin, E. (2000). Nurses experiences of being present with patients receiving a diagnosis of cancer. *Journal of Advanced Nursing* 32 (3): 611–618.

European Specialist Nurses Organizations (ESNO). (2015). Competences of the clinical nurse specialist (CNS): common plinth of competences for the common training framework of each specialty. Version 1, 17–10. https://esgena.org/assets/downloads/pdfs/general/esgena_esno_statement_competences.pdf.

Fernandez, C.V., Gao, J., Strahlendorf, C. et al. (2009). Providing research results to participants: attitudes and needs of adolescents and parents of children with cancer. *Clinical Oncology* 27 (6): 878–883.

Ferrell, B., Borneman, T., Williams, A.C. et al. (2020). Integrating palliative care for patients on clinical trials: opportunities for oncology nurses. *Asia-Pacific Journal of Oncology Nursing* 7 (3): 243–249.

Fisher, C.A., Griffith, C.A., Lee, H. et al. (2022). Extending the description of the clinical research nursing workforce. *Journal of Research in Nursing* 27 (1–2): 102–113.

Flocke, S.A., Antognoli, E., Daly, B.J. et al. (2017). The role of oncology nurses in discussing clinical trials. *Oncology Nursing Forum* 44 (5): 547–552.

French, C. and Stavropoulou, C. (2016). Specialist nurses' perceptions of inviting patients to participate in clinical research studies: a qualitative descriptive study of barriers and facilitators. *BioMed Central Medical Research Methodology* 16 (1): 1–12.

Gettrust, L., Hagle, M., Boaz, L., and Bull, M. (2016). Engaging nursing staff in research: the clinical nurse specialist role in an academic-clinical partnership. *Clinical Nurse Specialist* 30 (4): 203–207.

Gordon, J.M., Lorilla, J.D., and Lehman, C.A. (2012). The role of the clinical nurse specialist in the future of health care in the United States. *US Army Research* 196: 343–353.

Hackshaw, A. and Stuart, G.C.E. (2020). *Fast Facts: Clinical Trials in Oncology: The Fundamentals of Design, Conduct and Interpretation.* Oxford: S. Karger Publishers Ltd.

Harrop, E., Noble, S., Edwards, M. et al. (2016). I didn't really understand it, I just thought it'd help: exploring the motivations, understandings and experiences of patients with advanced lung cancer participating in a non-placebo clinical IMP trial. *Trials* 17 (1): 1–12.

Health Research Authority. (2021). Make it public: transparency and openness in health and social care research. https://www.hra.nhs.uk/planning-and-improving-research/policies-standards-legislation/research-transparency/make-it-public-transparency-and-openness-health-and-social-care-research (accessed 29 July 2022).

Hoffman, T., Bennett, S., and Del Mar, C. (2017). *Evidence-Based Practice across the Health Professions.* New South Wales: Elsevier.

Hong, M.N., Hayden, K.A.R., Bouchal, S., and Sinclair, S. (2021). Oncology clinical trials nursing: a scoping review. *Canadian Oncology Nursing Review* 31 (2): 137–149.

International Council for Harmonisation of Technical Requirements for Pharmaceuticals for Human Use (ICH). (2016). Integrated addendum to ICH E6(R1): Guidelines for Good Clinical Practice E6(R2). https://database.ich.org/sites/default/files/E6_R2_Addendum.pdf (accessed 29 July 2022).

Jonker, L. and Fisher, S.J. (2018). The correlation between National Health Service trusts' clinical trial activity and both mortality rates and care quality commission ratings: a retrospective cross-sectional study. *Public Health* 157: 1–6.

Jordan, Z., Lockwood, C., Munn, Z., and Aromataris, E. (2019). The updated Joanna Briggs Institute model of evidence-based healthcare. *International Journal of Evidence-Based Healthcare* 17 (1): 58–71.

Jylhä, V., Oikarainen, A., Perälä, M.-L., and Holopainen, A. (2017). *Facilitating Evidence-Based Practice in Nursing and Midwifery in the WHO European Region.* Denmark: World Health Organisation.

Kearns, C., Feighery, R., McCaffrey, J. et al. (2020). Understanding and attitudes toward cancer clinical trials among patients with a cancer diagnosis: National Study through cancer trials Ireland. *Cancers* 12 (7): 1–26.

Kerr, H. and Rainey, D. (2021). Addressing the current challenges of adopting evidence-based practice in nursing. *British Journal of Nursing* 30 (16): 970–974.

Kerr, H., Donovan, M., and McSorley, O. (2021). Evaluation of the role of the clinical nurse specialist in cancer care: an integrative literature review. *European Journal of Cancer Care* 30 (3): 1–13.

Kristensen, N., Nymann, C., and Konradsenet, H. (2016). Implementing research results in clinical practice – the experiences of healthcare professionals. *BioMed Central Health Services Research* 16 (48): 1–10.

La Salsa, C.A., Connors, P.M., Pedro, J.T., and Phipps, M. (2007). The role of the clinical nurse specialist in promoting evidence-based practice and effecting positive patient outcomes. *The Journal of Continuing Education in Nursing* 38 (6): 262–270.

Lancaster, N. and Dumville, J. (2019). Benefits of involving clinical nurse specialists in research. *Nursing Times* 115 (4): 34–36.

Lavender, V. and Croudass, A. (2019). The role of the nurse in supporting cancer clinical trials. *British Journal of Nursing* 28 (4): S14–S17. (oncology supplement).

Leary, A., Crouch, H., Lezard, A. et al. (2008). Dimensions of clinical nurse specialist work in the UK. *Nursing Standard* 23 (15–17): 40–44.

Mackey, A. and Bassendowski, S. (2017). The history of evidence-based practice in nursing education and practice. *Journal of Professional Nursing* 33 (1): 51–55.

Malik, G., Mc Kenna, L., and Plummer, V. (2015). Perceived knowledge, skills, attitude and contextual factors affecting evidence-based practice among nurse educators, clinical coaches and nurse specialists. *International Journal of Nursing Practice* 21 (2): 46–57.

Manne, S., Kashy, D., Albrecht, T. et al. (2015). Attitudinal barriers to participation in oncology clinical trials: factor analysis and correlates of barriers. *European Journal of Cancer Care* 24 (1): 28–38.

McGrath-Lone, L., Day, S., Schoenborn, C., and Ward, H. (2015). Exploring research participation among cancer patients: analysis of a national survey and an in-depth interview study. *BioMed Central Cancer* 15 (618): 1–12.

Miller, S.M., Hudson, S.V., Egleston, B.L. et al. (2013). The relationships among knowledge, self-efficacy, preparedness, decisional conflict and decisions to participate in a cancer clinical trial. *Psycho-Oncology* 22 (3): 481–489.

Moorcraft, S.Y., Marriott, C., Peckitt, C. et al. (2016). Patients' willingness to participate in clinical trials and their views on aspects of cancer research: results of a prospective patient survey. *Trials* 17 (17): 1–12.

Moorthy, V.S., Karam, G., Vannice, K.S., and Kieny, M.-P. (2015). Rationale for WHO's new position calling for prompt reporting and public disclosure of interventional clinical trial results. *PLoS Medicine* 12 (4): 1–4.

Murphy, M., McCaughan, E., Carson, M.A. et al. (2020). Nothing to lose: a grounded theory study of patients' and healthcare professionals' perspectives of being involved in the consent process for oncology trials with non-curative intent. *BMC Palliative Care* 19 (166): 1–10.

National Cancer Institute. (2020). Milestones in cancer research and discovery. https://www.cancer.gov/research/progress/250-years-milestones (accessed 29 July 2022).

Ness, E. (2020). The oncology clinical research nurse study co-ordinator: past, present, and future. *Asia-Pacific Journal of Oncology Nursing* 7 (3): 237–242.

Nursing and Midwifery Council. (2018). The code. Professional standards of practice and behaviour for nurses, midwives and nursing associates.

Oyer, R.A., Hurley, P., Boehmer, L. et al. (2022). Increasing racial and ethnic diversity in cancer clinical trials: an American Society of Clinical Oncology and Association of Community Cancer Centers Joint Research Statement. *Journal of Clinical Oncology* 40 (19): 2163–2171.

Ozdemir, B.A., Karthikesalingam, A., Sinha, S. et al. (2015). Research activity and the association with mortality. *PLoS One* 10 (2): 1–15.

Pearce, S., Brownsdon, A., Fern, L. et al. (2018). The perceptions of teenagers, young adults and professionals in the participation of bone cancer clinical trials. *European Journal of Cancer Care* 27 (6): 1–15.

Pii, K.H., Schou, L.H., Pii, K., and Jarden, M. (2019). Current trends in patient and public involvement in cancer research: a systematic review. *Health Expectations* 22 (1): 3–20.

Profetto-McGrath, J., Negrin, K.A., Hugo, K., and Balmer Smith, K. (2010). Clinical nurse specialists' approaches in selecting and using evidence to improve practice. *Worldviews on Evidence-Based Nursing* 7 (1): 36–50.

Purdom, M.A., Petersen, S., and Haas, B.K. (2017). Results of an oncology clinical trial nurse role delineation study. *Oncology Nursing Forum* 44 (5): 589–595.

Roberts, D. (2013). What's the problem with EBP? *Medical-Surgical Nursing* 22 (5): 279.

Santin, O., Treanor, C., Mills, M., and Donnelly, M. (2014). The health status and health service needs of primary caregivers of cancer survivors: a mixed methods approach. *European Journal of Cancer Care* 23 (3): 333–339.

Sawyer, C., Preston, L., Taylor, S. et al. (2021). Oncology patients' experiences in experimental medicine cancer trials: a qualitative study. *British Medical Journal Open* 11 (10): 1–9.

Siegel, R.L., Miller, K.D., Fuchs, H.E., and Jemal, A. (2022). Cancer statistics. *CA: A Cancer Journal for Clinicians* 72 (1): 7–33.

Smith, R. and Rennie, D. (2014). Evidence based medicine – an oral history. *British Medical Journal* 348: 365–367.

Thornton, J. (2017). Clinical trials: improving patient experience. *Cancer Nursing Practice* 16 (2): 16–22.

Treanor, C.J., Santin, O., Prue, G. et al. (2019). Psychosocial interventions for informal caregivers of people living with cancer. *Cochrane Database of Systematic Reviews* 176 (6): 1–113.

Ulrich, C.M., Zhou, Q., Ratcliffe, S.J. et al. (2012). Nurse Practitioners' attitudes about cancer clinical trials and willingness to recommend research participation. *Contemporary Clinical Trials* 33 (1): 76–84.

Ulrich, C.M., Knafl, K., Foxwell, A.M. et al. (2021). Experiences of patients after withdrawal from cancer clinical trials. *JAMA Network Open* 4 (8): 1–12.

Unger, J.M., Hershman, D.L., Till, C. et al. (2021). "When Offered to Participate": a systematic review and meta-analysis of patient agreement to participate in cancer clinical trials. *Journal of the National Cancer Institute* 113 (3): 244–257.

Wallace, I., Barratt, H., Harvey, S., and Raine, R. (2019). The impact of clinical nurse specialists on the decision making process in cancer multi-disciplinary team meetings: a qualitative study. *European Journal of Oncology Nursing* 43: 1–22.

Wilson, E., Elkan, R., and Cox, K. (2007). Closure for patients at the end of a cancer clinical trial: literature review. *Journal of Advanced Nursing* 59 (5): 445–453.

Wootten, A.C., Abbott, J.M., Siddons, H.M. et al. (2011). A qualitative assessment of the experience of participating in a cancer-related clinical trial. *Supportive Care in Cancer* 19 (1): 49–55.

World Medical Association. (2013). Declaration of Helsinki – Ethical principles for medical research involving human subjects, Brazil. https://www.wma.net/policies-post/wma-declaration-of-helsinki-ethical-principles-for-medical-research-involving-human-subjects (accessed 1 August 2022).

8

Symptom Management

Michelle Keenan and Helen Kerr

Abstract

Cancer and its treatment can cause multiple symptoms, which may lead to significant distress for patients and their families. Clinical nurse specialists (CNS)s have a vital role in the delivery of cancer care by providing supportive care and symptom advice. This requires CNSs to have the knowledge and skills to accurately assess, safely manage and evaluate interventions to alleviate symptoms. This can be challenging in cancer care due to patient complexity, multiple drug regimens and symptom burden. This chapter will discuss the role of the CNS in the assessment and management of four common symptoms that may be experienced by individuals with cancer: pain, breathlessness, nausea and vomiting and constipation. It will also highlight the need for CNSs to carefully consider contra-indications and side effects before advising on any pharmacological treatment and the importance of seeking additional support when symptoms are persistent or complex.

8.1 Introduction

Patients with cancer often experience symptoms that are disease or treatment-related and that can be complex and debilitating and may negatively affect quality of life (Verkissen et al. 2019). Patients with advanced cancer may present with multiple symptoms such as pain, fatigue, nausea, anorexia, depression and insomnia (Deshields et al. 2014; Grotmol et al. 2019). These symptoms can be challenging to treat, with 66% of patients in the last month of life requiring hospitalisation for acute management (Hjermstad et al. 2013). Clinical nurse specialists (CNS) play a vital role in the delivery of cancer care as they provide expertise in the management of symptoms while providing holistic and supportive care to patients and their families (Fulton et al. 2016; Kerr et al. 2021). The first author, Michelle

Keenan, is employed as a CNS in a hospital specialist palliative care team in Northern Ireland, which requires a high level of knowledge and skill in assessing and managing complex symptoms in patients with life-limiting conditions. The second author, Helen Kerr, is a senior lecturer at the School of Nursing and Midwifery, Queen's University Belfast, with a clinical nursing background in cancer and palliative care. This chapter will highlight the role of the CNS in the assessment, management and evaluation of four symptoms: pain, breathlessness, nausea and vomiting and constipation.

8.2 Pain

Pain is highly prevalent in individuals with cancer, affecting 66% of people with advanced disease (Van den Beuken-van Everdingen et al. 2016). The aetiology of cancer pain is often complex and multi-factorial due to disease burden, side effects of treatment and co-morbidities (Caraceni and Shkodra 2019). The experience of cancer pain is multidimensional and individual to the patient (Hui and Bruera 2014). Existential distress in individuals with cancer can often exacerbate their experience of pain (Huysmans et al. 2020). This requires CNSs to complete a holistic assessment, which should identify not only the physical symptoms but also the emotional, psychosocial and spiritual needs of the patient. This ensures that the experience of total pain is acknowledged and addressed.

Various tools are available that provide a structured pain assessment in determining the source of pain using mnemonics (Rayment and Bennett 2015; Quinn et al. 2017), such as PQRST (provocation, quality, radiation, severity and timing). When identifying the source of pain (e.g. nociceptive, neuropathic or combined), it is important to consider location, radiation, intensity, onset and duration of pain. In addition, exacerbating and alleviating factors should be considered, along with associated symptoms such as anxiety, depression and insomnia (Li et al. 2017). An effective assessment should also include a detailed medical treatment and analgesic history. A clinical examination, review of scans and consideration of appropriate investigations are also essential in determining or excluding the source of pain (Caraceni and Shkodra 2019).

For people with cognitive impairment, such as dementia, CNSs must also rely on observing emotional and behavioural manifestations of pain, as individuals may lose their ability to accurately self-report pain (Achterberg et al. 2020). A number of validated tools are available for assessing pain in cognitive impairment, such as the Abbey pain scale or Pain Assessment in Advanced Dementia (PAINAD) scale (Warden et al. 2003; Abbey et al. 2004); however, it is reported that these are underutilised in clinical practice (Burns and McIlfatrick 2015).

Untreated pain can manifest into behavioural disturbances such as agitation or aggression (Sampson et al. 2015), which causes distress not only to the individual but also to their family and caregivers (Lichtner et al. 2016). Therefore, it is vital that a CNS completes an effective, holistic and individualised pain assessment, as this will determine appropriate treatment options and analgesic choices.

When devising a treatment plan, it should be discussed, negotiated and agreed upon with the individual; their expectations and concerns should be addressed, as a lack of communication between the patient and healthcare professionals has been identified as a barrier to effective pain management (Zuccaro et al. 2012). This will include the CNS discussing treatment options, potential benefits and side effects with patients and, when consented, with their families if appropriate.

The pharmacological management of cancer pain should be a step-wise approach using the World Health Organisation (WHO) analgesic ladder (World Health Organisation 2003). Opioids are recommended in the pharmacological management of moderate to severe cancer pain and should be considered in combination with non-opioid analgesics, adjuvants and non-pharmacological therapies (National Institute for Health Care Excellence (NICE) 2021), such as transcutaneous electrical nerve stimulation (TENS), complementary therapies, relaxation or distraction (Hökkä et al. 2014). Unlike most analgesics, opioids have no ceiling dose and can be up-titrated without maximum dosing (Varilla et al. 2015). Oral opioids are often available in slow- and immediate-release preparations and provide pain relief within a 30–60 minute onset (Joint Formulary Committee 2022). Immediate-release opioids are used in the management of breakthrough pain, and the recommended dosing is normally one-sixth of the total 24-hour slow-release dose (Back et al. 2021). When adjusting the dose of slow-release opioids, the amount of breakthrough analgesia administered and the effectiveness and potential side effects should be considered. It is recommended that the up-titration of opioids should not exceed 30–50% of the total daily dose in 24 hours (Back et al. 2021). The up-titration of opioids should stop when pain is controlled or the individual is experiencing intolerable side effects (NICE 2012; Varilla et al. 2015).

Morphine sulphate is considered the gold standard opioid in the management of cancer pain (NICE 2012) and is considered cost-effective, easily accessible and available in various oral preparations. Common side effects include constipation, nausea, vomiting and drowsiness (Joint Formulary Committee 2022). Therefore, it is advisable to ensure that patients have access to an antiemetic and regular prophylactic laxative therapy (Back et al. 2021). Opioid-induced nausea will likely subside within five to seven days; however, opioid-induced constipation can remain problematic and should be reviewed daily.

Morphine is metabolised by the liver and excreted by the kidneys (Smith 2009), so careful titration should be considered in individuals with renal impairment or moderate to severe hepatic impairment (Wilcock et al. 2020). Renal impairment can increase the number of active morphine metabolites, which may lead to neurotoxicity such as myoclonus, confusion or drowsiness (Joint Formulary Committee 2022). It is vital that CNSs carefully monitor cerebral activity in opioid treatment and consider a dose reduction or opioid rotation to avoid these side effects, as severe opioid toxicity can lead to respiratory depression (Back et al. 2021). A dose reduction and careful titration may be required in older people or those who are opioid naïve. Morphine should be avoided in individuals with moderate to severe renal impairment and consideration given to alternative opioids, depending on the degree of impairment. Opioid rotation should also be considered in patients who experience intolerable adverse effects and unsuccessful pain control despite increasing titration (Back et al. 2021). Opioid conversion guidance should be used when switching opioids (NICE 2012), and it is recommended that clinicians dose-reduce by 25–50% for the first 24–48 hours when introducing an alternative opioid (Back et al. 2021). It is also important to ensure that patients have appropriate breakthrough analgesia when advising or prescribing a slow-release opioid.

Oxycodone is considered a 'second-line' opioid in the management of severe pain and has similar action and side effects to morphine (Guo et al. 2018). Similar to morphine, it is metabolised by the liver and excreted by the kidneys. Due to the risk of drug accumulation, it should be cautiously titrated in patients with mild to moderate renal impairment and avoided in patients with severe renal impairment (Ackroyd and Aman 2012). It is also contraindicated in moderate to severe hepatic impairment (Joint Formulary Committee 2022). Oxycodone is twice as potent as morphine; therefore, the CNS should always refer to opioid conversion guidance when considering switching from one opioid to another (McKie 2016; Back et al. 2021).

8.2.1 Renal Impairment

The presence of renal impairment should not delay the treatment of cancer pain. A CNS must recognise the risks of analgesic use and make adjustments to minimise potential side effects developing. This requires close monitoring of renal function and careful consideration of opioid choice, dose and frequency reduction.

Acute kidney injury (AKI) can be common in individuals with cancer and is reported to affect 50% of individuals (Cosmai et al. 2021). It often significantly affects prognosis and length of hospitalisation (Candrilli et al. 2008). In clinical practice, it is often observed in patients receiving systemic anticancer treatment due to nephrotoxic side effects or as a result of direct tumour invasion of the kidneys (Kitchlu et al. 2019). Other causes include dehydration due to sepsis, vomiting or diarrhoea, nephrotic syndrome and obstructive uropathy secondary to disease (Rosner and Dalkin 2012; Lameire et al. 2016; Folkard et al. 2020). For patients with rapidly deteriorating renal function, the CNS must assess for any reversible causes and consider a pre-emptive change in opioids and adjuvants.

The use of codeine, morphine or diamorphine is not recommended for severe pain in patients with renal failure (Ashley and Dunleavey 2019; Joint Formulary Committee 2022). Tramadol can be considered for mild to moderate pain (Coluzzi et al. 2020); and for severe pain, oxycodone or alfentanil should be considered (Back et al. 2021). The choice of opioid will be dependent on clinical condition and degree of renal impairment. Alfentanil is safe to administer in severe renal impairment as it is metabolised in the liver to non-toxic metabolites, which are excreted renally (Klees et al. 2005). However, alfentanil can only be administered parentally and has a short duration of action when given as breakthrough analgesia. Therefore, in clinical practice, it is often administered via continuous subcutaneous infusion with oxycodone for breakthrough analgesia. This can be problematic for patients who have ongoing cancer pain or chronic pain conditions or do not wish to have a syringe driver. A CNS should always seek guidance from specialist palliative care teams in the management of complex pain for patients with renal failure, for consideration of alternative opioids such as hydromorphone, subcutaneous fentanyl, transdermal fentanyl or buprenorphine. A CNS should also be mindful of the use of adjuvant analgesics in renal failure, such as non-steroidal anti-inflammatory drugs (NSAIDs), which are contra-indicated in patients with renal impairment (Ashley and Dunleavey 2019), and a dose reduction should be considered in neuropathic agents such as pregabalin or gabapentin (Lee et al. 2011; Ashley and Dunleavey 2019).

8.2.2 Hepatic Impairment

For individuals with cancer, liver impairment can be related to disease progression, anticancer treatment or other underlying conditions such as cirrhosis or hepatitis (Pinter et al. 2016). Liver metabolism is the main route of elimination for many drugs. Impairment can cause abnormal metabolism resulting in the accumulation of drug metabolites, increasing drug side effects. There are several factors to consider before choosing an analgesic, such as the patient's prognosis, the severity of the liver disease, liver function, internationalised normalised ratio (INR), and albumin and bilirubin levels (Bridgewater et al. 2014). Currently, there is no clear guidance on analgesic use in individuals with hepatic impairment; therefore, the CNS should seek guidance under the relevant drug in the British National Formulary (Joint Formulary Committee 2022).

A systematic review of the use of opioids in patients with cancer with hepatic impairment found that morphine is the preferred choice of opioid (Hughes et al. 2022); however, there is limited evidence to support this. As there is no clear guidance, all opioids should be used with caution in patients with hepatic impairment.

The general approach to pain management is to avoid hepatotoxic drugs such as NSAIDS, consider opioid reduction with extended dose intervals, and ensure close monitoring and regular review (Back et al. 2021). In acute liver failure, the use of regular immediate-release opioids, instead of controlled-release, should be used until the pain or liver function is stable (Joint Formulary Committee 2022). The use of transdermal patches should also be avoided until the liver function has stabilised (Soleimanpour et al. 2016). A CNS should also be mindful that although paracetamol is a relatively safe non-opioid analgesic, a dose reduction must be considered in hepatic impairment (Joint Formulary Committee 2022). For patients experiencing intolerable side effects or unresolved pain, the CNS should seek guidance from specialist palliative care for consideration of alternative opioids such as subcutaneous fentanyl. For the management of pain in patients with both renal and hepatic impairment, the CNS and medical team should always seek advice from specialist palliative care.

8.2.3 Neuropathic Pain

Neuropathic pain refers to 'pain caused by a lesion or disease of the somatosensory system' (Bouhassira 2019, p. 16). It is often characterized as paraesthesia, numbness and allodynia (Bouhassira 2019). Neuropathic pain is common in advanced cancer due to the direct invasion, compression, or irritation of peripheral or central nerves (Tomita et al. 2013). It is often difficult to treat as it does not normally respond to standard analgesics such as opioids (Jung et al. 2020). The NICE guidelines for the management of neuropathic pain recommend amitriptyline, duloxetine, pregabalin or gabapentin in pharmacological treatment (Tan et al. 2010). In clinical practice, pregabalin is often used first-line in specialist palliative care due to its efficacy and ease of titration. Pregabalin is a gabapentinoid licensed for the treatment of neurological disorders. In 2004, it was approved for the treatment of diabetic peripheral neuropathy and postherpetic neuralgia (Arnold et al. 2017), and it is now widely used in the treatment of other neuropathic pain. Due to drug misuse and increased mortality associated with pregabalin (Skopp and Zimmer 2012), it is now a class C controlled drug in the United Kingdom (UK).

Clinicians must be cautious about prescribing gabapentinoids and consider whether the potential risks outweigh the benefits (Derry et al. 2019); therefore, it is important that CNSs carefully evaluate for signs of drug abuse or dependence. The dosage of gabapentinoids such as pregabalin can be up-titrated depending on response and tolerability. The side effects include dizziness, headache, confusion, tremor, blurred vision, vertigo, ataxia and incoordination (Zaccara et al. 2011). The frequency and intensity of these effects are often increased in higher doses (Bafna et al. 2014). CNSs must also be aware of less common side effects such as peripheral oedema (Calkins et al. 2014), and caution must be taken with a patient with severe congestive heart failure (Ho et al. 2013). Abrupt withdrawal or rapid down-titration of pregabalin can cause insomnia, nausea, headache and diarrhoea (Naveed et al. 2018); therefore, it should be gradually down-titrated over a minimum of one week.

In clinical practice, regular review should be arranged to assess effectiveness and tolerability with every dose titration. Clinical judgement should be used when deciding to titrate slowly, and a dose reduction must be considered in individuals with renal impairment or receiving haemodialysis (Lee et al. 2011). If first-line treatment is not effective or intolerable, the CNS should seek advice from the medical team to consider switching to other recommended neuropathic agents. Pain secondary to nerve compression may benefit from corticosteroids such as dexamethasone (Wilcock et al. 2020; Back et al. 2021). CNSs should seek advice from specialist palliative care teams for pain management that is complex or persistent. In specialist palliative care, ketamine is often used under specialist supervision for complex neuropathic pain (Back et al. 2021).

Ketamine is an N-methyl D-aspartate (NMDA) receptor antagonist used when neuropathic pain has been unresponsive or poorly responsive to first-line conventional therapies. Although the efficacy of ketamine in the treatment of chronic and cancer pain has been widely debated (Velzen et al. 2021), it is often used in specialist palliative care. It is prescribed under the recommendation of a palliative medicine consultant and requires close monitoring of the individual, guided by the specialist palliative care team. Possible side effects include dysphoria, vivid dreams, hallucinations, hypertension, anxiety, tachycardia and cystitis (Joint Formulary Committee 2022). It is contraindicated in patients with raised intracranial pressure, uncontrolled hypertension, severe cardiac disease or cerebrovascular accident (CVA). Patients commencing ketamine will likely be on existing regular opioids; therefore, CNSs must be vigilant, as the introduction of ketamine can restore opioid sensitivity, increasing the risk of opioid toxicity (Lilius et al. 2015; Jonkman et al. 2017).

8.3 Breathlessness

Breathlessness is one of the most distressing symptoms for individuals with cancer (Solano et al. 2006), with intensity increasing in the last weeks to days of life (Hui et al. 2015). It is highly prevalent in advanced lung cancer, affecting 90% of individuals (Chan and Hughes 2015). There is a wide range of aetiology relating to disease progression, effects of cancer treatment, underlying co-morbidities, fear and anxiety (Cachia and Ahmedzai 2008). Dyspnoea can often lead to further symptom burden such as fatigue, depression, loss of appetite and functional decline (Currow et al. 2017). This not only affects the quality of life of patients but also increases the distress for family and/or caregivers (Farquhar et al. 2017).

Similar to pain, the experience of dyspnoea can be multidimensional and individual to the patient (Carel 2018), and this requires the CNS to complete a holistic assessment to address physical, psychosocial, spiritual and emotional needs. Clinical guidance is available on assessing and managing dyspnoea in patients with advanced cancer (Hui et al. 2020), with validated assessment tools available to provide a structured assessment (Birkholz and Haney 2018). This should include a comprehensive assessment of the onset, severity and frequency of symptoms, in addition to identifying exacerbating and alleviating factors, associated symptoms and impact on quality of life. A clinical examination should be considered to ascertain the extent and potential cause of the dyspnoea. For example, pallor may be suggestive of anaemia or cyanosis, and engorged veins of the neck or chest could indicate superior vena cava obstruction (SVCO). A CNS should observe the effectiveness of breathing at rest and during activity, including the rate, depth, oxygen saturation and expectoration of sputum.

Blood tests such as a full blood count (FBP) and imaging such as a chest X-ray or a computed tomographic pulmonary angiography (CTPA) (in a suspected pulmonary embolism) should also be considered. The CNS must identify potentially reversible causes such as infection, pleural effusions, anaemia, pulmonary embolism or exacerbation of heart failure (Back et al. 2021). Dyspnoea secondary to malignancy, such as tumour invasion, may benefit from further systemic cancer treatment (Ben-Aharon et al. 2012). Dyspnoea related to malignant pleural effusion or ascites may benefit from a paracentesis (Wittmer et al. 2020). Consideration of these invasive treatments will be dependent on prognosis, overall health, risk-to-benefit ratio and the wishes of the patient and their family (Akdeniz et al. 2021).

The management of dyspnoea often requires a multidisciplinary approach to improve a patient's coping ability (Shaw et al. 2019). CNSs should initially consider the use of a non-pharmacological intervention such as improving air circulation with a fan or window while encouraging relaxation and controlled breathing techniques (Kako et al. 2018; Malpass et al. 2018; Tan et al. 2019). In collaboration with the multidisciplinary team, they should discuss the individual's fears, expectations, personal capabilities and potential adaptations to daily living (Spathis et al. 2021). Dyspnoea can also be treated with supplemental oxygen therapy in individuals with hypoxemia (Abernethy et al. 2010), and in some cases, a therapeutic trial of non-invasive ventilation may be appropriate. Specialist palliative care guidance recommends opioids, benzodiazepines, bronchodilators or corticosteroids in the management of dyspnoea (Back et al. 2021).

Immediate-release oral morphine is considered the first-line opioid in the pharmacological management of dyspnoea (Barnes et al. 2016; Back et al. 2021). There is a wide variation of opioid regimes in clinical practice. The initial starting dose will depend on age, frailty, previous opioid use, co-morbidities and renal and liver function. NICE guidelines recommend a starting dose of 1–2 mg in opioid naïve individuals (NICE 2012).

There is no evidence to suggest that benzodiazepines have a direct effect on dyspnoea; however, they are often used to relieve associated anxiety or panic attacks (Simon et al. 2016). Benzodiazepines such as lorazepam, diazepam and midazolam are recommended in the management of dyspnoea-related anxiety (Back et al. 2021). As with opioids, a CNS should carefully consider the use of benzodiazepines. Common side effects include drowsiness, dizziness, fatigue, hypotension, low mood, muscle weakness and nausea (Joint Formulary Committee 2022). Benzodiazepines should also be used with caution in renal and hepatic impairment (Wilcock et al. 2020). Abrupt withdrawal can cause confusion and delirium (Joint Formulary Committee 2022); therefore, a slow reduction is advised in patients with long-term use. Benzodiazepines should also be used with caution in elderly individuals, as they are at greater risk of becoming ataxic and confused, leading to falls (Joint Formulary Committee 2022). This highlights the importance of regular monitoring and review by the CNS.

Corticosteroids may be offered for dyspnoea related to airway obstruction or inflammation (Joint Formulary Committee 2022), with reported benefit within three to five days (Back et al. 2021). Bronchodilators may also be beneficial in obstructive airways or bronchospasm (Joint Formulary Committee 2022). The CNS should also consider a timely referral to specialist palliative care, as early intervention has been known to improve dyspnoea and quality of life (Higginson et al. 2014).

8.4 Nausea and Vomiting

Nausea and vomiting are highly prevalent in patients with cancer, affecting 70% of individuals with advanced cancer (Hardy et al. 2018), and are often related to tumour location or cancer treatments (Dranitsaris et al. 2013; Farrell et al. 2013). Additional contributing factors include drugs, uraemia, constipation, systemic infection, electrolyte imbalances, and tumour invasion into the gastrointestinal tract, liver or central nervous system (O'Reilly et al. 2020). The cause of nausea and vomiting can be multi-factorial, and in some cases, the aetiology is unknown (Hardy et al. 2018).

Most clinical guidelines on the management of nausea and vomiting advocate an aetiology-based approach, which requires a systematic clinical assessment. CNSs should complete a detailed medical and treatment history including current medications, a clinical examination, appropriate bloods and investigations. Similar to the assessment of pain, it is important to ascertain symptom characteristics such as the onset, frequency, intensity, timing, and exacerbating and alleviating factors of nausea, in addition to the quantity, force and colour if the individual is vomiting. The features or patterns of nausea and vomiting can be indicative of the cause. For example, infrequent, large-volume vomitus; relief post-vomiting; reflux; or hiccups can be associated with gastric stasis. Clinical guidance is available in identifying patterns indicative of the causes of nausea and vomiting (Back et al. 2021).

A physical examination should be conducted to assess for signs of dehydration, infection, confusion, drowsiness or weakness. This should also include an examination of the abdomen to assess for tenderness and distension, which can be indicative of constipation, intestinal obstruction, organomegaly, ascites or disease progression. If faecal impaction is suspected, a rectal examination and imaging, such as an abdominal X-ray, should be considered. Further diagnostic imaging can be useful and should be discussed with the medical team. Blood tests to exclude hypercalcaemia, uraemia or infection should also be considered and discussed. Diagnostic investigations will be based on the stage of disease, prognosis, benefit to the patient and the wishes of the individual and their family (Wittenberg et al. 2018). Similar to the assessment of pain, existential distress in patients with cancer can often exacerbate their experience of nausea and vomiting (Baqutayan 2012); therefore, it is important for CNSs to identify the emotional, psychosocial and spiritual needs of the patient in the management of these symptoms.

Firstly, non-pharmacological management should be considered, such as avoiding strong smells or tastes, small but frequent meals, relaxation, distraction or the use of complementary therapies (Sheikhi et al. 2015). The pharmacological management of nausea and vomiting will depend on the identified aetiology. As a CNS, it is important to treat any reversible cause, such as hypercalcemia, infection or constipation. Specialist palliative care guidance on pharmacological management is available (Back et al. 2021); however, the effectiveness of these guidelines is dependent on a thorough clinical assessment to identify the underlying cause.

Nausea and vomiting affect 30–90% of individuals receiving moderate to high emetogenic chemotherapy regimens (Schwartzberg et al. 2014; Sekine et al. 2014), so the European Society of Medical Oncology (ESMO 2016) recommend pre-chemotherapy antiemetics based on the emetogenic risk of the cancer treatment. For most emetogenic chemotherapy, the use of ondansetron (5-HT3 receptor antagonist) or metoclopramide (dopamine antagonist) would be recommended. In higher-risk chemotherapy, additional antiemetic agents such as aprepitant (NK-1 receptor antagonist), dexamethasone or olanazapine may be considered in combination (Inoue et al. 2017; Vayne-Bossert et al. 2017).

Metoclopramide is a pro-kinetic antiemetic and is also useful in nausea and vomiting related to gastric stasis or constipation (Back et al. 2021). However, there is a risk of worsening bowel colic and extra-pyramidal side effects such as restlessness, akathisia and involuntary movements (Joint Formulary Committee 2022). Other antiemetics such as haloperidol, levomepromazine and olanzapine have similar extra-pyramidal effects and should not be routinely combined (Back et al. 2021). These side effects can be easily overlooked; therefore, CNSs must be vigilant and provide regular reassessment following the introduction of any antiemetic therapy. This should include assessment and review of current medications, as these antiemetics can enhance the extra-pyramidal side effects of other drugs such as tricyclic antidepressants and selective serotonin re-uptake inhibitors (SSRIs) (Back et al. 2021).

Metoclopramide should not be used concurrently with drugs with antimuscarinic properties, such as cyclizine or hyoscine butylbromide, as it will block the pro-kinetic action (Wilcock et al. 2020). Metoclopramide is contra-indicated in individuals with suspected bowel obstruction (Joint Formulary Committee 2022), and the CNS should always consult with the medical team to consider surgical or specialist palliative care advice, as the management of symptoms can often be complex. Metoclopramide should also be avoided in patients with Parkinson's disease, and a safer alternative should be considered, such as domperidone (Back et al. 2021). However, this can cause QTc prolongation (extended intervals between heartbeats) and should be used with caution in patients with cardiac disease (Joint Formulary Committee 2022). In patients with known Long QT Syndrome, CNSs should always seek guidance from a pharmacist, medical team or specialist palliative care as most antiemetics have a degree of QTc prolongation side effects (Gavioli et al. 2021). This highlights the importance of CNSs completing a detailed medical history and having the ability to recognise side effect profiles before advising on or prescribing any pharmacological treatment.

Levomepromazine is a broad-spectrum antiemetic recommended in specialist palliative care guidelines for nausea and vomiting of indeterminate or multiple causes (Twycross and Wilcock 2016). In clinical practice, it is often used when the first-line antiemetic option has failed. Sedation is a common side effect (Cox et al. 2015); therefore, close monitoring by the CNS is required when up-titrating. Levomepromazine also causes anticholinergic side effects such as dry mouth, urinary retention, agitation and restlessness. Cyclizine, which is useful for treatment of nausea and vomiting in intracranial disease or treatment (Back et al. 2021), has similar anticholinergic side effects and should not be in combination with levomepromazine. These antiemetics can also enhance the anticholinergic side effects of other medications, such as amitriptyline and hyoscine butylbromide (Back et al. 2021), and should be used with caution in cardiac disease (Joint Formulary Committee 2022).

The CNS must carefully consider the choice and route of antiemetics. In clinical practice, it is important to optimise the dose of the first-line antiemetic and give it regularly by the most appropriate route of administration. It is vital that the CNS regularly reviews and evaluates the effectiveness of the antiemetic therapy. If symptoms persist, a second-line antiemetic or a complementary combination can be considered. The CNS should liaise with the medical team and seek advice from specialist palliative care if symptoms remain uncontrolled or they are unsure of antiemetic choice.

8.5   Constipation

Constipation is highly prevalent in patients with advanced cancer (Clark et al. 2012) and can often be attributed to opioid use, disease progression, dehydration and fatigue (Muldrew et al. 2018). Despite the high risk of developing constipation, it is often not recognised and is undertreated (Cheng et al. 2013). Therefore, it is important for the CNS to regularly assess and review bowel patterns using assessment tools such as the Bristol Stool Chart (Blake et al. 2016). This should include the duration, frequency and consistency of stools, in addition to associated symptoms such as rectal discomfort, abdominal distension, excessive straining, incomplete evacuation, loss of appetite and nausea or vomiting (NICE 2021). CNSs should also identify potential risk factors that will exacerbate symptoms of constipation, including poor nutrition, reduced mobility or underlying clinical conditions such as inflammatory bowel disease, spinal cord injury or hypercalcaemia (Back et al. 2021). CNSs should also review the individual's cancer treatment, as some chemotherapy and targeted cancer drugs can cause constipation by disrupting the nerve supply to the bowel. CNSs should also identify any potential drugs with constipating side effects, such as opioids, antiemetics and antimuscinarics.

All individuals with cancer should be evaluated for constipation due to the wide variety of potential risk factors (Cheng et al. 2013). If constipation is suspected, an abdominal examination and possible digital rectal examination should be considered (Clark et al. 2016). An abdominal X-ray may also be useful if faecal loading is suspected.

Currently, there is no clear best-practice guidance on the pharmacological management of constipation, as national and regional guidelines vary. There is also limited evidence to suggest the use of one laxative over another (Muldrew et al. 2018); therefore, laxative choice is often dependent on clinician experience or patient preference. The CNS should evaluate a patient's bowel activity regularly and consider up-titration of laxative therapy in line with opioid titration (Back et al. 2021).

8.6   Conclusion

Effective symptom management is fundamental in improving the quality of life for individuals with cancer. CNSs play a vital role in the holistic assessment and support of patients and their families while providing advice on the alleviation of symptoms. This can be challenging, as individuals with cancer often experience multiple symptoms related to disease progression, co-morbidities and the effects of cancer treatments.

Effective symptom management relies on accurate holistic assessment and diagnosis, which requires CNSs to possess a high level of skill and expertise. Clinical guidance is available on the assessment and management of symptoms, and validated tools are available to provide a structured assessment. However, the effectiveness of these guidelines depends on a thorough clinical assessment to identify the aetiology. To ensure an accurate assessment, CNSs should complete a detailed medical and treatment history, current medications, clinical examination, appropriate bloods and investigations. Effective communication and collaboration with patients, their families and the multidisciplinary team can also ensure prompt identification and treatment of symptoms.

Before advising on any pharmacological management, CNSs must carefully consider contra-indications and side effect profiles. It is also vital that CNSs regularly review and evaluate the effectiveness of treatment. If symptoms are persistent or complex, CNSs should always seek additional guidance from the medical team or specialist palliative care. There should also be consideration of early palliative care support in patients with cancer, as it has been shown to improve the quality of life in patients with advanced progressive disease.

References

Abbey, J., Piller, N., De Bellis, A. et al. (2004). The Abbey pain scale: a 1-minute numerical indicator for people with end-stage dementia. *International Journal of Palliative Nursing* 10 (1): 6–13.

Abernethy, A.P., McDonald, C.F., Frith, P.A. et al. (2010). Effect of palliative oxygen versus room air in relief of breathlessness in patients with refractory dyspnoea: a double-blind, randomised controlled trial. *Lancet* 376 (9743): 784–793.

Achterberg, W., Lautenbacher, S., Husebo, B. et al. (2020). Pain in dementia. *PAIN Reports* 5 (1): 1–8.

Ackroyd, R. and Aman, S. (2012). Use of oxycodone and association with renal function. *British Medical Journal Supportive and Palliative Care* 2 (1): A62–A63.

Akdeniz, M., Yardımcı, B., and Kavukcu, E. (2021). Ethical considerations at the end-of-life care. *SAGE Open Medicine* 9: 1–9.

Arnold, L.M., Mccarberg, B.H., Clair, A.G. et al. (2017). Dose–response of pregabalin for diabetic peripheral neuropathy, postherpetic neuralgia, and fibromyalgia. *Postgraduate Medicine* 129: 921–933.

Ashley, C. and Dunleavey, A. (2019). *The Renal Drug Handbook*. Oxford: Radcliffe Medical Press.

Back, I., Watson, M., Armstrong, P., et al. (2021). Palliative care adult network guidelines. https://book.pallcare.info/index.php (accessed 22 July 2022).

Bafna, U., Rajarajeshwaran, K., Khandelwal, M., and Verma, A.P. (2014). A comparison of effect of preemptive use of oral gabapentin and pregabalin for acute post-operative pain after surgery under spinal anaesthesia. *Journal of Anaesthesiology and Clinical Pharmacology* 30 (3): 373–377.

Baqutayan, S.M. (2012). The effect of anxiety on breast cancer patients. *Indian Journal of Psychological Medicine* 34 (2): 119–123.

Barnes, P., McDonald, J., Smallwood, N., and Manser, R. (2016). Opioids for the palliation of refractory breathlessness in adults with advanced disease and terminal illness. *Cochrane Database Systematic Review* 3: 1–39.

Ben-Aharon, I., Gafter-Gvili, A., Leibovici, L., and Stemmer, S.M. (2012). Interventions for alleviating cancer-related dyspnea: a systematic review and meta-analysis. *Acta Oncologica* 51 (8): 996–1008.

Birkholz, L. and Haney, T. (2018). Using a dyspnea assessment tool to improve care at the end of life. *Journal of Hospice and Palliative Nursing* 20 (3): 219–227.

Blake, M.R., Raker, J.M., and Whelan, K. (2016). Validity and reliability of the Bristol stool form scale in healthy adults and patients with diarrhoea-predominant irritable bowel syndrome. *Alimentary Pharmacology and Therapeutics* 44: 693–703.

Bouhassira, D. (2019). Neuropathic pain: definition, assessment and epidemiology. *Revue Neurologique* 175: 16–25.

Bridgewater, J., Galle, P.R., Khan, S.A. et al. (2014). Guidelines for the diagnosis and management of intrahepatic cholangiocarcinoma. *Journal of Hepatology* 60 (6): 1268–1289.

Burns, M. and McIlfatrick, S. (2015). Nurses' knowledge and attitudes towards pain assessment for people with dementia in a nursing home setting. *International Journal of Palliative Nursing* 21 (10): 479–487.

Cachia, E. and Ahmedzai, S.H. (2008). Breathlessness in cancer patients. *European Journal of Cancer* 44 (8): 1116–1123.

Calkins, A., Shurman, J., Jaros, M. et al. (2014). Peripheral edema and weight gain in adult patients with painful diabetic peripheral neuropathy (DPN) receiving gabapentin enacarbil (GEn) or pregabalin enrolled in a randomized phase 2 trial (I6-1.004). *Neurology* 82 (10 Supplement): S369.

Candrilli, S., Bell, T., Irish, W. et al. (2008). A comparison of inpatient length of stay and costs among patients with hematologic malignancies (excluding Hodgkin disease) associated with and without acute renal failure. *Clinical Lymphoma and Myeloma* 8 (1): 44–51.

Caraceni, A. and Shkodra, M. (2019). Cancer pain assessment and classification. *Cancers* 11 (4): 1–13.

Carel, H. (2018). Breathlessness: the rift between objective measurement and subjective experience. *Lancet Respiratory Medicine* 6 (5): 332–333.

Chan, B.A. and Hughes, B.G. (2015). Targeted therapy for non-small cell lung cancer: current standards and the promise of the future. *Translational Lung Cancer Research* 4 (1): 36–54.

Cheng, C.W., Kwok, A.O.L., and Bian, Z.X. (2013). A cross sectional study of constipation and laxative use in advanced cancer patients: insights for revision of current practice. *Support Care Cancer* 21 (1): 149–156.

Clark, K., Smith, J.M., and Currow, D.C. (2012). The prevalence of bowel problems reported in a palliative care population. *Journal of Pain Symptom Management* 43 (6): 993–1000.

Clark, K., Lam, L.T., and Talley, N.J. (2016). Assessing the presence and severity of constipation with plain radiographs in constipated palliative care patients. *Journal of Palliative Medicine* 19 (6): 617–621.

Coluzzi, F., Caputi, F.F., Billeci, D. et al. (2020). Safe use of opioids in chronic kidney disease and hemodialysis patients: tips and tricks for non-pain specialists. *Therapeutics and Clinical Risk Management* 16: 821–837.

Cosmai, L., Porta, C., Foramitti, M. et al. (2021). Preventive strategies for acute kidney injury in cancer patients. *Clinical Kidney Journal* 14 (1): 70–83.

Cox, L., Darvill, E., and Dorman, S. (2015). Levomepromazine for nausea and vomiting in palliative care. *Cochrane Database Systematic Review* 11: 1–13.

Currow, D.C., Dal Grande, E., Ferreira, D. et al. (2017). Chronic breathlessness associated with poorer physical and mental health-related quality of life (SF-12) across all adult age groups. *Thorax* 72 (12): 1151–1153.

Derry, S., Bell, R.F., Straube, S. et al. (2019). Pregabalin for neuropathic pain in adults. *Cochrane Database Systematic Review* 1: 1–62.

Deshields, T.L., Potter, P., Olsen, S., and Liu, J. (2014). The persistence of symptom burden: symptom experience and quality of life of cancer patients across one year. *Support Care Cancer* 22: 1089–1096.

Dranitsaris, G., Bouganim, N., Milano, C. et al. (2013). Prospective validation of a prediction tool for identifying patients at high risk for chemotherapy-induced nausea and vomiting. *Journal of Supportive Oncology* 11 (1): 14–21.

ESMO (2016). MASSC and ESMO consensus guidelines for the prevention of chemotherapy and radiotherapy-induced nausea and vomiting: ESMO clinical practice guidelines. European Association of Medical Oncology. *Annals of Oncology* 13 (5): 119–127.

Farquhar, M., Penfold, C., Benson, J. et al. (2017). Six key topics informal carers of patients with breathlessness in advanced disease want to learn about and why: MRC phase I study to inform an educational intervention. *PloS one* 12 (5): 1–16.

Farrell, C., Brearley, S.G., Pilling, M., and Molassiotis, A. (2013). The impact of chemotherapy-related nausea on patients' nutritional status, psychological distress and quality of life. *Supportive Care in Cancer* 21 (1): 59–66.

Folkard, S.S., Banerjee, S., and Menzies-Wilson, R. (2020). Percutaneous nephrostomy in obstructing pelvic malignancy does not facilitate further oncological treatment. *International Urology and Nephrology* 52: 1625–1628.

Fulton, J.S., Mayo, A.M., Walker, J.A., and Urden, L. (2016). Core practice outcomes for Clinical Nurse Specialist: a revalidation study. *Journal of Professional Nursing* 32 (4): 271–282.

Gavioli, E.M., Guardado, N., Haniff, F. et al. (2021). The risk of QTc prolongation with antiemetics in the palliative care setting: a narrative review. *Journal of Pain and Palliative Care Pharmacotherapy* 35 (2): 125–135.

Grotmol, K., Lie, H., Loge, J. et al. (2019). Patients with advanced cancer and depression report a significantly higher symptom burden than non-depressed patients. *Palliative and Supportive Care* 17 (2): 143–149.

Guo, K.K., Deng, C.Q., Lu, G.J., and Zhao, G.L. (2018). Comparison of analgesic effect of oxycodone and morphine on patients with moderate and advanced cancer pain: a meta-analysis. *BMC Anesthesiology* 18 (132): 1–9.

Hardy, J., Skerman, H., Glare, P. et al. (2018). A randomized open-label study of guideline-driven antiemetic therapy versus single agent antiemetic therapy in patients with advanced cancer and nausea not related to anticancer treatment. *BMC Cancer* 18 (1): 1–9.

Higginson, I.J., Bausewein, C., Reilly, C.C. et al. (2014). An integrated palliative and respiratory care service for patients with advanced disease and refractory breathlessness: a randomised controlled trial. *Lancet Respiratory Medicine* 2 (12): 979–987.

Hjermstad, M.J., Kolflaath, J., Løkken, A.O. et al. (2013). Are emergency admissions in palliative cancer care always necessary? Results from a descriptive study. *British Medical Journal Open* 3: 1–8.

Ho, J.M., Tricco, A.C., Perrier, L. et al. (2013). Risk of heart failure and edema associated with the use of pregabalin: a systematic review. *Systematic Review* 2 (25): 1–8.

Hökkä, M., Kaakinen, P., and Pölkki, T. (2014). A systematic review: non-pharmacological interventions in treating pain in patients with advanced cancer. *Journal of Advanced Nursing* 70: 1954–1969.

Hughes, L.T., Raftery, D., Coulter, P. et al. (2022). Use of opioids in patients with cancer with hepatic impairment – a systematic review. *British Medical Journal Supportive and Palliative Care* 12 (2): 152–157.

Hui, D. and Bruera, E. (2014). A personalized approach to assessing and managing pain in patients with cancer. *Journal of Clinical Oncology* 32: 1640–1646.

Hui, D., Dos Santos, R., Chisholm, G. et al. (2015). Bedside clinical signs associated with impending death in patients with advanced cancer: preliminary findings of a prospective, longitudinal cohort study. *Cancer* 121 (6): 960–967.

Hui, D., Maddocks, M., Johnson, M.J. et al. (2020). ESMO Guidelines Committee. Management of breathlessness in patients with cancer: ESMO Clinical Practice Guidelines. *ESMO Open* 5 (6): e001038.

Huysmans, E., Leemans, L., Beckwée, D. et al. (2020). The relationship between cognitive and emotional factors and healthcare and medication use in people experiencing pain: a systematic review. *Journal of Clinical Medicine* 9 (8): 2–92.

Inoue, T., Kimura, M., Uchida, J. et al. (2017). Aprepitant for the treatment of breakthrough chemotherapy-induced nausea and vomiting in patients receiving moderately emetogenic chemotherapy. *International Journal of Clinical Oncology* 22: 600–604.

Joint Formulary Committee (2022). *British National Formulary 83*. London: BMJ Publishing and the Royal Pharmaceutical Society.

Jonkman, K., Dahan, A., van de Donk, T. et al. (2017). Ketamine for pain. *F1000 Research* 6: 1–11.

Jung, J.-M., Chung, C.K., Kim, C.H. et al. (2020). Comparison of the use of opioids only and pregabalin add-on for the treatment of neuropathic pain in cervical myelopathy patients: a pilot trial. *Scientific Reports* 10: 1–9.

Kako, J., Morita, T., Yamaguchi, T. et al. (2018). Fan therapy is effective in relieving dyspnea in patients with terminally ill cancer: a parallel-arm, randomized controlled trial. *Journal of Pain and Symptom Management* 56 (4): 493–500.

Kerr, H., Donovan, M., and McSorley, O. (2021). Evaluation of the role of the Clinical Nurse Specialist in cancer care: an integrative literature review. *European Journal of Cancer Care* 32 (3): 1–13.

Kitchlu, A., McArthur, E., and Amir, E. (2019). Acute kidney injury in patients receiving systemic treatment for cancer: a population-based cohort study. *JNCI Journal of the National Cancer Institute* 111: 727–736.

Klees, T.M., Sheffels, P., Dale, O., and Kharasch, E.D. (2005). Metabolism of alfentanil by cytochrome p4503a (cyp3a) enzymes. *Drug Metabolism and Disposition* 33 (3): 303–311.

Lameire, N., Vanholder, R., Van Biesen, W., and Benoit, D. (2016). Acute kidney injury in critically ill cancer patients: an update. *Critical Care* 20 (209): 1–12.

Lee, D.W., Lee, H.J., Kim, H.J. et al. (2011). Two cases of pregabalin neurotoxicity in chronic kidney disease patients. *NDT Plus* 4 (2): 138.

Li, X.M., Xiao, W.H., Yang, P., and Zhao, H.X. (2017). Psychological distress and cancer pain: results from a controlled cross-sectional survey in China. *Scientific Reports* 7 (39397): 1–9.

Lichtner, V., Dowding, D., Allcock, N. et al. (2016). The assessment and management of pain in patients with dementia in hospital settings: a multi-case exploratory study from a decision making perspective. *BMC Health Services Research* 16 (1): 1–21.

Lilius, T.O., Jokinen, V., Neuvonen, M.S. et al. (2015). Ketamine coadministration attenuates morphine tolerance and leads to increased brain concentrations of both drugs in the rat. *British Journal of Pharmacology* 172: 2799–2813.

Malpass, A., Feder, G., and Dodd, J.W. (2018). Understanding changes in dyspnoea perception in obstructive lung disease after mindfulness training. *British Medical Journal Open Respiratory Research* 5: 1–9.

McKie, J. (2016). What are the equivalent doses of oral morphine to other oral opioids when used as analgesics in adult palliative care? UK Medicines Information. https://www.sps.nhs.uk (accessed 12 June 2022).

Muldrew, D.H.L., Hasson, F., Carduff, E. et al. (2018). Assessment and management of constipation for patients receiving palliative care in specialist palliative care settings: a systematic review of the literature. *Palliative Medicine* 32 (5): 930–938.

National Institute of Clinical Excellence. (2012). Opioids in palliative care: safe and effective prescribing of strong opioids for pain in palliative care of adults. www.nice.org.uk (accessed 23 February 2022).

National Institute of Clinical Excellence. (2021). Palliative cancer care – pain. National Institute for Health and Clinical Excellence. http://cks.nice.org.uk/topics/palliative-cancer-care-pain (accessed 23 February 2022).

Naveed, S., Faquih, A.E., and Chaudhary, A.M.D. (2018). Pregabalin-associated discontinuation symptoms: a case report. *Cureus* 10 (10): 1–3.

O'Reilly, M., Mellotte, G., Ryan, B., and O'Connor, A. (2020). Gastrointestinal side effects of cancer treatments. *Therapeutic Advances in Chronic Disease* 27 (11): 1–9.

Pinter, M., Trauner, M., Peck-Radosavljevic, M., and Sieghart, W. (2016). Cancer and liver cirrhosis: implications on prognosis and management. *ESMO Open* 1 (2): 1–16.

Quinn, B., Luftner, D., Di Palma, M. et al. (2017). Managing pain in advanced cancer settings: an expert guidance and conversation tool. *Cancer Nursing Practice* 16 (10): 27–34.

Rayment, C. and Bennett, M.I. (2015). Definition and assessment of chronic pain in advanced disease. In: *Oxford Textbook of Palliative Medicine*, 5e (ed. N. Cherney, M. Fallon, S. Kaasa, et al.), 519–524. London: Oxford University Press.

Rosner, M.H. and Dalkin, A.C. (2012). Onco-nephrology: the pathophysiology and treatment of malignancy-associated hypercalcemia. *Clinical Journal of the American Society of Nephrology* 7 (10): 1722–1729.

Sampson, E.L., White, N., Lord, K. et al. (2015). Pain, agitation and behavioural problems in people with dementia admitted to general hospital wards: a longitudinal cohort study. *Pain* 156 (4): 675–683.

Schwartzberg, L., Barbour, S.Y., Morrow, G.R. et al. (2014). Pooled analysis of phase III clinical studies of palonosetron versus ondansetron, dolasetron, and granisetron in the prevention of chemotherapy-induced nausea and vomiting (CINV). *Support Care Cancer* 22 (2): 469–477.

Sekine, I., Okamoto, H., Horai, T. et al. (2014). A randomized phase III study of single-agent amrubicin vs. carboplatin/etoposide in elderly patients with extensive-disease small-cell lung cancer. *Clinical Lung Cancer* 15 (2): 96–102.

Shaw, V., Davies, A., and Ong, B.N.A. (2019). A collaborative approach to facilitate professionals to support the breathless patient. *British Medical Journal Supportive and Palliative Care* 9: 1–5.

Sheikhi, M.A., Ebadi, A., Talaeizadeh, A., and Rahmani, H. (2015). Alternative methods to treat nausea and vomiting from cancer chemotherapy. *Chemotherapy Research and Practice* 1–6.

Simon, S.T., Higginson, I.J., Booth, S. et al. (2016). Benzodiazepines for the relief of breathlessness in advanced malignant and non-malignant diseases in adults. *Cochrane Database Systematic Review* 10: 1–41.

Skopp, G. and Zimmer, G. (2012). Pregabalin – a drug with abuse potential? *Archives for Kriminologie* 229 (1–2): 44–54.

Smith, H.S. (2009). Opioid metabolism. *Mayo Clinic Proceedings* 84 (7): 613–624.

Solano, J.P., Gomes, B., and Higginson, I.J. (2006). A comparison of symptom prevalence in far advanced cancer, AIDS, heart disease, chronic obstructive pulmonary disease and renal disease. *Journal of Pain and Symptom Management* 31 (1): 58–69.

Soleimanpour, H., Safari, S., Shahsavari Nia, K. et al. (2016). Opioid drugs in patients with liver disease: a systematic review. *Hepatitis Monthly* 16 (4): 1–14.

Spathis, A., Burkin, J., Moffat, C. et al. (2021). Cutting through complexity: the breathing, thinking, functioning clinical model is an educational tool that facilitates chronic breathlessness management. *Primary Care Respiratory Medicine* 31 (25): 1–3.

Tan, T., Barry, P., Reken, S., and Baker, M. (2010). Pharmacological management of neuropathic pain in non-specialist settings: summary of NICE guidance. *British Medical Journal* 340: c1079.

Tan, S.B., Liam, C.K., Pang, Y.K. et al. (2019). The effect of 20-minute mindful breathing on the rapid reduction of dyspnea at rest in patients with lung diseases: a randomized controlled trial. *Journal of Pain and Symptom Management* 57 (4): 802–808.

Tomita, M., Koike, H., Kawagashira, Y. et al. (2013). Clinicopathological features of neuropathy associated with lymphoma. *Brain* 136: 2563–2578.

Twycross, R. and Wilcock, A. (ed.) (2016). *Introducing Palliative Care*. Padstow, Cornwall: Pharmaceutical Press.

Van den Beuken-van Everdingen, M.H., Hochstenbach, L.M., Joosten, E.A. et al. (2016). Update on prevalence of pain in patients with cancer: systematic review and meta-analysis. *Journal of Pain Symptom Management* 51 (6): 1070–1090.

Varilla, V., Schneiderman, H., and Keefe, S. (2015). No ceiling dose: effective pain control with extraordinary opiate dosing in cancer. *Connecticut Medicine* 79 (9): 521–524.

Vayne-Bossert, P., Haywood, A., Good, P. et al. (2017). Corticosteroids for adult patients with advanced cancer who have nausea and vomiting (not related to chemotherapy, radiotherapy, or surgery). *Cochrane Database Systematic Reviews* 7 (7): CD012002.

Velzen, M.V., Dahan, J.D.C., van Dorp, E.L.A. et al. (2021). Efficacy of ketamine in relieving neuropathic pain: a systematic review and meta-analysis of animal studies. *Pain* 162 (9): 2320–2330.

Verkissen, M.N., Hjermstad, M.J., Van Belle, S. et al. (2019). Quality of life and symptom intensity over time in people with cancer receiving palliative care: results from the international European palliative care cancer symptom study. *PLoS One* 14 (10): 1–16.

Warden, V., Hurley, A.C., and Volicer, L. (2003). Development and psychometric evaluation of the pain assessment in advanced dementia (PAINAD) scale. *Journal of the American Medical Directors Association* 4 (1): 9–15.

Wilcock, A., Howard, P., and Charlesworth, S. (ed.) (2020). *Palliative Care Formulary*. London: Pharmaceutical Press.

Wittenberg, E., Reb, A., and Kanter, E. (2018). Communicating with patients and families around difficult topics in cancer care using the COMFORT communication curriculum. *Seminars in Oncology Nursing* 34 (3): 264–273.

Wittmer, V.L., Lima, R.T., Maia, M.C. et al. (2020). Respiratory and symptomatic impact of ascites relief by paracentesis in patients with hepatic cirrhosis. *Archives of Gastroenterology* 57 (1): 64–68.

World Health Organization. (2003). WHO's pain ladder. www.who.int. (accessed 14 May 2022).

Zaccara, G., Gangemi, P., Perucca, P., and Specchio, L. (2011). The adverse event profile of pregabalin: a systematic review and meta-analysis of randomized controlled trials. *Epilepsia* 52 (4): 826–836.

Zuccaro, S.M., Vellucci, R., Sarzi-Puttini, P. et al. (2012). Barriers to pain management: focus on opioid therapy. *Clinical Drug Investigations* 22 (32 Suppl 1): 11–19.

9

Multidisciplinary Teamworking

Hinal Patel and Oonagh McSorley

Abstract

The multidisciplinary team (MDT) as a concept is viewed as a best practice or gold standard in cancer healthcare services globally. It evolved initially when (i) patient outcomes were seen to improve when based on available evidence; (ii) treatments for cancer such as surgery, radiotherapy and chemotherapy were combined; and (iii) the medical experts in these fields were working together. With the growing awareness that this approach improved patient care, disciplines such as nursing and allied health professionals were acknowledged as members of the MDT. The objective of the MDT is to consider all relevant treatment options; from these, an individual treatment plan is developed collectively. However, effective teamworking can be challenging due to organisational structures and demands. The clinical nurse specialist is a vital member of the MDT and is best placed to advocate for the patient. More research is required to ensure that the MDT and MDT meetings are effective in delivering the best treatment plans for individuals with cancer.

9.1 Introduction

Globally, the delivery of healthcare is experiencing multiple challenges and increasing demands as a result of ageing populations, chronic illness, complexity of ill health, lack of funding and, more recently, the COVID-19 global pandemic. Within this context, and driven by health policy, healthcare professionals are tasked with ensuring safe, quality health outcomes for individuals, which can be achieved through effective teamworking. In cancer care, the pathway to diagnosis and treatment can be complex; hence, consistency in care delivery is required to enhance patient outcomes. The multidisciplinary approach to care was designed to provide consistency in the quality of care delivered and improve survival rates

(Hoinville et al. 2019). The crucial role of the clinical nurse specialist (CNS) in delivering effective healthcare through their contribution to the multidisciplinary team (MDT) will be emphasised. Hinal Patel is a Clinical Nurse Specialist at University College London Hospitals NHS Foundation Trust, she works under the lymphoma sub-speciality in the CAR-T and autologous stem cell transplant team. Oonagh Mc Sorley is a lecturer at the School of Nursing and Midwifery, Queen's University Belfast and has a clinical background in cancer nursing.

9.2 The Multidisciplinary Team

Many terms in healthcare literature and policies are used interchangeably to describe the concept of a team: *interdisciplinary, multidisciplinary, multiprofessional* and *inter-professional*, among others. However, there is no consensus among healthcare professionals, policy-makers and academics on the meaning of these terms, leaving them open for interpretation (Chamberlain-Salaun et al. 2013; Martin et al. 2022). This debate warrants further discussion elsewhere; for the purposes of this chapter, the authors will use the description of the interdisciplinary team provided by Janssen et al. (2017), which describes it as co-operation between a group of professionals for a shared purpose that is then facilitated in healthcare by MDTs.

In cancer services, the MDT can be defined as specialised professionals working together in cancer care with the principal goal of improving patient care and treatment efficiency (Taberna et al. 2020). The MDT as a concept is viewed as a best practice or gold standard in cancer healthcare services globally, emerging initially in the United States of America (USA) in the 1980s and in the United Kingdom (UK), Europe and Australia from the late 1990s onwards (Patkar et al. 2011). As an example, the MDT developed in the UK following the publication of the Calman-Hine report (Department of Health 1995) and the National Cancer Plan (Department of Health 2000); both reports drove for timely, quality care for people with cancer, with the aim of reducing inequalities in care. These reports recognised that an integrated team approach and collaborative working could help to achieve better outcomes for individuals with a cancer diagnosis.

The MDT evolved initially when patient outcomes improved because treatments such as surgery, radiotherapy and chemotherapy were being combined based on the best available evidence; in addition, the medical experts in these fields were communicating and working together. With the growing awareness that multidisciplinary working improved patient care, disciplines such as nursing and allied health professionals involved in supportive care were invited to join the MDT (Taberna et al. 2020). Their addition to the team improved patients' quality of care by preventing and managing side effects of treatment and subsequently empowering patients in the decision-making processes before, during and after treatment (Punshon et al. 2017; Soukup et al. 2018).

Cancer MDTs can comprise oncologists and/or haematologists, surgeons, radiologists, nurses such as the CNS, pathologists and allied healthcare professionals who meet on a regular basis, often weekly or monthly in multidisciplinary meetings (MDMs). The team objective is to consider all relevant treatment options; from these, an individual treatment plan is developed collectively. It is mandatory in the context of the UK that MDMs occur (Department of Health 2004, 2013) to ensure that all individuals with cancer receive consistent quality care.

Interestingly, the MDT also have a governance role in overseeing and monitoring the impact of treatment decisions and ensuring the accountability of those decisions. However, for many years, this significant aspect of the MDM objective has been difficult to achieve due to a lack of time and resources (National Cancer Registration and Analysis Service 2010). More recently, it has been reported that MDMs cannot cope with the demand: each patient is allocated only a few minutes for discussion, which means all information is not considered and, therefore, time for reflection and evaluation is restricted (Cancer Research UK 2017). With the increase in cancer incidence and advances in technology and treatments, in addition to the complexity of individual cases, meaningful discussion and effective decision-making are vital within the MDT; therefore, it is important to reflect upon what makes a team effective and efficient.

9.2.1 Characteristics of an Effective Multidisciplinary Team

Prior to 2010, there was a lack of empirical evidence to demonstrate whether the MDT was effective (Soukup et al. 2018). The National Cancer Action Team (NCAT) developed an online survey that collected data from 2034 MDT members reporting on perceptions of the factors essential for an effective MDT (NCAT 2010). The results derived five main elements: the team, MDM organisational logistics, infrastructure for MDMs, person-centred clinical decision-making and team governance. Each of these elements could have its own chapter in this book; the next section summarises the pertinent points relating to the present National Health Service (NHS) culture in the context of the UK, which should be transferable to other contexts.

9.2.1.1 The Team

In the context of the UK, each individual who develops cancer will navigate their journey from referral, often from their general practitioner (GP)/primary physician, to diagnosis and treatment – this is often referred to as the *cancer pathway*. The MDT has a significant role in this pathway. In England, UK, for example, rapid cancer diagnostic and assessment pathways for lung, prostate and colorectal cancer have been published (NHS England 2018). Embedded in these pathways is the MDT, who have a significant level of expertise and specialisation of professionals within the team to ensure that knowledge of the disease, evidence-based treatments, and the patient's preference are represented, leading to a timely diagnosis and treatment plan. However, for the team to function effectively, this expert knowledge needs to be combined with effective working relationships based on respect, open communication and leadership (Soukup et al. 2018).

Furthermore, all members of the team must feel psychologically safe, which includes an opportunity to discuss their opinions and be comfortable reporting to their line manager when they have made an error without feeling insecure and embarrassed. This will lead to a supportive learning environment for development (Rosen et al. 2018). The NHS England and NHS Improvement (2019) highlight the importance of psychological safety in relation to delivering safe patient care. The NHS Health Education England (2021, p. 24) multidisciplinary toolkit summarises this issue as follows: 'It is essential within healthcare.... Psychological safety is seen as a key ingredient for patient safety and is created by compassionate leadership encouraging team members to pay attention to each other; to develop mutual understanding; to empathise and support each other. Feeling part of a team protects individuals against the demands of the organisation they work for and if they have clarity about their role in the team, they are less likely to burn out and more likely to operate in a safe way'.

Within the MDT, levels of hierarchy exist among different professions, and this can affect the individual member's sense of psychological safety, degree of participation and appreciation of contributions. The CNS is present to advocate for the patient's holistic needs. There is a paucity of research evaluating the contribution of the CNS in MDMs. The available research states that nurses and their knowledge are underrepresented in MDMs, and surgeons have a higher consideration for biomedical information (Atwal and Caldwell 2006; Lamb et al. 2013; Punshon et al. 2017). The CNS is faced with this underrepresentation alongside time constraints and increasing patient numbers that may restrict their ability to speak up and appropriately challenge in the context of the MDM (Punshon et al. 2017). This suggests that for some team members, psychological safety may be lacking within MDMs.

Another consideration that improves the functioning of the team, by ensuring that effective decisions are made is regular attendance by the core members of MDTs, such as surgeons, radiologists, oncologists and pathologists; this was one of the conclusions in a recent systematic review by Walraven et al. (2022). In this review, attendance rates at MDMs varied from 45% to 90%, and studies that reported low attendance rates among these core members also reported less efficient decision-making. Regular attendance may be difficult for many healthcare professionals to achieve due to staff shortages and competing demands on time.

An effective chairperson for the MDM is also recognised as an essential element in the clinical decision-making process (Lamb et al. 2011; Walraven et al. 2022). This role was traditionally held by the surgeon; however, it has been suggested that rotating the role of the chairperson among staff members and professions can increase team morale and reduce interprofessional conflict (Lamb et al. 2011). Furthermore, CNSs have demonstrated that patient outcomes are similar, if not better, when they chair the MDM instead of surgeons (McGlynn et al. 2017), demonstrating their value in the decision-making process. However, it is interesting to note that the CNS was not viewed as a core member in the Walraven et al. (2022) paper, especially concerning decision-making, suggesting that more evidence needs to be collected on the role and influence of the CNS in the MDM.

9.2.1.2 Multidisciplinary Meeting Organisational Logistics

NHS Trusts and other health organisations should support staff, including the CNS, by ensuring that they have protected time to attend and prepare for the MDT. Some evidence suggests that oncologists, pathologists and radiologists are more likely to attend and be better prepared for the MDM than other professionals (Soukup et al. 2016). For those who are not able to attain the relevant information and investigation results before the meeting or prepare sufficiently, this may be a barrier to attendance (Soukup et al. 2018). Lack of preparation time and unavailability of investigation results can also result in the development of a non-definitive care plan, rushed decision-making and poor morale, ultimately impacting the patient's care (Hoinville et al. 2019).

The increase in cancer caseloads, without a similar increase in resources and capacity, has resulted in a lack of time for each case to be discussed at the MDM, which again can lead to decisions not being made and treatment plans being delayed (Hoinville et al. 2019). Streamlining patient discussions by spending more time on complex cases has been suggested as a method to improve effectiveness; however, further evidence is required, as varying opinions among different professionals highlighted concerns around patient safety: i.e. those patients who are not discussed fully may receive sub-optimal care (Hoinville et al. 2019; Winters et al. 2021).

9.2.1.3 Infrastructure for the Multidisciplinary Meeting

The COVID-19 pandemic has advanced technological changes in how healthcare professionals communicate with each other in the workplace. Virtual conference calling is now an alternative to the traditional face-to-face clinic meeting (Walraven et al. 2022) for all healthcare professionals including the CNS. It has been suggested that this could help with the attendance issue as previously outlined and allow specialists from across the world to attend MDMs, which could help in reaching decisions on complex cases (Rajasekaran et al. 2021). Due to this shift towards online meetings, the physical environment – finding a suitably sized room to accommodate all attending the MDM, with the technology required to show scans and other investigations – has become less of an issue.

9.2.1.4 Person-Centred Clinical Decision-Making

The information provided at MDMs must be person-centred. Content should include the patient's co-morbidities, disease progression, frailty, preference regarding treatments and psycho-social needs. This information will facilitate the team to make clinical decisions that are acceptable to the patient (Soukup et al. 2018). Including timely and accurate person-centred information can be challenging, as patients' preferences may change according to circumstances, personal values and beliefs and the type of disease. The CNS plays a valuable role in this aspect of care. A recent integrative literature review (Kerr et al. 2021) demonstrated that the CNS had a positive outcome on patients' psychological needs and clinical outcomes, by managing pain and fatigue, in addition to general satisfaction with healthcare. This highlights that the CNS is well placed to be the patient's advocate within the MDT, as they will have developed a relationship with the individual and have a sense that they 'know' and can represent the patient holistically.

9.2.1.5 Team Governance

Team governance involves organisational support, which includes funding and resources; both issues are challenging in the current climate (Winters et al. 2021) but essential for MDTs and MDMs to function effectively (Soukup et al. 2018). Learning and development within the team should derive from the results of audits of the outcomes for patients arising from the decisions made at the MDM and data collected during team meetings (Soukup et al. 2018). It has been reported that there is a lack of regular and rigorous audits performed on MDMs, which could affect patient safety (Winters et al. 2021).

Clinical governance is adhered to by using agreed policies and guidelines about the structure and processes within the meeting, e.g. adhering to time schedules, using the correct forms to document data and evaluating the function of the meeting by using validated evaluation tools (Soukup et al. 2018; Walraven et al. 2022). However, from the literature, it remains unclear if any of these tools have demonstrated to optimise MDMs (Walraven et al. 2022).

Future developments to help with the functioning and effectiveness of the MDMs include computerised clinical decision-support systems (CDSSs). These systems consider the patient's data at a genomic and molecular level as well as information on novel treatments and clinical trials. Some may also contain electronic care records. These systems can aid in the decision-making process in MDMs (Winters et al. 2021).

9.3 The Role of the Clinical Nurse Specialist in Relation to the Multidisciplinary Team

The NCAT (2010) emphasises that leadership within the MDT and wider cancer team is one of the key contributions a CNS makes. The National Cancer Patient Experience Survey has highlighted that individuals with cancer who have access to a CNS generally report an enhanced experience during their care and a better understanding of their disease (Department of Health 2019). This highlights the importance of the CNS role and incorporates the 'no decision about me without me' approach.

Macmillan Impact Briefs (2015) outlines the CNS role as a key worker who manages the health concerns of individuals with cancer during and after their treatment. (The key worker role is the focus of Chapter 5 in this book). A CNS works as part of a MDT that supports other healthcare professionals in delivering effective, efficient services and improves the quality of care for those with cancer. The CNS manages their own caseload of patients, coordinates their care and ensures that the patient's needs are met and heard by the wider team. The CNS is often the patient's first point of contact, putting them in a valued position, as they are relied upon for healthcare advice and other matters concerning the patient.

Punshon et al. (2017) state that patient advocacy is a key component of the role of the CNS, something that is highly valued in practice. The CNS has a role in supporting the patient to understand their disease and treatment options and ensure that their concerns are listened to and wishes adhered to (Giesler et al. 2005). It has been suggested that a patient advocate should always be present during MDT meetings so the patient's point of view is always considered (Campagna 2013). However, findings from Lavender (2017) suggested that although CNSs are present during MDT discussions, they are often only observant and do not have much input. Theories such as person-centred care support the role of the CNS and the value of their role. However, as previously stated in this chapter, it has also been well-documented that although nurses try to act as patient advocates, in some instances they are unfortunately dismissed by more senior members of the MDT (Devitt et al. 2010; Lamb et al. 2011).

9.3.1 Challenges of the Clinical Nurse Specialist Working in a Team

Although multidisciplinary teamworking offers many benefits, such as sharing knowledge, enhancing skills, effective management and integrated care, there are also challenges. Four main themes can contribute to barriers experienced in relation to CNS contributions: authority over the treatment agenda, power dynamics, issues of understanding and implementing the role of the CNS and issues within the team (Amir et al. 2004; Willard and Luker 2007; Lanceley et al. 2008; Lamb et al. 2013; Rowlands and Callen 2013).

Evidence suggests that in some areas, CNSs do not feel valued as part of the wider team and are often left unheard (Taylor et al. 2014; Punshon et al. 2017). In group settings such as MDT meetings with other healthcare professionals, nurses may occasionally struggle to voice their thoughts and opinions due to traditional hierarchical structures. Some may assume that others with higher professional status may not value them or their input. Often, the CNS may have to be more assertive and find the confidence to advocate for the patient and for their voice to be heard. This theory is supported by Taylor et al. (2010), who outline that hierarchical boundaries and hostility between different professionals is the main cause of dysfunctional teams.

Willard and Luker (2007) have reported that one of the most important strategies CNSs use to gain acceptance and contribute is building effective relationships with key members of the MDT, mainly the senior clinicians, such as consultants leading the patient's care. Wallace et al. (2019) discuss the barriers to nurse participation in MDT meetings; these are well-identified and discussed earlier. However, they also provide insight into pathways that can be used by CNSs to strengthen their impact on the decision-making process, allowing the wider team to benefit from their knowledge and expertise. These processes include sharing person-centred information that only the CNS may be able to contribute because they are the patient's first point of contact and often the member of staff at the MDM who spends the most time with the patient. The CNS uses holistic assessment and care to identify any psycho-social needs and can confidently act as a patient advocate in this setting.

Asking relevant questions is another approach to address challenges for the CNS in the MDM, as this can prompt further discussion and influence the outcome. It may also facilitate other healthcare professionals in the meeting to contribute with their knowledge and expertise. These approaches enable the CNS to be the patient's advocate by asking questions the patient may wish to be addressed.

Another strategy is to provide practical suggestions that may influence the treatment and frame contributions to plan or change the course of action. Some examples of practical suggestions made by a CNS are accommodating the patients' needs without causing them too much disturbance, e.g. ad hoc clinic appointments, safety measures and raising awareness of specific issues that the patient is experiencing, considering social situations if patients need additional support and discussions on how they will cope with day-to-day activities. An additional strategy is using appropriate humour within the MDT to build rapport and de-escalate tense discussions. For example, if two colleagues disagree, humour can be used appropriately to diffuse a disagreement in an MDT meeting.

Overall, these strategies can influence discussions, contribute to decisions about treatment plans and promote teamwork. This demonstrates that being part of the MDT provides the CNS with the opportunity for discussion, questions and influence. Following is a personal reflection on the CNS role, written using Jasper's (2013) experience, reflection and action (ERA) model.

Personal Reflection on the CNS Role

The ERA Cycle (Jasper 2013) will be used to reflect on aspects of my role as a CNS and my experience of integrating into the role. The ERA cycle is a simple model of reflection with three stages: experience, reflection and action. It inspires a clear depiction of a situation, allowing a clear analysis of emotions and feelings and interpretation of it, resulting in a full assessment that will highlight what action should be taken as a result of an experience.

I joined the lymphoma CNS team in 2020, transferring from the clinical trials team where I worked as a research nurse in haematology. My role as a research nurse within the same hospital and department allowed me a smoother transition into the role of a CNS, and already having worked with members of the MDT helped me integrate into the team.

My experience in my role as a CNS is extremely rewarding, and I find that those we work with closely with on a day-to-day basis respect and value each other. In the department, each sub-disease group within haematology has a group of dedicated CNSs. Within the lymphoma team, we work very closely with a large group of consultants, registrars who rotate in and out of the service, support workers and the administrative team.

On reflection, when I initially transitioned over to this role, my previous experience allowed me to integrate into the team and the job role with great ease. However, I recognise that if I had come into the CNS post without the experience of being a key worker for patients or not having previously known the team, I might have found integration more challenging.

However, I have found the role of a CNS to be very complex, with a lack of clarity regarding what the role is and people's perceptions and expectations of it. It is important to outline the roles and responsibilities to other members of the team, especially those who do not work closely with us. As highlighted by Brault et al. (2014), it is crucial to have clarity about a role for effective interdisciplinary working. Professional roles must to be well-defined to avoid conflict and produce the most effective care and service delivery.

The action that was taken from this is having clarity on the role of a CNS. Highlighting its importance will allow future CNSs to better integrate into their roles and be fully aware of their responsibilities and how they improve the delivery of healthcare.

Hinal Patel

9.4 Conclusion

The MDT and MDMs remain the gold standard for decision-making with regard to the best treatment plans for individuals with cancer. The demands on health-care and those working within it influence how effectively the MDT will work together. Despite these demands, MDMs are generally reported to be positive, open forums that promote discussion from all participants. The CNS's role and influence within the MDT remains challenging but is crucial in ensuring that the patient's voice is heard and acceptable treatment plans are devised. Research and further discussion are required to clearly define the role of the CNS, but it remains a rewarding role within the MDT and healthcare and is beneficial to patients.

References

Amir, Z., Scully, J., and Borrill, C. (2004). The professional role of breast cancer nurses in multi-disciplinary breast cancer care teams. *European Journal of Oncology Nursing* 8: 306–314.

Atwal, A. and Caldwell, K. (2006). 'Nurses' perceptions of multidisciplinary teamwork in acute health-care. *International Journal of Nursing Practice* 12: 359–365.

Brault, I., Kilpatrick, K., D'Amour, D. et al. (2014). Role clarification processes for better integration of nurse practitioners into primary healthcare teams: a multiple-case study. *Nursing Research and Practice* 1–9.

Campagna, K.D. (2013). Who will be the patient advocate on a multidisciplinary team? *Hospital Pharmacy* 48 (2): 90–92.

Cancer Research UK. (2017). Meeting patients' needs: improving the effectiveness of multidisciplinary team meetings in cancer services.

Chamberlain-Salaun, J., Mills, J., and Usher, K. (2013). Terminology used to describe health care teams: an integrative review of the literature. *Journal of Multidisciplinary Healthcare* 6: 65–74.

Department of Health. (2000). The NHS cancer plan. London: Department of Health.

Department of Health. (2004). Manual for cancer services. London: Department of Health.

Department of Health. (2013). National peer review report: cancer services 2012/2013.

Department of Health. (2019). National cancer patient experience survey 2019. https://www.gov.uk/government/statistics/national-cancer-patient-experience-survey-2019 (accessed 15 September 2022).

Devitt, B., Philip, J., and McLachlan, S.A. (2010). Team dynamics, decision making, and attitudes toward multidisciplinary cancer meetings: health professionals' perspectives. *Journal of Oncology Practice* 6: e17–e20.

Expert Advisory Group on Cancer. (1995). A policy framework for commissioning cancer services – the Calman-Hine report. A report by the Expert Advisory Group on Cancer to the chief medical officers of England and Wales. Department of Health.

Giesler, R.B., Given, B., Given, C.W. et al. (2005). Improving the quality of life of patients with prostate carcinoma: a randomized trial testing the efficacy of a nurse-driven intervention. *Cancer* 104 (4): 752–762.

Hoinville, L., Taylor, C., Zasada, M. et al. (2019). Improving the effectiveness of cancer multidisciplinary team meetings: analysis of a national survey of MDT members' opinions about streamlining patient discussions. *British Medical Journal Open Quality* 8 (2): e000631.

Janssen, A., Brunner, M., Keep, M. et al. (2017). Interdisciplinary eHealth practice in cancer care: a review of the literature. *International Journal of Environmental Research and Public Health* 14 (11): 1–14.

Jasper, M. (2013). *Beginning Reflective Practice*. Andover: Cengage Learning.

Kerr, H., Donovan, M., and McSorley, O. (2021). Evaluation of the role of the clinical nurse specialist in cancer care: an integrative literature review. *European Journal of Cancer Care* 30 (3): 1–13.

Lamb, B.W., Brown, K.F., Nagpal, K. et al. (2011). Quality of care management decisions by multidisciplinary cancer teams: a systematic review. *Annals of Surgical Oncology* 18: 2116–2125.

Lamb, B.W., Taylor, C., Lamb, J.N. et al. (2013). Facilitators and barriers to teamworking and patient centeredness in multidisciplinary cancer teams: findings of a national study. *Annals of Surgical Oncology* 20: 1408–1416.

Lanceley, A., Savage, J., Menon, U., and Jacobs, I. (2008). Influences on multidisciplinary team decision-making. *International Journal of Gynecologic Cancer* 18: 215–222.

Lavender, V. (2017). Finding our voice in the MDT. *British Journal of Nursing* (Oncology Supplement) 26 (4): S3.

Macmillan Cancer Support. (2015). Cancer clinical nurse specialist. Macmillan Impact Briefs. https://www.macmillan.org.uk/documents/aboutus/research/impactbriefs/clinicalnursespecialists2015new.pdf (accessed 22 June 2022).

Martin, A.K., Green, T.L., McCarthy, A.L. et al. (2022). Healthcare teams: terminology, confusion, and ramifications. *Journal of Multidisciplinary Healthcare* 15: 765–772.

McGlynn, B., Johnston, M., and Green, J. (2017). A nurse-led multidisciplinary team approach in urology-oncology: addressing the new cancer strategy. *Journal of Clinical Urology* 10 (5): 449–456.

National Cancer Registration and Analysis Service. (2010). Multi-disciplinary teams. http://www.ncin.org.uk/cancer_type_and_topic_specific_work/multidisciplinary_teams/ (accessed 14 June 2022).

NHS England. (2018). Rapid cancer diagnostic and assessment pathways. https://www.england.nhs.uk/publication/rapid-cancer-diagnostic-and-assessment-pathways (accessed 31 August 2022).

NHS England and NHS Improvement (2019). The NHS patient safety strategy: safer culture, safer systems, safer patients. https://www.england.nhs.uk/wp-content/uploads/2020/08/190708_Patient_Safety_Strategy_for_website_v4.pdf (accessed 20 June 2022).

NHS Health Education England. (2021). Working differently together: progressing a one workforce approach. Multidisciplinary toolkit. https://www.hee.nhs.uk/sites/default/files/documents/HEE_MDT_Toolkit_V1.1.pdf (accessed 20 June 2022).

Patkar, V., Acosta, D., Davidson, T. et al. (2011). Cancer multidisciplinary team meetings: evidence, challenges, and the role of clinical decision support technology. *International Journal of Breast Cancer* 831605.

Punshon, G., Endacott, R., Aslett, P. et al. (2017). The experiences of specialist nurses working within the uro-oncology multi-disciplinary team in the United Kingdom. *Clinical Nurse Specialist* 31 (4): 210–218.

Rajasekaran, R.B., Whitwell, D., Cosker, T.D.A. et al. (2021). Will virtual multidisciplinary team meetings become the norm for musculoskeletal oncology care following the COVID-19 pandemic? – experience from a tertiary sarcoma Centre. *Biomedical Central (BMC) Musculoskeletal Disorders* 22 (18): 1–7.

Rosen, M.A., DiazGranados, D., Dietz, A.S. et al. (2018). Teamwork in healthcare: key discoveries enabling safer, high-quality care. *The American Psychologist* 73 (4): 433–450.

Rowlands, S. and Callen, J. (2013). A qualitative analysis of communication between members of a hospital-based multidisciplinary lung cancer team. *European Journal of Cancer Care* 22: 20–31.

Soukup, T., Petrides, K.V., Lamb, B.W. et al. (2016). The anatomy of clinical decision-making in multidisciplinary cancer meetings: a cross-sectional observational study of teams in a natural context. *Medicine* 95 (24): e3885.

Soukup, T., Lamb, B.W., Arora, S. et al. (2018). Successful strategies in implementing a multidisciplinary team working in the care of patients with cancer: an overview and synthesis of the available literature. *Journal of Multidisciplinary Healthcare* 19 (11): 49–61.

Taberna, M., Gil Moncayo, F., Jané-Salas, E. et al. (2020). The multidisciplinary team (MDT) approach and quality of care. *Frontiers in Oncology* 10 (85): 1–16.

Taylor, C., Munro, A.J., Glynne-Jones, R. et al. (2010). Multidisciplinary team working in cancer: what is the evidence? *British Medical Journal (Clinical Research Ed.)* 340: c951.

Taylor, C., Finnegan-John, J., and Green, J.S. (2014). 'No decision about me without me' in the context of cancer multidisciplinary team meetings: a qualitative interview study. *BMC Health Services Research* 14: 488.

Wallace, I., Barratt, H., Harvey, S., and Raine, R. (2019). The impact of clinical nurse specialists on the decision making process in cancer multidisciplinary team meetings: a qualitative study. *European Journal of Oncology Nursing* 43: 1–9.

Walraven, J., van der Hel, O.L., van der Hoeven, J. et al. (2022). Factors influencing the quality and functioning of oncological multidisciplinary team meetings: results of a systematic review. *Biomedical Central (BMC) Health Services Research* 22 (1): 1–27.

Willard, C. and Luker, K. (2007). Working with the team: strategies employed by hospital cancer nurse specialists to implement their role. *Journal of Clinical Nursing* 16 (4): 716–724.

Winters, D.A., Soukup, T., Sevdalis, N. et al. (2021). The cancer multidisciplinary team meeting: in need of change? History, challenges and future perspectives. *BJU International* 128 (3): 271–279.

10

Leadership and the Clinical Nurse Specialist

Ruth Thompson and Monica Donovan

Abstract

Leadership is essential at all levels of practice in healthcare, yet it is a difficult concept to define. There is a growing expectation for nurses to demonstrate leadership; however, to do so, clinical nurse specialists (CNS)s must recognise themselves as leaders and be able to articulate this aspect of their role. Understanding the difference between formal and informal leadership is the first step in recognising the leadership potential of the CNS. Few studies have focused on the leadership aspect of the CNS role, and as a result, there is little consensus on what it means and how it should be operationalised. Viewing CNS leadership through the lens of 'clinical' and 'professional' leadership enables the delineation of this important aspect of the CNS role.

10.1 Introduction

The role of the clinical nurse specialist (CNS) is multifaceted and encompasses several components. There is a consensus within the nursing professions that leadership is one component that defines the advanced practitioner's role; the others are consultant, clinician, educator and researcher (De Grasse and Nicklin 2001). Beauman (2006, p. 22) highlights an overlap in these sub-roles, stating, 'One cannot educate effectively without being a clinical expert, one cannot implement research without education, and one cannot consult without knowledge of research and clinical expertise', and argues that none of these roles can be performed effectively without leadership. This chapter presents definitions of leadership and provides an overview of the importance of self-recognition of leadership for the CNS. Leadership in the context of the CNS role is difficult to delineate; however, this will be discussed under two distinct

The Role of the Clinical Nurse Specialist in Cancer Care, First Edition. Edited by Helen Kerr.
© 2024 John Wiley & Sons Ltd. Published 2024 by John Wiley & Sons Ltd.
Companion website: www.wiley.com/go/kerr

headings – clinical leadership and professional leadership – in an attempt to enable CNSs to articulate their leadership role.

Ruth Thompson is one of the authors and her role has changed recently. Please change this in the introduction to 'Ruth Thompson is Associate Director of Nursing Policy and Practice at the Royal College of Nursing, and was previously the Interim Clinical Manager for Cancer Services in a Health and Social Care Trust in Northern Ireland. The second author, Monica Donovan, has worked as a cancer nurse for almost 20 years and has occupied formal leadership positions in cancer services. Monica is now a lecturer in adult nursing in the School of Nursing and Midwifery, Queen's University Belfast, and co-ordinates a leadership module for nurses and other healthcare professionals.

10.2   Leadership

Leadership is a highly desirable and highly valued commodity in all industries (Northouse 2019), yet it is one of the most difficult concepts to define due to its complex nature. Northouse (2019) also argues that attempting to define the concept of leadership is similar to trying to define concepts such as democracy, love and peace. Individuals intuitively know the meaning of such words; however, they can mean different things to different people. Many years ago, having completed a review of the leadership research literature, Stogdill (1974, p. 7) claimed there were as 'many definitions of leadership as those who have tried to define it'. Kouzes and Posner (2012) describe leadership as a set of skills and abilities that a person embodies; however, Daft (2015) believes leadership is more than a set of skills: it is a set of powerful personal qualities such as integrity, humility, courage and enthusiasm. Such definitions represent leadership as a generic concept; however, leadership is context-specific and needs to be understood in terms of its professional and organisational contexts (Turnbull-James 2011). In nursing, those in advanced nursing practice roles are increasingly identified as leaders who have progressed into areas of higher-level practice, improving care quality and outcomes (Leggat et al. 2015; Thompson et al. 2019; Evans et al. 2020).

10.3   Self-Recognition of the Clinical Nurse Specialist as a Leader

In the last decade, there has been a growing expectation that all nurses should be leaders (Nursing and Midwifery Council 2018). Anecdotal evidence suggests that CNSs do not always recognise themselves as leaders and often fail to appreciate the enhanced skill set developed in their careers before embarking on the CNS role. This view is perhaps predetermined by the lack of self-recognition of nurses as leaders in general. Historically, nurses have been taught to follow, not lead; and until recently, the concept of nursing leadership has largely been associated with nurse executives and formal leadership roles (AL-Dossary 2017). Research has predominantly focused on first-line managers/executives and has explored attributes, traits, competencies, roles and styles, and impact (Austin et al. 2003). AL-Dossary (2017) further highlight that nursing leadership has rarely been associated with bedside nursing practice.

Few studies have explored nurses' self-perceptions of leadership; however, one study by Booher et al. (2021) explored the perception of leadership with clinical nurses at the bedside in relation to patient care and outcomes. All participants in this study identified qualities they admired in leaders, such as integrity, compassion, good communication, vision, caring and self-awareness. The authors report that almost 50% did not initially view themselves as leaders until they realised that they often demonstrated those same leadership qualities in providing nursing care to patients and families. Booher et al. (2021) concluded that nurses assume a formal title is required to be a leader. This lack of self-recognition of leadership in nursing can help to explain why some nurses who progress to an advanced level do not consider themselves leaders.

It is essential that CNSs recognise themselves as leaders. Daft (2015, p. 6) believes that 'to see our own opportunities for leadership and recognize the leadership of people we interact with every day, we must stop equating leadership with greatness and public visibility'. Understanding the difference between formal and informal leadership roles is a first step in recognising the leadership potential of the CNS. Formal leaders such as managers and lead nurses gain authority by formal appointment. Northouse (2019) describes this as 'assigned leadership', where leadership is based on the position occupied in an organisation. Furthermore, leadership is often associated and confused with management, contributing to its vagueness. In contrast, registered nurses at the bedside attain authority informally from acceptance and support by followers who trust them, a phenomenon described as 'emergent leadership' (de Souza and Klein 1995) or 'informal leadership'. The emergent leader can be the most influential member of a group or an organisation, regardless of the individual's title.

CNSs have an informal leadership role that is no less important in achieving successful patient outcomes than those in formal leadership positions. The level of recognition as a leader may depend on the level of experience of those who occupy the CNS role. Nurses need to accept that leadership is a core activity of their role at all levels – once this is acknowledged, the transition to advanced roles will be easier (Wood 2021). Furthermore, they need to acknowledge their role as leaders to themselves, patients, other healthcare professionals and healthcare executives (Larsson and Sahlsten 2016).

10.4 Leadership in the Context of the Clinical Nurse Specialist

It is important to explore leadership in professional and organisational contexts, not just in terms of leader competencies, behaviours, attributes and values (Turnbull-James 2011). The advanced practitioner is considered a key leadership position of influence for innovation, improving clinical practice, healthcare delivery and advancing the nursing profession (Delamaire and Lafortune 2010). Advanced practice nurses (APNs) have completed graduate education, possess an expert level of knowledge and complex decision-making skills, have additional responsibility for practice innovation and strategic professional development and are considered to be particularly well suited for the leadership role (Finkelman 2013; Elliott et al. 2016; Lamb et al. 2018). Interestingly, however, in an integrative review by Kerr et al. (2021) to identify components of the CNS in cancer care, leadership did not emerge as a core component. There are many explanations for this finding by Kerr et al. (2021), one of which may be that leadership often threads through many care delivery processes and is not always apparent or tangible (Whitehead et al. 2017). As a result, the contribution that APNs make to the healthcare system is often misunderstood because what they do is considered clinical practice rather than leadership.

The leadership component of the APN role is challenging, to say the least. Few studies have focused on the leadership aspect of the APN role, and as a result, there is little consensus on what it means and how it should be operationalised. One exception is a large case study conducted across 13 sites in Ireland, involving 13 CNSs and advanced practitioners (clinical midwife specialists and APN's) (Begley et al. 2010). An important finding of this study was the identification of multiple activities that focused on two areas of leadership: clinical and professional. Further, Lamb et al. (2018) used a qualitative descriptive methodology informed by a well-established leadership framework to explore APNs' perceptions of their leadership. Two similar overarching themes were identified: 'patient-focused leadership' and 'organisation and system-focused leadership'. Patient-focused leadership, as described by APNs, includes capabilities intended to directly impact patients and families and can be aligned to 'clinical leadership'. 'Organisation and system-focused leadership' includes capabilities that are intended to directly impact nurses and other healthcare providers, the organisation or larger healthcare system and can be aligned to 'professional leadership'.

Viewing leadership through the lens of 'clinical' and 'professional' leadership is a good place to start to understand it in the context of the CNS role. By considering 'clinical' and 'professional' leadership, the CNS should be able to clearly articulate this important component of their role.

10.4.1 Clinical Leadership

Healthcare delivery is becoming more complex, with more demanding and high-acuity patients, shorter lengths of stay, staffing shortages and recovery from the challenges presented by the COVID-19 pandemic. Clinical leadership has been highlighted as a necessity for the provision of safe and efficient care in governmental reports (Francis 2013; Keogh 2013; Kirkup 2015) and the academic literature (Mianda and Voce 2018). Furthermore, it is linked to job satisfaction and retention of frontline healthcare providers (Edmonstone 2009; Casey et al. 2011; Daly et al. 2014). The need to foster clinical leadership development has been embedded into health policy in the United Kingdom (UK) (NHS England 2019) and other jurisdictions (Fealy et al. 2015; Pizzirani et al. 2019), where the need for training and development in clinical leadership for the health workforce has been emphasised to produce effective improvements in care quality and outcomes (Dunigan et al. 2020). Therefore, clinical leadership is required at all levels, not least in advanced nursing practice.

Organisational power or a leadership title is not required to identify as a clinical leader (Boamah 2019) because clinical leadership focuses on patients and healthcare teams rather than formal leadership positions (AL-Dossary 2017). While there is consensus as to the importance of clinical leadership as a way of ensuring optimal care and overcoming issues in the healthcare environment, as with 'leadership', there is less agreement on a clear definition of the concept (Davidson et al. 2006; Howieson and Thaigarajah 2011). Clinical leadership is described as clinical healthcare staff undertaking the roles of leadership: using their clinical skills to ensure that the needs of the patient are the central focus of the organisation's aims and objectives (Jonas et al. 2011). Clinical leaders are experts in their field, effective communicators and clinically knowledgeable; they demonstrate competence and provide guidance and support to patients and their families (Lett 2002). These characteristics are inherent to CNS practice. Studies have identified common characteristics of clinical leadership in advanced nursing practice, which include clinical embeddedness, expertise, critical thinking, decision-making, visibility within care environments, role modelling, facilitation of care, working within and across professional boundaries and concern with improving care quality (Santiano et al. 2009; Elliott et al. 2013; Walsh et al. 2015; Giles et al. 2018). Most importantly, in nursing, clinical leadership involves influencing and co-ordinating patient care processes with the healthcare team for the purpose of achieving positive patient outcomes (Boamah 2019).

There are many components to the clinical leadership enacted by the CNS, but exploring them all individually would be beyond the scope of this chapter. Two core components of the CNS clinical leadership role are clinical expert and coordination of care and will be considered together.

10.4.1.1 Clinical Expertise and Coordination of Care

Clinical expertise is considered an essential component of clinical leadership (Mannix et al. 2013). Interest in clinical nursing expertise grew following the seminal work of Benner (1983). Benner described expert nurses as those who can make judgements by fluidly connecting prior knowledge and skills to new situations and being able to seamlessly draw on practical and theoretical knowledge of the clinical issues before them. The clinical nurse expert is also described as someone who demonstrates superior performance in their everyday work life. In fact, it is difficult to separate the concept of clinical expertise from clinical leadership because the clinical expert in their field of practice is one who is approachable, a role model and an effective communicator and can motivate others by matching their values and beliefs about nursing care to their practice (Stanley 2006). It is argued that clinical expertise and clinical leadership are inextricably linked.

The effect of a cancer diagnosis and living with and beyond cancer can be so profound for individuals and their families that it can threaten their physical, emotional, psychological, spiritual and social wellbeing (Charalambous 2019). Patients living with and beyond cancer rely on the cancer CNS to advocate for them, communicate effectively, enable shared decision-making, provide symptom management and provide knowledge and education about treatments and their side effects (Krishnasamy et al. 2021). Other healthcare professionals within the multidisciplinary team (MDT) also rely on the CNS for mentoring, teaching, guidance and communication (Begley et al. 2012). It is exactly this clinical expertise that makes the CNS an effective leader (Beauman 2006), because they have the knowledge and skills to meet the unique care needs of the individual with cancer and enhance the cancer workforce to improve overall care.

Expertise is an integral part of leadership in that leaders are challenged to master situations in an ever-changing environment. Over the past decade, cancer CNSs have witnessed new paradigms in the treatment of cancer, including anticancer agents and technologies. These have brought unanticipated and unfamiliar biopsychosocial consequences, a change in patient demographics and an increasing cohort of those diagnosed with cancer presenting with multiple co-morbidities. Most recently, the challenges presented by the COVID-19 pandemic have led to significant changes in service delivery. As a result, the CNS has had to quickly develop new knowledge and skills and adapt to new and unfamiliar situations, which closely align to Benner's definition of an expert nurse as someone who has an intuitive grasp of each situation, operates from a deep understanding of the total situation and demonstrates high proficiency through flexibly and fluidly applying their knowledge (Benner 1983). Therefore, clinical expertise is not an end product but a constantly evolving aspect of the CNS's leadership role.

The clinical expertise of the CNS also places them in a perfect position to co-ordinate the care of the person living with and beyond cancer. The care of many individuals with cancer involves multimodal cancer therapies, treatment of co-morbidities, multiple healthcare providers and often various sites of care delivery; therefore, the coordination of cancer care is essential to high-quality healthcare. Healthcare delivered by nurses in advanced roles, such as CNSs, has positively impacted cancer care coordination (Gorin et al. 2017). Coordination of cancer care depends on effective information exchange and regular communication between patients and physicians, family members, support staff and services and even community organisations (McDonald et al. 2010). As previously mentioned, research into the clinical aspect of CNSs working in advanced practice roles is limited; however, a few studies have highlighted the value of APN roles in collaboration with the MDT in improving patient outcomes such as patient satisfaction, reduced waiting times and the development of services in response to patient needs (Santiano et al. 2009; Begley et al. 2010; Elliott et al. 2013; Higgins et al. 2014; Coyne et al. 2016).

10.4.2 Professional Leadership

Ackerman et al. (1996) identified professional leadership in their proposed framework for advanced practice and reported that this type of leadership operates at a higher level than clinical leadership and is more externally focused, crossing boundaries of the local service into the national and international arena. They also argue that this type of leadership enabled clinicians to influence others with higher seniority, help shape and influence healthcare and healthcare reform and contribute to the advancement of nursing practice and knowledge (De Grasse and Nicklin 2001).

The National Cancer Action Team (2010) recognise that CNSs have influence and credibility across the care pathway. They increasingly take on a leadership role in refining systems and smoothing care pathways, making a demonstrable contribution to the effectiveness of patient experience and safety. This demonstrates the professional leadership aspect of the CNS role. As previously discussed, Lamb et al. (2018) describe this as organisation- and system-focused leadership. This role requires CNSs to develop services at a strategic level and act as change agents and innovators (Elliott et al. 2016). In doing so, CNSs can impact outcomes not only for service users and other healthcare professionals but also for healthcare services (Begley et al. 2010).

As senior nurses, CNSs adeptly respond to complex clinical challenges, which can provide insight when dealing with a range of difficult situations. Within this realm of leadership, the CNS requires extensive knowledge of service provision and skills to collaborate with other stakeholders and influence practice. The professional leadership skills required include negotiation, facilitation, partnership working, leading by example and quality improvement methodology.

Again, there are numerous facets to this type of leadership, but for the purposes of this chapter, three components of professional leadership will be examined:

enhancing practice, service improvement and innovation, and collaborative working. They are inextricably linked to the components of clinical leadership already discussed, as one can influence another.

10.4.2.1 Enhancing Practice

As professional leaders, CNSs act as role models. As such, they hold high standards, support colleagues and are acutely aware of their scope of practice (Royal College of Nursing 2021). In leading by example, CNSs should display values and behaviours that exemplify high-quality nursing practice and professionalism. This element of leadership focuses on influence rather than position or power. Due to their high level of expertise, CNSs build trust and respect from colleagues, and as a result of their credibility, they are usually held in high esteem by peers (Elliott et al. 2013). Effectiveness as a role model can also help encourage and motivate others to promote excellence in practice and create a culture of holistic and ethical standards within organisations (Heinen et al. 2019). In 2015, Macmillan Cancer Support developed a standardised role description for band 7 cancer CNSs across the United Kingdom (UK). The first core responsibility within this document is the need to act as a role model to demonstrate these high standards and provide leadership to others. CNSs can exhibit excellence in practice to colleagues in a number of ways but more commonly encourage others through mentorship and coaching (Lamb et al. 2018).

Begley et al. (2010) reported in their study that there was evidence that practitioners in specialist roles showed leadership through being role models for enhancing practice by creating a positive milieu towards ongoing development: keeping up-to-date with new practice development and research evidence, attending courses and conferences, and networking with other professional colleagues within and outside their own services. In doing so, they integrate their role firmly within the healthcare system.

CNSs also guide, initiate and provide leadership in policy-related activities to influence practice, health services and public policy (Heinen et al. 2019; Wood 2021). In addition, Elliott et al. (2013) noted their role in leading audits; and along with data collection and collation, they are often involved in monitoring organisational performance standards, thus providing information to inform practice development.

10.4.2.2 Service Improvement and Innovation

The demands of clinical practice can often limit time for other activities; however, the CNS is uniquely positioned to recognise where change could be instigated to improve practice. Macmillan Cancer Support (2015) identified that the CNS can use insight from patient experience to lead service redesign and implement improvements to ensure that services are responsive to patient needs. Their role enables them to identify gaps in services, but as leaders, these issues can become opportunities to find solutions to facilitate improvements in quality of care provision.

As advanced practitioners, CNSs have extensive knowledge of operational systems within the organisation in which they work (Heinen et al. 2019). Such insights can enable a whole-system, strategic approach and understanding, and help shape the culture of the organisation.

An economic modelling analysis by Macmillan Cancer Support (2010), focusing on the role of the CNS, suggested that service improvements along the cancer pathway could release about 10% of cancer expenditure in the Manchester area, UK. This work was focused on individuals with breast and lung cancer, but it was believed that if extrapolated to a national level, the economic benefits would be significant. Service improvement can in turn lead to increased productivity and efficiency.

10.4.2.3 Collaborative Working

CNSs are often part of a number of teams and liaise with colleagues from numerous departments and across various sectors. Therefore, their coordination of care impacts not only patients but also teams and service as a whole. This provides the opportunity to share expertise and influence others. Heinen et al. (2019) described how CNSs employ consultative and leadership skills with intra-professional and inter-professional teams to create change in healthcare and within complex healthcare delivery systems. The Royal College of Nursing (2010) reported that cancer CNSs have clearly demonstrated their commitment to work collaboratively with their colleagues to ensure that patients have access to best practice, equity of care and continuity of care throughout their cancer journey. This links directly to coordination of care, discussed previously under clinical leadership.

Although CNSs aim to improve services for patients, they also work in partnership with patients and service users to gain feedback on their experience, thus using this insight to drive innovation and change (Macmillan Cancer Support 2020). CNSs also often hold office within a range of local and national committees and represent the nursing profession (Macmillan Cancer Support 2020) by using their skills, knowledge and expertise.

10.5 Conclusion

This chapter focused on the leadership aspect of the CNS role. The importance of CNSs' self-recognition of their leadership capacity and potential has been highlighted, with an emphasis on the informal leader. The chapter has viewed leadership in the context of the CNS through the lens of clinical and professional leadership. It has provided an overview of theories and styles that underpin leadership practice and will enable CNSs to further explore and develop their leadership style and behaviours.

References

Ackerman, M.H., Norsen, L., Martin, B. et al. (1996). Development of a model of advanced practice. *American Journal of Critical Care* 5 (1): 68–73.

AL-Dossary, R.N. (2017). Leadership in nursing. In: *Contemporary Leadership Challenges* (ed. A. Alvinius). London: IntechOpen https://doi.org/10.5772/65308.

Austin, S., Brewer, M., Donnelly, G. et al. (2003). Five keys to successful nursing management. In: *Why Leadership Is Important to Nursing* (ed. G.F. Donnelly), 57–80. Springhouse, PA: Lippincott Williams and Wilkins.

Beauman, S.S. (2006). Leadership and the clinical nurse specialist: from traditional to contemporary. *New-Born and Infant Reviews* 6 (1): 22–24.

Begley, C., Murphy, K., Higgins, A. et al. (2010). *An Evaluation of Clinical Nurse and Midwife Specialist and Advanced Nurse and Midwife Practitioner Roles in Ireland (SCAPE)*. Dublin: National Council for the Professional Development of Nursing and Midwifery in Ireland.

Begley, C., Elliott, N., Lalor, J. et al. (2012). Differences between clinical specialist and advanced practitioner clinical practice, leadership, and research roles, responsibilities, and perceived outcomes (the SCAPE study). *Journal of Advanced Nursing* 69 (6): 1323–1337.

Benner, P. (1983). Uncovering the knowledge embedded in clinical practice. *Journal of Nursing Scholarship* 15 (2): 36–41.

Boamah, S.A. (2019). Emergence of informal clinical leadership as a catalyst for improving patient care quality and job satisfaction. *Journal of Advanced Nursing* 75 (5): 1000–1009.

Booher, L., Yates, E., Claus, S. et al. (2021). Leadership self-perception of clinical nurses at the bedside: a qualitative descriptive study. *Journal of Clinical Nursing* 30 (11–12): 1573–1583.

Casey, M., McNamara, M., Fealy, G., and Geraghhty, R. (2011). 'Nurses' and midwives clinical leadership development needs: a mixed methods study. *Journal of Advanced Nursing* 67: 1502–1513.

Charalambous, A. (2019). Individualised nursing care in cancer care. In: *Individualized Care* (ed. R. Suhonen, M. Stolt, and E. Papastavrou), 131–139. Cham: Springer.

Coyne, I., Comiskey, C.M., Lalor, J.G. et al. (2016). An exploration of clinical practice in sites with and without clinical nurse or midwife specialists or advanced nurse practitioners, in Ireland. *BMC Health Service Research* 16 (151): 1412–1418.

Daft, R.L. (2015). *Management*, vol. 12. Mason, Ohio South-Western: Cengage Learning.

Daly, J., Jackson, D., Mannix, J. et al. (2014). The importance of clinical leadership in the hospital setting. *Journal of Healthcare Leadership Health* 6: 75–83.

Davidson, P., Elliott, D., and Daly, J. (2006). Clinical leadership in contemporary clinical practice: implications for nursing in Australia. *Journal of Nursing Management* 14 (3): 180–187.

De Grasse, C. and Nicklin, W. (2001). Advanced nursing practice: old hat, new design. *Canadian Journal of Nursing Leadership* 14 (4): 7–12.

Delamaire, M. and Lafortune, G. (2010). Nurses in advanced roles: a description and evaluation of experiences in 12 developed countries. Organisation for Economic Co-operation and Development (OECD) working paper 54.

Dunigan, M., Drennan, J., and McCarthy, J.C. (2020). Impact of clinical leadership in advanced practice roles on outcomes in healthcare: a scoping review. *Journal of Nursing Management* 29 (4): 613–622.

Edmonstone, J. (2009). Evaluating clinical leadership: a case study. *Leadership Health Service* 22: 210–224.

Elliott, N., Higgins, A., Begley, C. et al. (2013). The identification of clinical and professional leadership activities of advanced practitioners: findings from the specialist clinical and advanced practitioner evaluation study in Ireland. *Journal of Advanced Nursing* 69 (5): 1037–1050.

Elliott, N., Begley, C., Sheaf, G., and Higgins, A. (2016). Barriers and enablers to advanced practitioners' ability to enact their leadership role: a scoping review. *International Journal of Nursing Studies* 60: 24–45.

Evans, C., Poku, B., Pearce, R. et al. (2020). Characterising the evidence base for advanced clinical practice in the UK: a scoping review protocol. *British Medical Journal Open* 10 (5): e036192.

Fealy, G.M., McNamara, M.S., Casey, M. et al. (2015). Service impact of a national clinical leadership development programme: findings from a qualitative study. *Journal of Nursing Management* 23 (3): 324–332.

Finkelman, A. (2013). The clinical nurse specialist: leadership in quality improvement. *Clinical Nurse Specialist* 27 (1): 31–35.

Francis, R. (2013). *Report of the Mid Staffordshire NHS Foundation Trust Public Inquiry*. London: The Stationery Office. https://assets.publishing.service.gov.uk/government/uploads/system/uploads/attachment_data/file/279118/0898_ii.pdf (accessed 20 June 2022).

Giles, M., Parker, V., Conway, J., and Mitchell, R. (2018). Knowing how to get things done. Nurse consultants as clinical leaders. *Journal of Clinical Nursing* 27 (9–10): 1981–1993.

Gorin, S.S., Haggstrom, D., Han, P.K. et al. (2017). Cancer care coordination: a systematic review and meta-analysis of over 30 years of empirical studies. *Annals of Behavioral Medicine* 51 (4): 532–546.

Heinen, M., van Oostveen, C., Peters, J. et al. (2019). An integrative review of leadership competencies and attributes in advanced nursing practice. *Journal of Advanced Nursing* 75 (11): 2378–2393.

Higgins, A., Begley, C., Lalor, J. et al. (2014). Factors influencing advanced practitioners' ability to enact leadership: a case study within Irish healthcare. *Journal of Nursing Management* 22 (7): 894–905.

Howieson, B. and Thaigarajah, T. (2011). What is clinical leadership? A journal-based meta-review. *International Journal of Clinical Leadership* 17: 7–18.

Jonas, S., McCay, L., and Keogh, B. (2011). The importance of clinical leadership. In: *The ABC of Clinical Leadership* (ed. T. Swanick and J. McKimm). Wiley-Blackwell, BMJ Books.

Keogh, B. (2013). Review into the quality of care and treatment provided by 14 hospital trusts in England: Overview report. Department of Health. https://www. nhs.uk/nhsengland/bruce-keogh-review/documents/outcomes/keogh-review-final-report.pdf (accessed 23 June 2022).

Kerr, H., Donovan, M., and McSorley, O. (2021). Evaluation of the role of the clinical nurse specialist in cancer care: an integrative literature review. *European Journal of Cancer Care* 30 (3): 1–13.

Kirkup, B. (2015). *The Report of the Morecambe Bay Investigation*. London: The Stationery Office. https://www.gov.uk/government/publications (accessed 28 June 2022).

Kouzes, J.M. and Posner, B.Z. (2012). *Leadership the Challenge: How to Make Extraordinary Things Happen in Organizations*, 5e. San Francisco: Jossey-Bass.

Krishnasamy, M., Webb, U.M., Babos, S.L. et al. (2021). Defining expertise in cancer nursing practice. *Cancer Nursing* 44 (4): 314–322.

Lamb, A., Martin-Misener, R., Bryant-Lukosius, D., and Latimer, M. (2018). Describing the leadership capabilities of advanced practice nurses using a qualitative descriptive study. *Nursing Open* 5: 400–413.

Larsson, I.E. and Sahlsten, M.J.M. (2016). The staff nurse clinical leader at the bedside: Swedish registered nurses' perceptions. *Nursing Research and Practice.*

Leggat, S.G., Balding, C., and Schiftan, D. (2015). Developing clinical leaders: the impact of an action learning mentoring programme for advanced practice nurses. *Journal of Clinical Nursing* 24 (11–12): 1576–1584.

Lett, M. (2002). The concept of clinical leadership. *Contemporary Nurse* 12 (1): 16–21.

Macmillan Cancer Support. (2010). Demonstrating the economic value of co-ordinated cancer services; an examination of resource utilisation in Manchester. www.macmillan.org.uk/documents/aboutus/commissioners/ monitorresearchinmanchesterbriefing.pdf (accessed 24 August 2022).

Macmillan Cancer Support. (2015). Cancer Clinical Nurse Specialists. www. macmillan.org.uk/Documents/AboutUs/Research/Impactbriefs/ImpactBriefs-ClinicalNurseSpecialists2014 (accessed 22 July 2022).

Macmillan Cancer Support. (2020). Macmillan competency framework for nurses. https://www.macmillan.org.uk/healthcare-professionals/news-and-resources/ guides/competency-framework-for-nurses (accessed 22 July 2022).

Mannix, J., Wilkes, L., and Jackson, D. (2013). Marking out the clinical expert/clinical leader/clinical scholar: perspectives from nurses in the clinical arena. *BMC Nursing* 12 (12): 1–8.

McDonald, K., Schultz, E., and Albin, L. (2010). *Care Coordination Atlas Version 3.* Rockville, MD: Agency for Healthcare Research and Quality.

Mianda, S. and Voce, A. (2018). Developing and evaluating clinical leadership interventions for frontline healthcare providers: a review of the literature. *BMC Health Services Research* 18 (1): 747.

National Cancer Action Team (2010). *Excellence in Cancer Care: the contribution of the Clinical Nurse Specialist.* NCAT.

NHS England 2019: kingsfund.org.uk/projects/positions/NHS-*leadership*-culture (accessed 06 June 2022)

Northouse, P.G. (2019). *Leadership: Theory and Practice*, 8e. SAGE.

Nursing and Midwifery Council. (2018). The code. Professional standards of practice and behaviour for nurses, midwives and nursing associates. https://www.nmc.org.uk/globalassets/sitedocuments/nmc-publications/revised-new-nmc-code.pdf (accessed 03 November 2022).

Pizzirani, B., O'Donnell, R., Skouteris, H. et al. (2019). Clinical leadership development in Australian healthcare: a systematic review. *Internal Medicine Journal* 50 (12): 1451–1456.

Royal College of Nursing (2010). Specialist nurses: changing lives, saving money.

Royal College of Nursing (2021) Five ways to embrace your inner leader. https://www.rcn.org.uk/magazines/Bulletin/2021/Feb/Five-ways-to-embrace-your-inner-leader (accessed 03 November 2022).

Santiano, N., Young, L., Baramy, L.-S. et al. (2009). How do CNCs construct their after hours support role in a major metropolitan hospital. *Collegian Royal College of Nursing, Australia* 16 (2): 85–97.

de Souza, G. and Klein, H.J. (1995). Emergent leadership in the group goal-setting process. *Small Group Research* 26 (4): 475–496.

Stanley, D. (2006). Recognizing and defining clinical nurse leaders. *British Journal of Nursing* 15: 108–111.

Stogdill, R.M. (1974). *Handbook of Leadership. A Survey of Theory and Research.* New York: The Free Press.

Thompson, J., McNall, A., Tiplady, S. et al. (2019). Whole systems approach: advanced clinical practitioner development and identity in primary care. *Journal of Health Organization and Management* 33 (4): 443–459.

Turnbull-James, K. (2011). *Leadership in Context: Lessons from New Leadership Theory and Current Leadership Development Practice.* London: The King's Fund https://www.kingsfund.org.uk (accessed 23 May 2022).

Walsh, K., Bothe, J., Edgar, D. et al. (2015). Investigating the role of clinical nurse consultants in one health district from multiple stakeholder perspectives: a cooperative inquiry. *Contemporary Nurse* 51 (2–3): 171–187.

Whitehead, D., Welch, D.P., and McNulty, D. (2017). *Leadership and the Advanced Practice Nurse, the Future of a Changing Healthcare Environment.* Philadelphia, PA: F.A. Davis Company.

Wood, C. (2021). Leadership and management for nurses working at an advanced level. *British Journal of Nursing* 30 (5): 282–286.

11

Nurse-Led Clinics

Shelley Mooney and Helen Kerr

Abstract

Nurse-led clinics play a significant role in cancer follow-up reviews and consultations, and support the delivery of effective cancer services. The clinical nurse specialist is one of the advanced practice nurse roles that pioneered the development of nurse-led clinics. Nurse-led clinics have reported positive outcomes for patients, the healthcare professional undertaking the clinic and the healthcare organisation.

11.1   Introduction

This chapter will focus on the emergence and evolvement of nurse-led clinics in cancer services. The background to the introduction of nurse-led clinics within healthcare will be outlined, followed by the pragmatic matters to be considered when introducing a nurse-led clinic in any service area. There will be a focus on the advanced nursing skills required to successfully implement nurse-led clinics and the range of approaches used. Various benefits of nurse-led clinics for patients, the healthcare professional and the healthcare organisation will be outlined, in addition to potential barriers and suggestions to address them. The importance of service evaluation and the future of nurse-led clinics will also be explored. The chapter will conclude with recommendations on how nurse-led clinics can be embedded into routine practice.

The first author, Shelley Mooney, works as a band 7 uro-oncology clinical nurse specialist (CNS) in the Northern Ireland (NI) Cancer Centre, Belfast, providing direct patient care to individuals with a diagnosis of prostate or bladder cancer, which includes being responsible for nurse-led clinics. This author commenced this post in 2017, having previously worked in an inpatient oncology ward for five years as a band 5 registered nurse. The second author, Helen Kerr, is a senior lecturer at the School of Nursing and Midwifery, Queen's University Belfast, with a clinical background in cancer and palliative care nursing.

11.2 Nurse-Led Care and the Launch of Nurse-Led Clinics in Healthcare

The evolvement of the broad term *nurse-led care* has been in response to the high demand for long-term holistic support and ongoing follow-up (Vinall-Collier et al. 2016). Two decades ago, Corner (2003) suggested that nurse-led care involved nurses being delegated to accomplish specific tasks previously undertaken by medical staff. This view may be considered contentious, as Hamric and Tracy (2019) state that advanced nursing roles and responsibilities are not a substitution for medical practice. Lai et al. (2017) suggest there is no clear and consistent definition of the broad terminology of nurse-led care but suggest that nurse-led care involves clinics led by registered nurses who are able to work autonomously delivering person-centred care within their area of practice and make evidence-based clinical decisions independently. Nurse-led care is often provided by an advanced nurse practitioner (NP) in their speciality and uses a holistic approach to patient care that takes account of the individual's physical, psychological, social and spiritual needs (Ndosi et al. 2014).

One component of nurse-led care is the establishment and maintenance of nurse-led clinics. Due to the diversity of nurse-led clinics, they are difficult to define; however, Wong and Chung (2006) state that a nurse-led clinic is a formalised and structured healthcare delivery mode that encompasses a nurse and a client, in which a client as an individual alongside their family has healthcare needs that can be addressed by a nurse. Nurse-led clinics first emerged in the United States of America (USA) in the 1990s and the United Kingdom (UK) in the early 2000s (McLachlan et al. 2019) in a range of chronic conditions such as cardiology and diabetes. According to Wiles et al. (2001), nurse-led clinics were introduced in the UK to provide intermediate care to patients discharged from hospital but still needing support to regain their maximum health. Nurse-led clinics can also support intermediate care after the acute phase of a disease (Wong and Chung 2006). As a result of their introduction, nurse-led clinics freed up inpatient hospital beds for those requiring acute medical attention and enabled patients to receive ongoing care in an outpatient or community setting.

Nurse-led clinics are now a crucial component of healthcare provision, as they offer an alternative to traditional physician-led models of care and provide safe, high-quality care (Connolly and Cotter 2021). Nurse-led clinics are often the responsibility of an advanced practice nurse, such as an NP or a CNS. The development of advanced practice nurses was an important milestone in the professional development of the nursing discipline throughout the twentieth century and has become a global trend in the twenty-first century. Nurse-led clinics serviced by advanced practice nurses have become common international practice since the 1990s (Shiu et al. 2011). According to Randall et al. (2017), nurse-led clinics are now established worldwide in various clinical settings and are reported as an effective method of patient assessment and care.

11.3 Components of a Nurse-Led Clinic

Hatchett (2016) outlines that nurse-led clinics involve nurses having their own patient workload, which requires increased autonomy and often using advanced clinical skills such as physical assessment, diagnosis and medication management. For a registered nurse to lead their own clinic, they must demonstrate advanced competence to practice in a specific healthcare area and practice either independently and/or interdependently with other members of a healthcare team in at least 80% of their work (Wong and Chung 2006). Nurse-led clinics are reported to be commonly focused on treating and managing chronic conditions (Randall et al. 2017). According to the International Council of Nursing (ICN) (2021), key to nurse-led clinics is the central role of the CNS, who has an understanding of the patient and their condition and can develop a trusting relationship with the patient. To effectively lead a clinic, the majority of the caseload should be protocolised, which empowers the nurse to lead the clinic without the need for support from other healthcare professionals; however, there will be situations where unique patient cases present, requiring support from other healthcare professionals and leading to opportunities for further learning and development.

In the context of cancer care, the National Cancer Plan in the UK (Department of Health 2000) stated that cancer services needed to be re-designed to make the best use of skills within the cancer workforce and ensure that patients and their families had appropriate and timely access to supportive aftercare. Thus, support and follow-up after treatment were important in the development of cancer services, and as a result, numerous nurse-led activities emerged, such as nurse-led clinics (Cox and Wilson 2003). Furthermore, an ambitious strategy launched by the Independent Cancer Taskforce (2015) aimed to transform cancer care between 2015 and 2020 through alternative models of patient care after cancer treatment, such as follow-up carried out by a specialist nurse. Nurse-led follow-up was identified as a suitable means of follow-up in cancer care, and its acceptability has been widely demonstrated in lung, breast, prostate and bladder cancer (Smits et al. 2015) and continues to be developed in other tumour sites. Nurse-led clinics are now embedded into routine clinical practice in cancer care for a range of tumour sites.

Nurse-led clinics differ in purpose and functionality. Whilst some nurse-led clinics are focused on patient assessment and management, others focus on the CNS being in a more supportive role. Nurse-led clinics may include health assessments to manage a patient's health condition and symptoms, health education to facilitate compliance and a healthy lifestyle, and co-ordination of care using a holistic approach (Wong and Chung 2006). Within cancer care, a diverse range of nurse-led clinics may be available throughout the patient pathway, and often the disease site dictates what type of nurse-led clinic is suitable for which patient group. Depending on the tumour site, a nurse-led clinic may be available when the individual receives a diagnosis; for other tumour sites, the nurse-led clinic may be available at treatment review, during radiotherapy or systemic anti-cancer therapy (SACT), post-treatment follow-up, or for a holistic needs assessment (HNA) to be completed. According to Campbell et al. (2000), whilst the primary aim of a nurse-led radiotherapy review clinic was to monitor radiation reactions and tolerance to treatment and manage radiotherapy-related toxicities, it also provided the nurse with an opportunity to assess the patient for physical, psychological and social problems, contributing to a holistic approach to care.

The Macmillan Cancer Support Recovery Package and National Health Service (NHS) England highlight the potential benefits of risk-stratifying follow-up of individuals with cancer (Macmillan Cancer Support 2015; NHS England 2016). In terms of post-treatment follow-up, certain disease sites, such as prostate and breast cancer, have large cohorts of patients who require long-term follow-up over many years (National Institute of Clinical Excellence 2021). In response to UK national guidelines, many nurses now provide this routine follow-up to bridge gaps where medical follow-up may be ceasing due to high clinical demands for increasing new patient diagnoses and the development of new treatment modalities (Sheppard 2007).

11.4 Introducing a Nurse-Led Clinic

Introducing a nurse-led clinic requires meticulous planning and takes time to 'pull together' (Jones et al. 2016). Hatchett (2008) identifies a 10-step process when establishing a new service. In summary, these 10 key steps include building a business case, defining aims and objectives, establishing patient criteria, planning publicity, determining the clinic location, gaining support from colleagues, planning professional development, considering medicine management if appropriate, planning audit and evaluation and, finally, facilitating ongoing improvement. Following these 10 steps enhances a nurse's ability to introduce and effectively establish a nurse-led clinic.

Prior to embarking on any new developments within healthcare, Judd (2009) outlines the importance of establishing whether there is a service need, which involves pre-determining which patient groups are appropriate. This can be facilitated with discussions with relevant clinical team members to identify current gaps in practice to determine whether a nurse-led clinic would be a suitable solution to address the service need. In terms of appropriate patient groups, patients with straightforward protocolised follow-up are often deemed suitable to attend a nurse-led clinic. These clinics have strict inclusion and exclusion criteria; therefore, only patients who meet these criteria should be referred.

Furthermore, clear communication with all multidisciplinary team members is crucial in the initial planning stage, and those influenced by the service change should be included in these discussions in addition to the planning processes. This should include management, relevant healthcare professionals and administrative teams. Setting up a nurse-led clinic in any speciality may pose challenges due to a potential change in practice. Hatchett (2005) states that ensuring all staff influenced by the change are kept informed and that their opinions are valued, should lead to a smoother transition to change when introducing a new clinic. A team approach is also required, which includes all stakeholders, such as administrative staff and both medical and nursing healthcare professionals. A team approach will facilitate administrative staff and healthcare professionals to provide their valuable input, contributing to the smooth introduction of a nurse-led clinic (Hatchett 2005).

A hierarchy of support is crucial, including the logistics and costs associated with introducing a nurse-led clinic. Indirect costs may include room allocation, information technology support and clinical supervision for nursing staff provided by medical staff such as oncologists. In addition to these indirect costs, direct costs include CNS staffing for the nurse-led clinic. A nurse-led clinic is often embedded into the CNS's current job plan; therefore, finances to support this component of the role are allocated from this budget with no additional cost (Moore 2018).

When logistics such as room allocation have been considered and a hierarchy of support is secured, Judd (2009) suggests the need for a robust protocol to support advanced nursing practice independently. Initial standard operating procedures and protocols must be developed alongside an assessment record. An assessment record acts as a template to guide the nurse when assessing patients to ensure that all required information is included to reduce the risk of omitting vital data. These documents should be developed within the team with refinements provided by oncologists and agreement with written information approval groups (or equivalent) and document control (Jones et al. 2016).

Robust protocols are essential to deliver independent nurse-led clinics. Protocols must cover expected patient presentations and potential non-expected presentations associated with the condition that may arise, alongside an action plan. The importance of these protocols is to assist and direct nurses in their clinical decision-making. Protocols must be agreed upon by the referring clinicians and validated by the hospital's Clinical Governance Committee (or equivalent). However, Judd (2009) advises that nurses must be cautious not to 'fit the patient to the protocol', so the nurse in charge of the clinic must draw on their knowledge and expertise when presented with new situations and acknowledge and work within their limitations. Furthermore, Gousy and Green (2015) highlight that a person-centred approach is a vital component of nurse-led clinics to ensure that the clinic is designed to meet the needs of the person and not limited to the clinical diagnosis.

Nursing documentation is essential in the nurse-led clinic, as it provides evidence regarding the patient's progress and/or any complications that require further interventions (Leahy et al. 2013). Individualised assessment records specific to each cancer site may be developed and used for nurse-led clinics to record symptoms reviewed, blood test results and any follow-up plans (Robertson et al. 2013). In 2016, a Regional Information System for Oncology and Haematology (RISOH) (Northern Ireland Cancer Network 2022) was introduced in NI: it is an online system for documenting patient information. Within RISOH, healthcare professionals can type freehand or complete a template questionnaire about their contact with patients. The online information is available for all healthcare professionals within oncology and haematology. This up-to-date, real-time, accurate documentation enhances patient safety and promotes clear communication between teams. In addition, template questionnaires are an excellent resource for recently appointed CNSs responsible for nurse-led follow-up clinics, as they ensure that all relevant patient information is available.

11.5 Nursing Skills Required to Introduce and Establish a Nurse-Led Clinic

All registered nurses must demonstrate competencies in a range of skills, such as communication and clinical skills. Nurses who work in advanced practice roles must also demonstrate expertise in the four pillars of advanced practice (Lee et al. 2020): clinical, research, education and management/leadership. Furthermore, Wong and Chung (2006) highlight that CNSs must possess credibility in a relevant speciality area; be capable of contributing to enhancing the quality of service; be competent in project management, research, leadership and people skills; and possess the personal qualities of creativity, flexibility, confidence, assertiveness and perceptiveness.

Prior to embarking on setting up a nurse-led clinic, it is crucial that the CNS is competent in the required clinical skills specific to the proposed clinic, such as abdominal examinations, digital rectal examination, etc. This will require an assessment of the skills required to facilitate the specific nurse-led clinic, and attendance at additional training and educational sessions is likely to be required. The availability of clinical supervision will support the determination of the skills required and a pathway to becoming competent.

Research and education are two additional essential skills, and according to Kerr et al. (2021), it is imperative that CNSs in cancer care are involved in the design, implementation and evaluation of research in order to embed research and evidence-based care into clinical practice. (Evidence-based practice is the focus of Chapter 7 of this book.) Leadership skills are paramount for delivering excellent patient care, collaborating with other healthcare professionals, implementing innovations in clinical practice and enhancing evidence-based practice (Heinen et al. 2019). By developing these advanced practice skills, CNSs are better equipped with the knowledge and expertise required to successfully introduce and establish a nurse-led clinic in their area of clinical practice. (Leadership in the CNS role is the focus of Chapter 10 of this book.)

11.6   Approaches to Delivering a Nurse-Led Clinic

Prior to the COVID-19 pandemic, which commenced in 2019, nurse-led clinics were largely delivered in a hospital or clinical setting. This face-to-face mode of delivery provided the nurse with the opportunity to physically assess the patient, which is essential for certain types of nurse-led clinics such as those involved in prescribing cancer treatments. Face-to-face assessment is paramount prior to prescribing treatments such as chemotherapy and immunotherapy, as it provides the assessor with the opportunity to 'eyeball' the patient, carry out any necessary physical examinations and ensure that the patient is tolerating treatment despite what the blood results and scans portray. However, for routine follow-up based largely on blood results such as tumour markers, a face-to-face appointment is not always essential; other modes can be considered, such as telephone or virtual nurse-led clinics. Virtual clinics enable patients to have their care assessed and managed by a healthcare professional without the requirement to attend a hospital appointment in person. Two modes available for virtual clinics are telephone calls and video consultations using an online platform such as Skype. According to Greenhalgh et al. (2016), telephone consultations require considerable skill and judgement because of the lack of visual cues and therefore may not be suitable for all nurse-led clinics. Consequently, remote video consultations between patients and healthcare professionals are becoming increasingly acceptable (Greenhalgh et al. 2016).

According to Day and Kerr (2012), nurse-led virtual clinics can be used efficiently for various chronic conditions such as cancer. An integrative review carried out by Almeida and Montayre (2019) reported a strong preference towards nurse-led virtual clinics, as patients appreciated the opportunity to be assessed and cared for remotely instead of in a busy and rushed clinic environment. Travelling to an oncology outpatient appointment may also be physically demanding for patients and their families, time-consuming and costly; as a result, virtual or telephone clinics are an increasingly preferred mode of care delivery for some patients when appropriate (Barsom et al. 2021).

11.7   Patient Outcomes Related to Nurse-Led Clinics

Nurse-led clinics have demonstrated many holistic benefits for patients. They are often undertaken by CNSs, who may be known to patients already as their key worker, contributing to the provision of continuity of care. According to Ling et al. (2013), the key worker role was originally conceived as the appointment of a specified healthcare professional from a patient's care team who acts as a point of contact between hospital and community staff and promotes continuity and co-ordination of care for individuals with a cancer diagnosis. Therefore, a therapeutic relationship may already be formed with the CNS as key worker prior to a patient attending a nurse-led clinic, which has been demonstrated to improve patient experience and promote continuity of care (Jones et al. 2016). This should contribute to patients feeling more at ease in discussing any concerns they may have and streamline patient care.

Loftus and Weston (2001) acknowledge that nurse-led clinics not only reduce patient waiting times but also offer holistic assessment, screening and monitoring, thus facilitating compliance, co-ordinating the care pathway and ensuring consistency of contact with healthcare professionals. According to Rush et al. (2019), in a systematic review of nurse-led cardioversion clinics, there was a significant mean reduction of 10 weeks in wait time across included studies for nurse-led clinics compared to physician-led clinics, highlighting a benefit to the patient related to being reviewed sooner.

Molassiois et al. (2020) report that nurse-led clinics in cancer care have demonstrated improved clinical outcomes such as emotional wellbeing, quality of life and physical symptoms such as fatigue, as well as ensuring that patient information needs are more fully met. An umbrella review focused on assessing the effectiveness of nurse-led clinics on healthcare delivery reported that all nine studies included in the review demonstrated improvements in patient outcomes such as adherence to medication and disease management (Connolly and Cotter 2021), suggesting that nurse-led clinics are effective across a variety of settings and health issues. This umbrella review primarily included studies focused on cardiovascular disease, atrial fibrillation, chronic obstructive pulmonary disease, diabetes and chronic kidney disease.

Moore (2018) highlights that nurse-led clinics enhance the patient experience whilst meeting individuals' holistic needs and are associated with fewer hospital appointments. Despite less input from the medical team, the CNS facilitating nurse-led clinics usually has rapid access to the medical team if required and carries out clinics with indispensable skills and competencies. Wong and Chung (2006) state that the quality of care provided through nurse-led clinics compared to physician care was, in fact, better for record-keeping, information provided to patients and levels of communication. In summary, nurse-led clinics have demonstrated improvements in providing a high standard of person-centred care with reported benefits for the patient.

11.8   Benefits of Nurse-Led Clinics for the Registered Nurse

In addition to nurse-led clinics contributing to positive outcomes for the patient, there are also reported benefits for the nurse leading the clinics. Gousy and Green (2015) highlight the importance of nurse-led clinics in terms of professional development by enabling CNSs to work autonomously and become more competent in new areas of expertise. CNSs are often involved in identifying ways in which patient care can be reshaped, providing opportunities for expanding the CNS roles by strategically contributing to the development of services. However, this contribution may blur professional boundaries between nursing and medicine (Judd 2009), and nurses must ensure that they always work within their limitations. Due to variations in the CNS roles and responsibilities in facilitating nurse-led clinics across different tumour sites and clinical teams, there should be clarity in job descriptions, with ongoing discussions among the healthcare team as the role evolves. This will identify what the CNS role involves in the nurse-led clinic, leading to a greater understanding and recognition of the CNS role (Trisyani and Windsor 2019). Whilst one rationale for establishing nurse-led clinics is to meet the needs of a service and deliver care to meet patient needs, it also provides opportunities for professional development and advancing skills (Moore et al. 2002; Beaver et al. 2009; Sheppard et al. 2009; Kimman et al. 2011; Strand et al. 2011).

Loftus and Weston (2001) acknowledge that the aim of nurse-led clinics is to improve patients' quality of life rather than simply fill a void due to a medical staffing crisis. Initiating and facilitating a nurse-led clinic offers nurses an opportunity to develop a variety of transferable skills, in addition to developing advanced skills such as clinical assessment, history taking and medication management. Additionally, the ability to manage time and patient caseloads is a valued skill within a highly pressured health service that the nurse can develop and can continue to use throughout their career progression (Hatchett 2016).

11.9   Benefits of Nurse-Led Clinics for the Healthcare Organisation

Nurse-led clinics are an excellent example of how the role of the CNS has developed to meet the demands of cancer care in the twenty-first century (Fishburn and Fishburn 2021). With more diagnoses and advances in treatment modalities, there are increased burdens on medical teams due to high volumes of patients. According to Moore (2018), nurse-led clinics release medical consultant time for reviewing more individuals with complex needs, thus improving service access and enabling more cost-effective service. Furthermore, nurse-led clinics improve service delivery, are more efficient, and increase patient satisfaction, as they are often tailored to their individual needs (Casey et al. 2017). Whilst patient care costs are much lower in nurse-led care compared to physician-led care due to substantial differences in salaries, Verschuur et al. (2008) report in a randomised trial that reduced costs have also been linked to nurses being more responsive to individual needs and reducing the burden of unnecessary hospital visits and investigations for patients.

11.10   Challenges to Implementing Nurse-Led Clinics

Whilst there are many benefits to nurse-led clinics in relation to assessing and providing holistic patient care, in addition to developing the role of the CNS and improving the delivery of healthcare, there are also challenges to implementing nurse-led clinics effectively into clinical practice. According to Jones et al. (2016), two main barriers to implementing nurse-led clinics are a lack of clinic space due to room shortages in hospital settings and insufficient administrative support. To address these, it is essential to complete a scoping exercise prior to establishing a nurse-led clinic. Managerial support will be required to ensure that these challenges are proactively addressed.

One approach to address room shortages in a clinical setting is to consider establishing a telephone or virtual clinic as an alternative to face-to-face clinics, if appropriate. Such clinics may include follow-up appointments after treatment for certain cancers measured by tumour markers, such as prostate, testicular and colorectal cancer. This allows the initiation of new clinics to meet ongoing service demands without the need for a clinical room, as clinics can be delivered in either office space or in alternative setting remotely.

Administrative support may be assisted by using online questionnaire templates such as those available through the RISOH IT system (previously introduced) to record clinical assessments. Questionnaires are completed by the nurse after the patient consultation. This contributes to less administrative support being required for a nurse-led clinic, as it reduces the need for dictating clinic letters; these can be printed directly from RISOH and sent to the appropriate healthcare professionals. Additionally, in NI, information on RISOH can be made easily available on a patient's electronic care record (ECR), enabling primary care to have immediate access to relevant oncology information. ECR is a tool used to improve the quality and safety of patient care: it brings together key information from health and social care records and positions it in a single secure computer system for all healthcare professionals to access.

Whilst nurse-led clinics within cancer care are well established, concerns exist about future demand for follow-up exceeding the current supply of CNSs.

If possible, CNSs should not work in isolation in a nurse-led clinic setting and should ensure good communication skills to enable safe working within a multi-disciplinary team, reviewing and making appropriate referrals when necessary (Hatchett 2016). This team approach ensures that robust systems are in place, should individual staffing roles change or a change in circumstances occur; the nurse-led clinic can continue in its current format, and patient care can be maintained and delivered efficiently.

11.11 Nurse-Led Clinic Service Evaluation

After a nurse-led clinic is established, an evaluation is recommended to review its successes and identify any emerging problems (Judd 2009). Clear aims and objectives of the nurse-led clinic are vital in measuring the clinic's value (Hatchett 2016). Aims and objectives may relate to reducing patient waiting times for clinic appointments, providing holistic support to patients, or prescribing medications and managing treatment toxicities. Evaluation of services is crucial to measure outcomes, and this can be achieved through audits, questionnaires and feedback.

Audits identify CNS caseload in numerical values and are useful in identifying the impact of a nurse-led clinic on reducing patient waiting times. Questionnaires to service users can assess patient satisfaction. Feedback from medical teams is crucial in identifying any issues and recognising the benefits of the nurse-led clinic, such as reducing waiting lists, which provides more time for medical consultants to review individuals presenting with challenging complexities. A service evaluation of specialist nurse telephone follow-up of individuals with bowel cancer after surgery was completed by assessing patient satisfaction in 30 patients using a questionnaire (Mole et al. 2019). The results highlighted that this innovative approach to patient care was well-liked by patients and cost-effective for the health service and increased outpatient medical capacity to see more individuals who required more complex care. Therefore, this model of nurse-led care is one option for providing a solution to reducing outpatient appointments in the future.

11.12 Future of Nurse-Led Clinics

There is an increased trend towards telephone consultations in the NHS in the context of the UK, which can benefit the patient – they are potentially more convenient, reducing travel for hospital appointments and avoiding the challenges of securing parking (Greenhalgh et al. 2016). Telephone follow-up is an innovative approach to healthcare delivery that is advantageous for continuity of care, improved accessibility, improved economic efficiency and superior patient satisfaction with information, which reduces anxiety (Gilmartin et al. 2019). According to Casey et al. (2017), patients may find attending hospital appointments problematic in terms of time, loss of control and anxiety due to travelling to and from appointments, financial costs of parking and waiting in overcrowded waiting rooms to attend consultations that may only last a few minutes. Therefore, hospital-based care may not always be the best option for patients, particularly individuals with chronic conditions such as cancer.

Prior to the COVID-19 pandemic, telephone consultations were delivered in some cancer disease-specific sites, but they were not universal. Virtual consultations became a routine approach for many healthcare organisations during the COVID-19 pandemic, demonstrating a new mode of facilitating consultations with patients. The virtual platform contributes to patient safety, especially those who are clinically vulnerable or immuno-compromised. These service developments promote continuity of patient care for those requiring ongoing treatment or follow-up post-treatment and can support patients who are shielding from the COVID-19 virus by limiting their exposure to a hospital setting where they may be subjected to the risk of community transmission (International Council of Nurses 2020). As a result, there is the potential for continued growth in the demand for nurse-led clinics post-COVID-19 in an attempt to reduce patient waiting times, resources and costs whilst keeping patient safety at the forefront (Connolly and Cotter 2021). However, there may be challenges to telephone consultations for individuals with a hearing impairment or language barriers due to ethnicity (Fishburn and Fisburn 2021); consequently, some individuals may prefer to attend face-to-face consultations.

11.13 Reflection on the Role as a Uro-Oncology CNS Undertaking Nurse-Led Clinics

Whilst CNS roles exist in urology in the surgical setting, the uro-oncology CNS role occupied by the first author was introduced for individuals with prostate and bladder cancer in an oncology setting in a hospital in Belfast, NI. Oncology nurse practitioners (ONPs) were in post prior to the introduction of the uro-oncology CNS role, with established nurse-led review clinics for individuals with prostate cancer as part of their follow-up; however, this is now the responsibility of the uro-oncology CNS.

The uro-oncology CNS role incorporates many vital aspects to ensure that holistic person-centred care is achieved. This role involves attending two new patient diagnostic clinics each week and acting as a key worker for individuals with a prostate or bladder cancer diagnosis, ensuring that each person has a point of contact for any questions or concerns. As a key worker, this role acts as a direct link between the patient and the medical team. (The key worker role is the focus of Chapter 5 of this book.) This role also involves being a non-medical prescriber (NMP), working alongside an oncologist on a weekly basis, assessing patients and prescribing SACT such as chemotherapy, immunotherapy and hormonal therapy. (Non-medical prescribing is also the focus of Chapter 12 in this book.)

An HNA clinic is facilitated by the uro-oncology CNS, providing an opportunity for patients to openly discuss their physical, emotional, social, spiritual, sexual and psychological wellbeing, and includes support and signposting to relevant resources. Three nurse-led review clinics for individuals with prostate cancer are facilitated weekly by the uro-oncology CNS for individuals who have completed radiotherapy or brachytherapy treatment and require follow-up care for a minimum of five years post-diagnosis.

The uro-oncology CNS role is multi-dimensional, supported by a range of transferable skills. The role contributes to service development, providing opportunities for professional development. A service evaluation carried out by the first author demonstrated patient satisfaction with telephone nurse-led review clinics in comparison to face-to-face. The evaluation found that patients preferred a telephone review, as they felt more comfortable discussing sensitive issues such as sexual dysfunction on the telephone and preferred to undertake the review in the comfort of their own home to reduce travel, time and personal cost.

11.14   Conclusion

Within cancer services, a range of nurse-led clinics are facilitated throughout the patient pathway depending on the disease site, and these are often undertaken by a CNS. Establishing a new nurse-led clinic requires careful planning, clear communication between multidisciplinary team members and a hierarchy of support. CNSs must possess advanced nursing skills and have the knowledge required to work at a higher level and display autonomy. Nurse-led clinics have demonstrated many benefits to patients, healthcare workers and the healthcare organisation. Patients report them to be beneficial because of the therapeutic relationship already established with the CNS as their key worker and the improved clinical outcomes. Nurse-led clinics provide CNSs with opportunities for personal and professional development. They also have the potential to provide enhanced service delivery more cost-effectively for the healthcare organisation, which improves patient experiences. CNSs can face challenges in initiating and developing nurse-led clinics; however, if a service need has been identified and a hierarchy of support is available, these can be addressed. Finally, considering alternative modes of working when introducing a nurse-led clinic is important, with increasing evidence of the positive experiences of telephone and virtual consultations.

References

Almeida, S. and Montayre, J. (2019). An integrative review of nurse-led virtual clinics. *Nursing Praxis in New Zealand* 35 (1): 18–28.

Barsom, E.Z., Jansen, M., Tanis, P.J. et al. (2021). Video consultation during follow up care: effect on quality of care and patient- and provider attitude in patients with colorectal cancer. *Surgical Endoscopy* 35: 1278–1287.

Beaver, K., Tysver-Robinson, D., Campbell, M. et al. (2009). Comparing hospital and telephone follow-up after treatment for breast cancer: randomised equivalence trial. *British Medical Journal* 338: 1–9.

Campbell, J., German, L., Lane, C., and Dodwell, D. (2000). Radiotherapy outpatient review: a nurse-led clinic. *Clinical Oncology* 12: 104–107.

Casey, R.G., Powell, I., Braithwaite, M. et al. (2017). Nurse-led phone call follow-up clinics are effective for patients with prostate cancer. *Journal of Patient Experience* 4 (3): 114–120.

Connolly, C. and Cotter, P. (2021). Effectiveness of nurse-led clinics on healthcare delivery: an umbrella review. *Journal of Clinical Nursing* 00 (1): 1–8.

Corner, J. (2003). The role of nurse-led care in cancer management. *Lancet Oncology* 4 (10): 631–636.

Cox, K. and Wilson, E. (2003). Follow-up for people with cancer: nurse-led services and telephone interventions. *Journal of Advanced Nursing* 43 (1): 51–61.

Day, K. and Kerr, P. (2012). Telemedicine: rethinking healthcare roles for smarter care. *Health Care and Informatics Review* 16 (2): 8–16.

Department of Health. (2000). The NHS cancer plan. London: DoH.

Fishburn, A. and Fishburn, N. (2021). Establishing a nurse-led thyroid cancer follow-up clinic. *British Journal of Nursing (Oncology Supplement)* 30 (4): S28–S35.

Gilmartin, M., Leaver, N., Hall, G. et al. (2019). Patient perception of telephone follow-up after resection for colorectal cancer: is it time for an alternative to the outpatient clinic? *Patient Experience Journal* 6 (1): 81–86.

Gousy, M. and Green, K. (2015). Developing a nurse-led clinic using transformational leadership. *Nursing Standard* 29 (30): 37–41.

Greenhalgh, T., Vijayaraghavan, S., Wherton, J. et al. (2016). Virtual online consultations: advantages and limitations (VOCAL) study. *British Medical Journal Open* 6 (1): 1–13.

Hamric, A.B. and Tracy, M.G. (2019). A definition of advanced practice nursing. In: *Hamric and Hanson's Advanced Practice Nursing: An Integrative Approach*, 6e (ed. M.F. Tracy and E.T. O'Grady), 202–251. Missouri: Elsevier.

Hatchett, R. (2005). Key issues in setting up and running a nurse-led cardiology clinic. *Nursing Standard* 20 (14–16): 49–53.

Hatchett, R. (2008). Nurse-led clinics: 10 essential steps to setting up a service. *Nursing Times* 104 (4): 62–64.

Hatchett, R. (2016). How to set up a nurse-led clinic. *Nursing Standard* 30 (37): 64–65.

Heinen, M., van Oostveen, C., Peters, J. et al. (2019). An integrative review of leadership competencies and attributes in advanced nursing practice. *Journal of Advanced Nursing* 75 (11): 2378–2392.

Independent Cancer Taskforce. (2015). Achieving world-class cancer outcomes: a strategy for England 2015–2020. https://www.england.nhs.uk/wp-content/uploads/2017/10/national-cancer-transformation-programme-2016-17-progress.pdf (accessed 11 November 2021).

International Council of Nurses. (2020). Oncology services during the COVID-19 pandemic: Ireland. https://www.icn.ch/news/international-nurses-day-2020-case-study-week-17 (accessed 7 March 2022)

International Council of Nurses. (2021). Guiding breast cancer patients through care management, China. https://www.icn.ch/news/guiding-breast-cancer-patients-through-care-management-china (accessed 7 March 2022).

Jones, S., Thomas, T., and Lavelle, E. (2016). Nurse-led clinic for men receiving targeted therapies for metastatic hormone-relapsed prostate cancer. *Cancer Nursing Practice* 15 (5): 32–36.

Judd, J. (2009). The practical issues of establishing paediatric orthopaedic nurse led clinics and judging success through parent satisfaction. *Journal of Orthopaedic Nursing* 13 (2): 63–69.

Kerr, H., Donovan, M., and McSorley, O. (2021). Evaluation of the role of the clinical nurse specialist in cancer care: and integrative literature review. *European Journal of Cancer Care* 30 (3): 1–13.

Kimman, M.L., Dirksen, C.D., Voogd, A.C. et al. (2011). Nurse-led telephone follow-up and an educational group programme after breast cancer treatment: results of a 2 × 2 randomised controlled trial. *European Journal of Cancer* 47 (7): 1027–1036.

Lai, X.B., Ching, S.S.Y., and Wong, F.K.Y. (2017). Nurse-led cancer care: a scope review of the past years (2003–2016). *International Journal of Nursing Sciences* 4 (2): 184–195.

Leahy, M., Krishnasamy, M., Herschtal, A. et al. (2013). Satisfaction with nurse-led telephone follow-up for low to intermediate risk prostate cancer patients treated with radical radiotherapy. A comparative study. *European Journal of Oncology Nursing* 17 (2): 162–169.

Lee, G., Hendriks, J., and Deaton, C. (2020). Advanced nursing practice across Europe: work in progress. *European Journal of Cardiovascular Nursing* 19 (7): 561–563.

Ling, J., McCabe, K., Brent, S., and Crosland, A. (2013). Key workers in cancer care: patient and staff attitudes and implications for role development in cancer services. *European Journal of Cancer Care* 22 (5): 691–698.

Loftus, L.A. and Weston, V. (2001). The development of nurse-led clinics in cancer care. *Journal of Clinical Nursing* 10: 215–220.

Macmillan Cancer Support. (2015). The recovery package. https://www.macmillan. org.uk/documents/aboutus/health_professionals/macvoice/sharinggoodpractice_ therecoverypackage.pdf (accessed 11 December 2021).

McLachlan, A., Aldridge, C., Lee, M. et al. (2019). The development and first six years of a nurse-led chest pain clinic. *The New Zealand Medical Journal* 132 (1489): 39–47.

Molassiois, A., Liu, X., and Kwok, S.W. (2020). Impact of advanced nursing practice through nurse-led clinics. In the care of cancer patients: a scoping review. *European Journal of Cancer Care* 30 (1): 1–17.

Mole, G., Murali, M., Carter, S. et al. (2019). A service evaluation of specialist nurse telephone follow-up of bowel cancer patients after surgery. *British Journal of Nursing* 28 (19): 1134–1138.

Moore, L. (2018). Nurse-led cancer care clinics: an economic assessment of breast and urology clinics. *Cancer Nursing Practice* 17 (1): 34–41.

Moore, S., Corner, J., Haviland, J. et al. (2002). Nurse led follow up and conventional medical follow up in management of patients with lung cancer: randomised trial. *British Medical Journal* 325 (7373): 1–7.

National Institute for Health and Care Excellence. (2021). Prostate cancer: diagnosis and management. www.nice.org.uk/guidance/ng131/chapter/recommendations (accessed 7 March 2022).

Ndosi, M., Lewis, M., Hale, C. et al. (2014). The outcome and cost-effectiveness of nurse-led care in people with rheumatoid arthritis: a multicentre randomised controlled trial. *Annals of the Rheumatic Diseases* 73: 1975–1982.

NHS England. (2016). Innovation to Implementation: stratified pathways of care for people living with cancer – 'A how to guide'. https://www.england.nhs.uk/ publication/innovation-to-implementation-stratified-pathways-of-care-for-people-living-with-or-beyond-cancer-a-how-to-guide (accessed 11 December 2021).

Northern Ireland Cancer Network. (2022). Other areas of work. https://nican.hscni. net/info-for-professionals/nican-work-programmes (accessed 15 March 2022).

Randall, S., Crawford, T., Currie, J. et al. (2017). Impact of community based nurse-led clinics on patient outcomes, patient satisfaction, patient access and cost effectiveness: a systematic review. *International Journal of Nursing Studies* 73: 24–33.

Robertson, A.F., Windsor, P.M., and Smith, A. (2013). Evaluation of a nurse-led service for follow-up of patients with prostate cancer. *International Journal of Urological Nursing* 7 (2): 92–97.

Rush, K.L., Burton, L., Schaab, K., and Lukey, A. (2019). The impact of nurse-led atrial fibrillation clinics on patient and healthcare outcomes: a systematic mixed studies review. *European Journal of Cardiovascular Nursing* 18 (7): 526–533.

Sheppard, C. (2007). Breast cancer follow-up: literature review and discussion. *European Journal of Oncology Nursing* 11: 340–347.

Sheppard, C., Higgins, B., Wise, M. et al. (2009). Breast cancer follow up: a randomised controlled trial comparing point of need access versus routine 6-monthly clinical review. *European Journal of Oncology Nursing* 13 (1): 2–8.

Shiu, A.T.Y., Lee, D.T.F., and Chau, J.P.C. (2011). Exploring the scope of expanding advanced nursing practice in nurse-led clinics: a multiple-case study. *Journal of Advanced Nursing* 68 (8): 1780–1792.

Smits, A., Lopes, A., Das, N. et al. (2015). Nurse-led telephone follow-up: improving options for women with endometrial cancer. *Cancer Nursing* 38 (3): 232–238.

Strand, E., Nygren, I., Bergkvist, L., and Smedh, K. (2011). Nurse or surgeon follow-up after rectal cancer: a randomized trial. *Colorectal Disease* 13 (9): 999–1003.

Trisyani, Y. and Windsor, C. (2019). Expanding knowledge and roles for authority and practice boundaries of Emergency Department nurses: a grounded theory study. *International Journal of Qualitative Studies on Health and Well-Being* 14 (1): 1–12.

Verschuur, E.M.L., Steyerberg, E.W., Tilanus, H.W. et al. (2008). Nurse-led follow-up of patients after oesophageal or gastric cardia cancer surgery: a randomised trial. *British Journal of Cancer* 100: 70–76.

Vinall-Collier, K., Madill, A., and Firth, J. (2016). A multi-centre study of interactional style in nurse specialist- and physician-led rheumatology clinics in the UK. *International Journal of Nursing Studies* 59: 41–50.

Wiles, R., Postle, K., Steiner, A., and Walsh, B. (2001). Nurse-led intermediate care: an opportunity to develop enhanced roles for nurses? *Journal of Advanced Nursing* 34: 813–821.

Wong, F.K.Y. and Chung, L.C.Y. (2006). Establishing a definition for a nurse-led clinic: structure, process and outcome. *Journal of Advanced Nursing* 53 (3): 358–369.

12

Non-Medical Prescribing

Laura Croan and Barry Quinn

Abstract

This chapter explores the background and development of non-medical prescribing through supplementary prescribing and patient group directives to the rapid recent growth of independent prescribing. It discusses the skills and experiences necessary to embark on a non-medical prescribing course and the importance of adhering to the Royal Pharmaceutical Society Prescribing Framework to ensure safe practice. This chapter also addresses the benefits and challenges of non-medical prescribing through case studies and summarises how this element of advanced practice can be amalgamated into a clinical nurse specialist role.

12.1   Introduction

This chapter will focus on the important role of independent prescribing as part of the evolving scope of practice within clinical nurse specialisms. The nurse prescriber has a fundamental role as part of the response to the growing and changing needs of global health and social care (Noblet et al. 2018; International Council of Nursing [ICN] 2020). There will be an exploration of developments that have led to the current approach to independent prescribing and how these advanced clinical skills will become an increasing part of the clinical nurse specialist (CNS) role. The chapter will then focus on two case studies from clinical practice to illustrate the central role prescribing plays as part of the specialist nurse role and some important issues to consider.

The role of the independent prescriber in specialist nursing has evolved to become an important component of nursing practice in meeting the individual receiving treatment, care and support (World Health Organisation [WHO] 2021).

The Role of the Clinical Nurse Specialist in Cancer Care, First Edition. Edited by Helen Kerr.
© 2024 John Wiley & Sons Ltd. Published 2024 by John Wiley & Sons Ltd.
Companion website: www.wiley.com/go/kerr

Laura Croan has 18 years of experience working in haematology, has been an independent prescriber for 9 years, worked as a lymphoma CNS for 7 years and is currently training to be an advanced nurse practitioner. Barry Quinn has worked in the field of cancer and palliative care for over 30 years in London, United Kingdom (UK) in a variety of roles, including consultant nurse for cancer. He is an independent prescriber and currently a senior lecturer at Queen's University Belfast.

12.2 Background

While changes in health and social care may vary in different regions of the world, there is global growth in the number of people living longer with multiple and sometimes complex co-morbidities (Quinn 2022). Alongside this reality is a predicted shortage of nurses and doctors (WHO 2021). Moving forward, CNSs will be required not only to have expert knowledge of their own specialist area of practice (cardiology, dementia, renal, mental health, learning disability, cancer, childhood diseases) but also to be knowledgeable about other co-morbidities and social factors that will impact the individual who needs nursing support and for whom the specialist nurse will prescribe (Hand 2019).

Across the world, nurses working in specialist roles continue to have a key role in creatively responding to the person and family in need through their advanced skills and by expanding their scope of practice. This reality is reflected in the key pillars required of all CNSs or advanced nurse practitioners: being able to work at an advanced level of clinical practice; an ability to lead and respond to the global, social, political, economic and technological challenges; facilitating education and learning; and delivering advance clinical nurse practice based on evidence research and development (ICN 2020).

In recognition of these growing global needs and changes required within the nursing workforce, the WHO (2021), the ICN (2020), the Nursing and Midwifery Council (NMC) of the UK (NMC 2018a,b; 2019), the Royal College of Nursing (RCN) of the UK (2018) and many other national and global professional nursing bodies predict that nurses will need to be better prepared to deliver care to meet these changing and diverse needs. This includes the increasing need for many nurses working in specialist and advanced roles to undertake an expanded scope of practice, including that of the independent prescriber.

Whether working as part of a community, a hospital or a combined hospital/community service, there will be an increasing need for suitably skilled nurses to lead services, where nurses work with other members of the multiprofessional team to deliver care in a more holistic and person-focussed manner (WHO 2021). An increasing number of CNSs working as prescribers will be involved in prescribing treatments to treat the underlying illness or condition, prescribing medicines to deal with the side effects of treatments and complications of disease, or prescribing supportive drugs to help individuals live with chronic and advancing illness (RCN 2018).

12.3 Developments in Nursing Practice and the Role of Prescribing

In 2018, the NMC (2018a), in the context of the UK, recognised that with more people presenting with a range of complex and indeed multiple conditions and more nursing care being delivered in community settings, there was a need for nurses to be prepared with an increasing set of skills and competencies to meet these demands. This included a commitment to delivering high-quality nursing care in a range of settings aimed at supporting people in need while promoting better health and responding to personal choice. In recognition of this reality, today, newly registered/ qualified nurses are being educated and trained to have a higher level of proficiency in skills such as assessment, diagnostics, care planning and management, pharmacology and leadership (NMC 2019). All these skills, which are also essential to nurse prescribers, suggest that more and more nurses will be required to take on the role of the specialist and advanced nurse while working as an independent prescriber.

The central role of prescribing in nursing has continued to grow in response to local, regional and national need. Previously in the UK, in order to become a community prescriber or an independent prescriber, nurses needed at least two or three years of clinical practice (NMC 2018b, 2019). However, current requirements no longer focus on years of experience but on the skills required, including clinical and health assessment, diagnostics, care management, planning and evaluating care, all core components of preregistration nurse education (NMC 2019). Nurses working in specialist roles will be vital in leading and role-modelling these skills required to respond to the increasing and complex needs of those within the health and social care system.

12.3.1 Community Nurse Prescribing

The recognition of the vital role of independent prescribing within nursing began with a community-based focus. In 1986, a community nursing review, The Cumberlege Report, undertaken by the Department of Health and Social Security (DHSS) (1986), recognised that community-based nurses were spending extended periods requesting prescriptions from doctors, including dressings and ointments, when it was argued that these nurses knew more than community doctors about the suitability of these products for the healthcare needs of those they nursed and supported. The UK Department of Health agreed that a limited number of products could be prescribed by these experienced community nurses as part of their service. Over the next decade, this approach to community nurse prescribing was piloted and subsequently extended to a number of community services within the UK. An evaluation report (Luker et al. 1997) and another report in 2004 (McKenna and Keeney 2004) demonstrated that this approach to prescribing not only benefited the patient and carer but also enhanced the work of nurses, doctors and community services. By the end of the decade, community nurse-led prescribing, although limited to certain treatments, was widespread within the UK.

12.3.2   Clinical Management Plans

In another development, the clinical management plan (CMP), also known as supplementary prescribing, was introduced to help support better prescribing and care. The CMP was introduced to enhance the care of people living with chronic diseases including asthma, heart disease and mental illness (James 2006). It is described by the National Institute for Health and Care Excellence (NICE), UK (2015) as an agreed partnership between the patient, the doctor and a supplementary prescriber. Following an initial assessment by a doctor, the nurse or allied health professional can prescribe for the patient using an agreed patient-specific CMP (Table 12.1). This is usually focused on prescribing for non-acute medical conditions and/or health needs affecting the chronically ill patient. Once again, this innovative approach to prescribing focuses on better supporting the person in need and in a timelier manner.

12.3.3   Patient Group Directives

Another change to improving patient care and prescribing practice came with the development of patient group directives (PGDs) (NICE 2017). Unlike CMPs, these are not patient-specific. Today, they are used extensively in clinical areas including emergency departments, urgent care centres and other domains of specialist practice where the individual patient may not be identified before presenting for

Table 12.1   The clinical management plan.

- The patient/carer agrees to the arrangement.
- Benefit to the patient and the service.
- Good communication and access to the patient's record.
- Supplementary prescribing supports but does not replace multidisciplinary care.
- The independent and supplementary prescriber will need training.
- The prescriber must be registered on their appropriate professional register.
- Prescribing and dispensing responsibilities should, where possible, be separate – patient safety and governance.
- Written instruction – supply/administration of licensed (or, in exceptional circumstances, off-label) medicines in an identified clinical situation.

Source: NICE (2015).

treatment. The supply and administration of medicines under PGDs are reserved for situations where the PGD offers an advantage for patient care without compromising safety (NICE 2017). This includes consistency with appropriate professional teamworking and accountability. The PGD is drawn up locally by doctors, pharmacists, other health professionals and health and social care agencies. It must meet certain legal criteria, including being signed by a doctor and a pharmacist, and be approved by the organisation in which it is to be used. Only named professionals can administer or supply medicines under an agreed PGD (NICE 2017).

12.3.4 The Growth of Independent Prescribing

Alongside CMPs and PGDs, other developments in prescribing emerged. In recognition of the growing need for better prescribing, the National Prescribing Centre (2001) recommended that suitably qualified nurses and pharmacists should be able to prescribe any licensed medicine for any medical condition within their area of competence. This meant the scope of prescribing practice was being broadened, leading the way for suitably trained nurses and pharmacists to undertake specific training and work as independent prescribers. In each of these developments, the focus was in response to patient needs and on implementing a more person-centred approach to care and better use of personnel and resources, including better use of patient, nurse, allied health professional and doctor time.

The competency framework for prescribers in the UK was first published by the National Prescribing Centre (2012). In 2016, NICE agreed that the Royal Pharmaceutical Society (RPS) (2016) would take the lead on maintaining and updating these competencies in collaboration with, and with endorsement by, other prescribing professions, including the NMC, the nursing and midwifery professional body in the UK. The Competency Framework, which is aimed at all prescribers, sets out what good prescribing looks like. Focusing on the consultation and governance processes, the framework helps to inform and improve practice, ensuring a high standard of care and safety for the patient and the prescriber (Table 12.2). Although the competencies have been set out under the consultation and governance processes, none stand alone, and each set of competencies is necessary to ensure safety and best practice.

The RPS recognised that broadening the scope of prescribing practice had the potential to improve the quality of peoples' lives and healthcare outcomes. However, it was recognised that this approach needed to be undertaken safely, ensuring that each prescriber was able to remain competent to prescribe or not prescribe the correct medicines for each patient and that the increased responsibility of prescribing should not be underestimated (RPS 2016). Recently, the RPS have revised and updated the Competency Framework (2021), which continues to support and guide prescribers in expanding their knowledge, skills, motives and personal traits to continually improve their performance and work safely and effectively (RPS 2021).

Table 12.2 Prescribing in practice.

The consultation

- Assessment: person-centred, focusing on the physical, emotional, social and spiritual aspects of care
- Evidence-based treatment/support options: non-pharmacological, pharmacological, co-morbidities, existing medication, impact on quality of life
- Present options and reach a shared decision: working with the patient/carer, consider diversity, values, beliefs and expectations
- Prescribe: medicine/s with awareness of its actions, indications, dose, contraindications, interactions, cautions, side effects and potential for misuse
- Provide information: patient/carer's understanding of plan, monitoring and follow-up, empower patient/carer (deterioration or no improvement)
- Monitor and review: plan and adapt in response to monitoring, patient's condition and preferences.

Clinical governance

- Safety: scope of practice, recognises limits of own knowledge and skill
- Professional: decisions based on the person
- Competency: patient and peer review feedback, prescribing practice and audit
- Teamwork: support and supervision for role as a prescriber, organisational policies and procedures

---

Source: Adapted from Royal Pharmaceutical Society (2021).

The RPS Competency Framework underpins the professional responsibility required of all those who prescribe as part of their role. Prescribers can use the framework to support their practice, including self-assessment and clinical reflection, and it guides the prescriber when required to expand or change their prescribing. The competencies also help guide regulators, education providers, professional organisations and specialist groups to inform and support constancy in standards, training, guidance and prescribing advice. Each nurse who is a prescriber is also required to adhere to the core principles of their professional code of practice (Table 12.3).

Table 12.3 Principles of professional nursing.

- Maintaining a person-centred approach
- Confidentiality
- Good communication
- Leadership
- Reflecting on practice
- Maintaining competency
- Professional development
- Working within their scope of practice
- Networking for support and learning

Source: NMC (2018a); ICN (2020); WHO (2021).

12.4   Preparing to Prescribe

All nurses wishing to undertake prescribing as part of their specialist role are required to undertake an approved prescribing course (ICN 2020). Topics may include pharmacotherapeutics, prescribing in practice and health assessment. Each nurse prescriber who has achieved a recognised prescribing qualification is required to be registered as an independent prescriber on the NMC register and on the local register of the Trust where they work. This is vital for patient and prescriber safety and to ensure adherence to clinical governance. Each prescriber is expected to undertake training related to their prescribing role at least annually and to participate in audits and peer reviews of their prescribing practice (NMC 2018b; RPS 2021). In the UK, nurse prescribers are expected to reflect on their prescribing role as part of their professional revalidation process (NMC 2018b).

Today, although non-medical prescribing has become globally accepted, nurse and allied health professional prescribers in the UK are pioneering this role extension and have some of the most extended prescribing rights in the world (Courtenay et al. 2011). Under the RPS competencies, each prescriber is required to have their advanced role of prescribing written into their job description (ICN 2020; RPS 2021).

A helpful tool, 'Preparing to Prescribe', has been devised and is widely available online to guide those who wish to undertake prescribing as part of their role to ensure that the organisation is able to provide suitable support and effective implementation of the new prescribing qualification (Carey and Stenner 2020). The toolkit comprises questions for guidance, links to current regulations and support, and signposting for those wishing to embark on a prescribing course.

12.5   Benefits and Challenges of Non-Medical Prescribing

Reflecting on the competencies defined by the RPS (2021), CNSs are in an ideal position to provide the service of independent prescribing. The CNS is required to have expertise in their chosen speciality; many have undertaken training in advanced communication skills, have enhanced adherence to medication regimes and deliver more person-centred informed decision-making (Nuttall 2013). Nurses in these roles also have experience in performing complex holistic patient assessments and providing information needs and consequently have the opportunity to develop therapeutic relationships to augment a patient's level of engagement in their care (Kerr et al. 2021). Further reports claim that patients have expressed that they are more at ease talking to nurses, with a feeling of person-centredness and being treated with compassion (Cannaby et al. 2020).

Many CNSs have previously reported frustrations with delays in the prescribing process, waiting for a doctor to prescribe for the management plan the nurse and patient have agreed on or advising junior medical staff on what to prescribe in specialised situations (Omer et al. 2021). Skilled nurses not only provide more streamlined care through fulfilling their patient review in its entirety with prescribing skills but also provide more continuity of care and continue to develop the essential therapeutic relationship to improve medication adherence (Graham-Clarke et al. 2018; Noblett et al. 2018). A number of reviews into patient satisfaction of nurse prescribers have remained positive; and research suggests that non-medical prescribing is safe and effective and can provide beneficial clinical outcomes, with multiple case studies demonstrating that specialist nurses can improve the management of symptoms and provide rapid appropriate prescribing (Abuzour et al. 2018; Noblett et al. 2018; Kerr et al. 2021).

Although patients have reported positive perspectives regarding their encounters with nurse prescribers, there is still a lack of understanding in the general public, which may account for some of the scepticism about nurse prescribers' knowledge and expressions of feeling safer when medication is prescribed by a doctor (Graham-Clarke et al. 2018; Omer et al. 2021). Some of the literature has reported issues with non-medical prescribers gaining professional credibility on attaining their prescribing qualification, with a lack of support from their nursing colleagues and the medical team, or experiences of an obstructive work environment (Creedon et al. 2015; McHugh et al. 2020). Prescribing is a skill traditionally performed only by doctors; therefore, when nurse prescribers amalgamate their newly acquired abilities into the team, there can be some role ambiguity and blurring of duties or being referred to as a 'mini-doctor' rather than considered an advanced nurse; however, reports demonstrate that these attitudes are quickly disappearing (Nuttall 2013; McHugh et al. 2020).

When building the prescribing qualification into a CNS role, it is important for nurses to remember the hidden workload of prescribing and be mindful of the additional time to review interactions with an often long list of already prescribed medications, provide the patient with adequate information regarding the drugs prescribed and monitor medications prescribed or make referrals to do so (Creedon et al. 2015).

12.6   Deciding to Become a Non-Medical Prescriber

When contemplating whether to become a prescriber, it is important for each nurse to consider whether it is the right decision for them and their role. CNS roles are diverse, with many varying responsibilities within differing subspecialties (Kerr et al. 2021). It has been demonstrated that having access to nurses working in specialist roles is associated with enhanced patient experiences and better psychological outcomes (Alessy et al. 2021); therefore, these nurses are in a prime position to improve service delivery by expanding their professional skills to non-medical prescribing (Graham-Clarke et al. 2018).

Before embarking on a prescribing qualification, it is imperative that each nurse evaluate their role and consider whether becoming a prescriber will benefit the service user, the role and the specialist service (Hand 2019; NMC 2019).

It may be helpful to consider:

- Why do you want to prescribe?
- How will it advance your service?
- What patient group will you be prescribing for? Where will you be prescribing: primary, secondary, or tertiary care?
- What will you be prescribing?
- What is your scope of practice?
- Who can support you in this new and developing role (peers, doctors, management)?
- How will this new skill be amalgamated into your current role?
- Are clinical governance, policies and protocols in place?

Case Study 1   Communication in Non-medical Prescribing

Jack (pseudonym) (he/him) was a 75-year-old man who lived with his wife (she/her) and who continued to work as a farmer on a small piece of land with his two sons. Following multiple investigations, Jack was diagnosed with chronic lymphocytic leukaemia (CLL) but initially did not require treatment and remained on an active monitoring program for the first five years. Three months before his consultation with his CNS, Jack's disease had progressed, and he had been commenced on ibrutinib, a tyrosine kinase inhibitor (TKI) – a drug that has the ability to block cancer growth – as a systemic anti-cancer treatment (SACT).

Jack's past medical history included hypertension, and he had previously undergone a total right knee replacement. Jack was taking ramipril 5 mg once a day, co-codamol 8/500 up to four times a day as required, ibrutinib 420 mg once a day and prophylactic medications to reduce infection (aciclovir 400 mg twice daily and co-trimoxazole 480 mg twice daily on Monday, Wednesday and Friday). Jack reported not taking any other 'over-the-counter' medications and had an intolerance to bisoprolol.

Jack attended the clinic with a one-week history of diarrhoea and abdominal pain. He was assessed by the CNS, who focused on his gastro-intestinal symptoms. A full review of prescribed and 'over-the-counter' medications was addressed, but Jack reported that he was not taking any new medications. Jack had a sensitivity to pollen but no dietary intolerances. An infection was ruled out following negative blood and faecal samples. Ibrutinib is known to cause some gastro-intestinal disturbance.

Jack's condition was discussed between the CNS and Jack's medical consultant. The consultant agreed with the CNS that the ibrutinib treatment was the likely cause of Jack's abdominal symptoms. In consultation with Jack, the CNS and consultant agreed to pause the treatment, with a plan to review Jack in three weeks.

Three weeks later, Jack came back to the clinic for his review with his wife; however, his abdominal symptoms had not settled, despite stopping the anti-cancer drug. During the consultation, Jack's wife asked the CNS if Jack should stop his 'Chinese herbs', which he had purchased on the internet (not 'over the counter'), as Jack had read that these herbs were 'good for treating cancer'. Jack, his wife and his medical team were unsure of the content of these herbs, and in consultation with Jack, he was advised to stop the herbs immediately. Within one week, Jack's symptoms subsided, and his ibrutinib treatment was recommended with no further gastro-intestinal symptoms.

This case study illustrates the importance of clear communication within the prescribing consultation, an important component of the RPS competencies (2021). Jack did not think to declare the 'Chinese herbs', as he did not consider herbs a medication, and he had not bought them 'over a counter', as the CNS had asked. Nevertheless, these herbs were potent enough to give Jack significant side effects and caused his treatment to be needlessly interrupted, and further delay of his anti-cancer treatment might have impacted Jack and his survival.

To prescribe safely and effectively, it is essential that any prescriber keep up to date and maintain competence not only in medications but also in disease management and conditions (McHugh et al. 2020). A comprehensive systematic literature review highlighted that the fear of prescribing errors due to a restricted ability to undertake frequent continuous professional development (CPD) was a common source of anxiety for non-medical prescribers (Creedon et al. 2015). The skill of clinical reasoning and communication guiding decision-making during a patient consultation has been strongly linked with a background of expert knowledge paired with continuous learning (Abuzour et al. 2018).

It has become an increasing practice in many parts of the world for a review of a patient's health to be completed by telephone or video link (Richardson et al. 2020). However, while this has benefits, the lack of 'hands-on' clinical assessment makes for a challenging patient assessment and a source of anxiety for clinicians (Churchouse et al. 2021).

Case Study 2   Potential Difficulties with Remote Monitoring

Miriam (pseudonym) (she/her) was a 69-year-old lady who lived with her husband (he/him) and two dogs and was diagnosed with mantle cell lymphoma (low-grade lymphoma) four years previously. Miriam had gained remission with intravenous SACT at diagnosis but unfortunately relapsed and was commenced on ibrutinib (TKI), which had been well-tolerated for over two years. Miriam also had a medical history of depression and anxiety and type 2 diabetes mellitus, which was diet controlled. Miriam was taking citalopram 20 mg once daily, ibrutinib 420 mg once a day and prophylactic medication to reduce infection (aciclovir 400 mg twice daily and co-trimoxazole 480 mg twice daily on Monday, Wednesday and Friday). Miriam reported that her only allergy was a rash secondary to penicillin.

Miriam was on a 12 weekly telephone review with home delivery of medication since April 2020 due to COVID-19 restrictions. At her most recent telephone review with her CNS, Miriam's haemoglobin had dropped to 92 g/l (previous baseline 124 g/l). There was a slight drop in her mean corpuscular volume (MCV) level, which often suggests an element of iron deficiency, but no change in the rest of her bloods results.

During the telephone review, Miriam stated that she was experiencing some tiredness but no other symptoms suggestive of anaemia. Miriam reported that she had no gastro-intestinal symptoms, no change in diet, no new medications and no symptoms of bleeding. Miriam reported that she had no weight loss, night sweats, infections or swollen glands that may have been suggestive of malignant disease.

The CNS, working with the medical team, made a differential diagnosis of iron deficiency due to the drop in Miriam's haemoglobin and MCV, cause yet unknown. The CNS was aware that a secondary cancer can appear during cancer treatment, and the nurse was concerned for Miriam. The CNS asked Miriam to attend the clinic for a face-to-face assessment and further investigations.

When Miriam was reviewed in the clinic, the CNS observed that Miriam had developed a 3 cm right-sided neck node and had lost some weight. The CNS, along with Miriam's consultant, were concerned about progressive disease. A computerised tomography (CT) scan was requested, as well as additional bloods to assess for iron or vitamin deficiency and a referral to the gastro-intestinal team to rule out any additional cause for her anaemia, such as gastro-intestinal blood loss.

In discussing this with the CNS at the clinic, Miriam expressed her fear of coming back to hospital during a global pandemic and of requiring potentially 'stronger' treatment that would make her feel unwell and increase her risk of infection. Miriam admitted that she had chosen not to share her symptoms with her medical or nursing team and felt her current treatment would be enough to keep her disease under control. Being able to see Miriam face-to-face enabled the CNS to observe Miriam and pick up on her symptoms and concerns. While a video call could have improved the consultation, such calls still reduce the human connection between the nurse and the patient and restrict the essential skill of observing the patient as they enter the consultation. During the pandemic and the switch to telephone review, Miriam felt isolated and scared of the potential changes to her healthcare and did not know what to expect when she returned to the unit. In the face-to-face consultation, the CNS was able to allay Miriam's fears, providing prescribing information and support. Following a confirmation of disease progression, Miriam was commenced on a new treatment regimen and went into disease remission.

The recent rapid move to additional telemedicine clinics highlighted some issues surrounding confidentiality, governance, effective communication, shared decision-making and safety netting. Consequently, the Health & Care Professionals Council (2021) developed their guidance. High-level principles for good practice in remote consultations and prescribing underpin telemedicine and ensure effectiveness and governance. All these guidelines, the use of forums for peer support and the use of online non-medical prescribing toolkits can help maintain competence and safeguard both new and experienced prescribers.

12.7 Conclusion

Alistair Campbell (1984) previously described the role of the healthcare professional as one of a skilled companion. The nurse, the doctor, the allied health professional and the prescriber are called on to use their clinical knowledge and expertise alongside the gift of being a companion and providing support to those in need. Similarly, Quinn et al. (2017) suggest that in managing or treating any condition or concern, there is a need for the practitioner/prescriber to pay attention to the individual, see beyond the symptom and recognise the impact the condition or symptom has on the individual's life. West and Chowla (2017) describe the ongoing need for a more compassionate approach to care, which involves being present and open to hear and acknowledge the distress of those in need. Similarly, it requires the prescriber to be open and willing to listen, to be present and to learn from those they care for.

The role of the nurse prescriber within the CNS role requires the prescriber to move beyond a medical focus of care to explore the personal meaning of symptoms for the individual (Quinn 2022). It requires a more person-centred approach, where the prescriber listens to what is important for the individual and is willing to walk alongside them. Sheila Cassidy, a doctor and a prescriber, in her book *Sharing the Darkness* (Cassidy 1988), reflecting on the role of healthcare professionals in supporting people with advanced disease and facing death, suggests that those who are ill know the limitations of nursing and healthcare practice but are asking healthcare practitioners to stay with them and support them at difficult and uncertain times. It means being prepared to work as a member of the team as a compassionate prescriber, including responding to diverse needs within community and hospital settings and, most importantly, responding to the person in need.

References

Abuzour, A.S., Lewis, P.J., and Tully, M.P. (2018). A qualitative study exploring how pharmacist and nurse independent prescribers make clinical decisions. *Journal of Advanced Nursing* 74 (1): 65–74.

Alessy, S.A., Lüchtenborg, M., Rawlinson, J. et al. (2021). Being assigned a clinical nurse specialist is associated with better experiences of cancer care: English population-based study using the linked National Cancer Patient Experience Survey and Cancer registration dataset. *European Journal of Cancer Care* 30 (6): 1–11.

Campbell, A. (1984). *Moderated Love: A Theology of Professional Care*. London: SPCK.

Cannaby, A.M., Carter, V., Rolland, P. et al. (2020). The scope and variance of clinical nurse specialist job descriptions. *British Journal of Nursing* 29 (11): 606–611.

Carey, N. and Stenner, K. (2020). Preparing to prescribe: an online implementation tool kit for non-medical prescribers. *Journal of Prescribing Practice* 2 (10): 532–533.

Cassidy, S. (1988). *Sharing the Darkness*. London: Darton, Longman and Todd.

Churchouse, W., Griffiths, B., Sewell, P. et al. (2021). Remote consultations, prescribing and virtual teaching during the COVID-19 pandemic. *Journal of Prescribing Practice* 3 (7): 264–272.

Courtenay, M., Carey, N., and Stenner, K. (2011). Non medical prescribing leads views on their role the implementation of non-medical prescribing from a multi-organisational perspective. *BMC Health Services Research* 11: 1–10.

Creedon, R., Byrne, S., Kennedy, J., and McCarthy, S. (2015). The impact of nurse prescribing on the clinical setting. *British Journal of Nursing* 24 (17): 878–885.

Department of Health and Social Security (1986). *Neighbourhood Nursing – A Focus for Care. Report of the Community Nursing Review Cumberlege Report*. London: HMSO.

Graham-Clarke, E., Rushton, A., Noblet, T., and Marriott, J. (2018). Facilitators and barriers to non-medical prescribing – a systematic review and thematic synthesis. *PLoS One* 13 (4): 1–18.

Hand, P.R. (2019). Non-medical prescribing of systemic aanti-cancertherapy in a multidisciplinary team oncology clinic. *British Journal of Nursing* 28 (11): 715–720.

Health & Care Professionals Council. (2021). High level principles for good practice in remote consultations and prescribing. https://www.hcpc-uk.org/standards/ meeting-our-standards/scope-of-practice/high-level-principles (accessed 23 January 2022).

International Council of Nurses. (2020). Guidelines on advanced practice nursing. https://www.icn.ch/system/files/documents/2020-04/ICN_APN%20Report_EN_ WEB.pdf (accessed 14 September 2022).

James, J. (2006). A review of non-medical prescribing: current practice and future developments. *European Diabetes Nursing* 3 (1): 46–51.

Kerr, H., Donovan, M., and McSorley, O. (2021). Evaluation of the role of the clinical nurse specialist in cancer care: an integrative literature review. *European Journal of Cancer Care* 30 (3): 1–13.

Luker, K., Austin, L., Willcock, J. et al. (1997). 'Nurses' and GPs' views on the nurse prescribers' formulary–evaluation of nurse prescribing. *Nursing Standard* 11 (22): 33–38.

McHugh, A., Hughes, M., Higgins, A. et al. (2020). Non-medical prescribers: prescribing within practice. *Journal of Prescribing Practice* 2 (2): 68–77.

McKenna, H. and Keeney, S. (2004). Community nursing: health professional and public perceptions. *Journal of Advanced Nursing* 48 (1): 17–25.

National Institute for Health and Clinical Excellence. (2015). Medicines optimisation: the safe and effective use of medicines to enable the best possible outcomes. https://www.nice.org.uk/guidance/ng5 (accessed 7 August 2022).

National Institute for Health and Clinical Excellence. (2017). Patient group directions. https://www.nice.org.uk/guidance/mpg2 (accessed 24 July 2022).

National Prescribing Centre. (2001). Maintaining competency in prescribing. An outline framework to help nurse prescribers.

National Prescribing Centre. (2012). A single competency framework for all prescribers.

Noblet, T., Marriott, J., Graham-Clarke, E. et al. (2018). Clinical and cost-effectiveness of non-medical prescribing: systematic review of randomised controlled trials. *PLoS One* 13 (3): 1–15.

Nursing and Midwifery Council. (2018a). Standards of proficiency for registered nurses. https://www.nmc.org.uk/standards/standards-for-nurses/standards-of- proficiency-for-registered-nurses (accessed 7 August 2022).

Nursing and Midwifery Council. (2018b). Part 3: Standards for prescribing programmes. https://www.nmc.org.uk/globalassets/sitedocuments/education- standards/programme-standards-prescribing.pdf (accessed 7 August 2022).

Nursing and Midwifery Council (2019). Becoming a prescriber. https://www.nmc.org. uk/education/becoming-a-nurse-midwife-nursing-associate/becoming-a-prescriber (accessed 7 August 2022).

Nuttall, D. (2013). Self-assessing competence in non-medical prescribing. *Nurse Prescribing* 10 (11): 510–514. https://www.magonlinelibrary.com/doi/abs/ 10.12968/npre.2013.11.10.510.

Omer, U., Veysey, M., Crampton, P., and Finn, G. (2021). What makes a model prescriber? A documentary analysis. *Medical Teacher* 43 (2): 198–207.

Quinn, B. (2022). How should nurses assess and manage pain in a person with cancer? *Cancer Nursing Practice* 14 (18).

Quinn, B., Luftner, D., Di Pala, M. et al. (2017). Managing pain in the advanced cancer setting. *Cancer Nursing Practice* 16 (10): 27–34.

Richardson, E., Aissat, D., Williams, G.A., and Fahy, N. (2020). Keeping what works: remote consultations during the COVID-19 pandemic. *Eurohealth* 26 (2): 73–76.

Royal College of Nursing. (2018). RCN standards for advanced level nursing practice. https://www.rcn.org.uk/Professional-Development/publications/pub-007038 (accessed 7 August 2022).

Royal Pharmaceutical Society. (2016). A competency framework for all prescribers.

Royal Pharmaceutical Society. (2021). A competency framework for all prescribers. https://www.rpharms.com/resources/frameworks/prescribing-competency-framework/competency-framework (accessed 7 August 2022).

West, M. and Chowla, R. (2017). Compassionate leadership for compassionate health care. In: *Compassion: Concepts, Research and Applications* (ed. P. Gilbert), 237–257. London: Routledge.

World Health Organisation. (2021). The WHO global strategic directions for nursing and midwifery (2021–2025). https://www.who.int/publications/i/item/ 9789240033863 (accessed 7 August 2022).

13

Cancer in the Adolescent and Young Adult

Kerrie Sweeney and Helen Kerr

Abstract

Adolescents and young adults with cancer are a distinct group with specific needs unique to their physical and psycho-social development. This period of life can be challenging at the best of times, as young people develop their own independence in life, but a cancer diagnosis can result in additional significant challenges, posing a risk of isolation, psychological distress, educational or vocational failure as well as leading to long-term health concerns in adult life.

This chapter will discuss some of the key skills and attributes of the clinical nurse specialist (CNS) required to provide age-appropriate care for this patient group, such as person- and family-centred individualised holistic care, acting as a key worker, collaborative multidisciplinary working, age-appropriate communication, improvements to the hospital environment and opportunities for peer support. The CNS is in a key position to advocate for the needs of teenagers and young adults, enhancing outcomes for young people.

13.1 Introduction

This chapter will focus on the skills and attributes required by the clinical nurse specialist (CNS) to support adolescents and young adults (AYAs) with cancer, including a discussion on some of the key priorities of care. The first author, Kerrie Sweeney, works as a teenage and young adult (TYA) CNS in the Northern Health and Social Care Trust (NHSCT), Northern Ireland (NI). This post is funded by the Teenage Cancer Trust (TCT), one of the United Kingdom's (UK) leading AYA cancer charities that funds many CNS and youth support co-ordinator posts across the UK in addition to providing age-appropriate environments and support

The Role of the Clinical Nurse Specialist in Cancer Care, First Edition. Edited by Helen Kerr.
© 2024 John Wiley & Sons Ltd. Published 2024 by John Wiley & Sons Ltd.
Companion website: www.wiley.com/go/kerr

for young people and professionals. The second author, Helen Kerr, is a senior lecturer at the School of Nursing and Midwifery, Queen's University Belfast, with a clinical nursing background in cancer and palliative care.

Within NI, the regional TYA cancer service supports young people aged 13 years up to their 25th birthday with any cancer diagnosis. Although the term *TYA* is generally used to describe this group of patients in the context of the UK, the term *adolescent and young adult* (AYA) is generally used globally, so the latter will be predominately used in this chapter.

Cancer is rare in the AYA age group. However, within the four countries of the UK, there are approximately 2110 diagnoses per year in the 15–24 year age group, with five-year survival figures estimated at 87% (Public Health England 2021). Approximately 75 young people within this age range are diagnosed each year within NI (Cancer Research 2021). The regional TYA cancer service across all of NI was launched in 2017 to ensure that specialist support was available to all AYAs throughout NI. The TYA CNSs in NI provide support as part of a wider multidisciplinary team to any AYA who presents to any of the Health and Social Care Trusts (HSCTs) in NI as an inpatient or outpatient or to community teams.

Within NI, there are six HSCTs: Belfast, Southern, Northern, Western and South-Eastern HSCTs and the NI Ambulance Service, which provides support to all of NI. The wider NI TYA cancer team currently consists of CNSs, specialist social workers, ward support specialists and a community worker. Teenagers aged 13–15 years old are usually treated within paediatric cancer services at the Royal Belfast Hospital for Sick Children, NI, whilst young adults who are diagnosed or who relapse from 16 years or over are usually treated within adult services across NI. The majority of AYAs in NI are treated within the main Cancer Centre located in the capital city of Belfast, NI. However, approximately half of all AYAs are diagnosed and treated in one of the regional cancer units throughout NI.

13.2 Background to Adolescent and Young Adult Cancer Services

AYAs can develop a wide range of cancers, which may cross between paediatric and adult protocols. Some more common cancer types in the AYA age group include leukaemia, central nervous system and brain tumours, lymphomas, germ cell cancers and malignant melanoma (Public Health England 2021). Whilst there are some specific 'true' AYA cancers, others involve late presentation of paediatric cancers or early presentation of adult cancers and may include some carcinomas, lymphoma or bone tumours (Barr et al. 2006; Carr et al. 2013; Smith et al. 2016). Close working relationships between adult and paediatric clinicians are therefore vital to ensure appropriate treatment plans (Ferrari 2014; Osborn et al. 2019). Some evidence suggests AYAs experience poorer outcomes than younger children and older adults; for example, acute lymphoblastic leukaemia and sarcoma are associated with higher survival rates when diagnosed in children than AYAs (Carr et al. 2013; Wilhelm et al. 2014; Stark et al. 2015). AYAs have a unique biology that differs from older adults or children and can result in specific challenges from a pharmacology and drug toxicity perspective as well as pose a risk of the development of distinct late effects later in life (Stark et al. 2015).

The period of adolescence into young adulthood is associated with rapid physical, psychological, social and cognitive development (Ginsberg et al. 2006; World Health Organisation 2017). Smith et al. (2016) discuss that this development includes rapid physical changes driven by hormones and changes within the brain itself and continues through adolescence into adulthood, until the late twenties or early thirties. They also discuss psycho-social development, as young people are developing their own self-identity, beliefs and independence and may be developing intimate relationships and relying on peers rather than families for support. This normal physical and psycho-social development can be difficult for any young person to navigate, and a cancer diagnosis can result in immense challenges (Smith et al. 2016). Young people may be faced with complex and lengthy treatment regimens such as chemotherapy, immunotherapy, radiotherapy, stem cell transplants or surgery, which have the potential to impact normal physical development, growth and puberty. Additionally, cancer poses a risk of educational or vocational failure, which may result in feelings of loneliness and isolation as young people observe their peers moving on with their lives (Smith et al. 2016). Levels of distress in AYAs with cancer have been indicated to be more directly associated with psycho-social concerns than specific variables related to cancer type or stage (Kwak et al. 2013; McCarthy et al. 2016).

Traditional models of care struggle to meet the evolving autonomy and psychosocial needs of young people. Paediatric services are traditionally family-orientated, with a strong focus on family member involvement in decision-making (Ferrari et al. 2017; Osborn et al. 2019). Adult services, whilst promoting more individual patient autonomy, can still be challenging for young people, as many will benefit from a level of family or professional support to help in advocating for their healthcare needs and supporting them to navigate the complex healthcare systems (Sansom-Daly et al. 2016; Osborn et al. 2019). Furthermore, psycho-social concerns tend to be addressed with a more reactive approach in adult services compared to paediatric services, which may not suit the complex needs of AYAs (Osborn et al. 2019). Therefore, it is now well-recognised that young people with cancer have specific and unique needs that differ from younger children and older adults, and AYA specialist services have evolved globally in response to provide specialist support.

Within the UK, several guidance documents set out requirements for AYA care. In 2005, the National Institute for Health and Care Excellence (NICE) (2005) published 'Improving Outcomes in Children and Young People with Cancer'. This best practice guidance addresses children and young people with cancer up to the age of 24 years. Some of the key recommendations include co-ordinated care, services close to the patient's home, the availability of a key worker, delivery of age-appropriate care, availability of specialist multidisciplinary staff and accessibility to clinical trials. NICE (2014) published further recommendations in 2014 by developing quality standards for 'Cancer Services for Children and Young People', promoting measurable quality care with respect to priorities of care, such as availability of clinical trials and fertility preservation. The National Cancer Peer Review Team – National Cancer Action Team (2011) published 'Teenage and Young Adult Measures' in 2011, which set out standards for benchmarking AYA services across the UK. NHS England (2013/2014) set out AYA service specifications (currently under review) outlining recommendations in relation to the organisation and delivery of AYA services in England, UK. Similar guidance is available in different geographical contexts.

Within the UK and worldwide, the role of the non-statutory/voluntary sector has been crucial in the creation and establishment of AYA services (Lea et al. 2018; Osborn et al. 2019). Presently, within NI, funding for the AYA cancer service is provided solely from charitable organisations such as TCT, Young Lives vs Cancer, Friends of the Cancer Centre, Cancer Fund for Children and The Children's Cancer Unit Charity. TCT was one of the first UK charities to drive AYA services across the UK in the 1990s, establishing specialist units for this group of patients (Lea et al. 2018). Similarly, in other parts of the world, non-statutory organisations play a vital role in supporting the delivery of AYA services: for example, CanTeen Australia in Australia and Canada's, Canadian Partnership Against Cancer (Osborn et al. 2019). Such organisations also provide vital practical support and information to young people and their families and provide support and networks for professionals. The non-statutory and voluntary sectors play a vital role in driving policy and guidance for AYA care. TCT, for example, published a best practice document entitled 'A Blueprint of Care' to support AYA services within the UK, providing recommendations and advice when working with the AYA age group (Smith et al. 2016).

The term *age-appropriate care* is widely used to describe delivery of AYA services (NICE 2005, 2014); however, there is no standard definition of this term. Lea et al. (2018) carried out a mixed-methods study across 29 UK hospitals – using semi-structured interviews involving young people with cancer and AYA healthcare professionals along with a literature review to establish what encompasses age-appropriate care for AYAs – that led to seven key components. These include best treatment, healthcare professional knowledge, communication, interactions and relationships, recognising individuality, empowering young people, and promoting normality and the environment. These components can be used as a framework for AYA CNSs and wider teams to plan age-appropriate AYA service delivery. A joined-up approach to care is recommended between site-specific and AYA cancer teams, allowing AYAs to be supported by professionals with expertise in specific cancer types as well as those with expertise in their age group (NICE 2005; Marris et al. 2011; Lea et al. 2018).

13.3 Person-Centred Adolescent and Young Adult Care

The AYA population are a heterogeneous and diverse group; therefore, approaches to AYA care must facilitate flexibility and individualised care. Young people differ in terms of cultural, sexual and gender identity (Hammond 2017). In addition, they may differ in terms of their independent living ability. Whilst some young people may live independently from a young age, others may remain at home with parents for much longer into adulthood, perhaps focusing on their career or education before establishing their own homes and families (Fry et al. 2018). The CNS must recognise and adapt to meet the range of needs of this divergent population. A person-centred approach to care is, therefore, essential.

Person-centred care is defined as care that places the individual first, with a focus on respect, empowerment and holistic individualised care (Morgan and Yoder 2012). Lea et al. (2018) report that AYA professionals and young people alike value the importance of individualised care. TCT advocate for this approach in their 'Blueprint of Care' document, where they recommend viewing the AYA as a young person first, getting to know their interests and hobbies, rather than exclusively focusing on their cancer diagnosis (Smith et al. 2016). This approach to care and communication can help foster therapeutic relationships through building rapport, dialogue and trust between young people and professionals (Smith et al. 2016; Vindrola-Padros et al. 2016; Ferrari et al. 2017). The AYA CNS can help to promote therapeutic relationships by focusing on person-centred care, patient involvement and the care context (Kitson et al. 2013; Lea et al. 2018).

13.4 Support for Family and Significant Others

Person-centred approaches in AYA care must include the young adult's support networks such as family, siblings, friends and partners (Osborn et al. 2019). AYAs often rely heavily on these networks for support during a cancer diagnosis and treatment. The impact of an AYA cancer diagnosis on the whole family is well-recognised, with individuals experiencing varying levels of distress (Osborn et al. 2019). Additionally, families may face particular financial or employment concerns, as it is not uncommon for parents or carers to have to take time off work to facilitate appointments, stay with a young person during a hospital admission or care for the young person at home during treatment. The AYA CNS and wider team have a role in supporting the wider AYA network, which may include siblings or their own children, friends and partner; identifying any concerns, such as educational or psychological needs; and ensuring the availability of appropriate support or signposting to other agencies (Smith et al. 2016). It is therefore essential that the AYA CNS adopts a flexible, person-centred, family-focused, individualised approach to care that reflects the unique needs of each individual AYA and their family.

13.5 Holistic Care

It is recommended that each young person be allocated a key worker (NICE 2005). The AYA CNS usually occupies the role as a key worker, which may involve adopting a collaborative approach along with site-specific CNSs. (The key worker role is the focus of Chapter 5 of this book.) This role has overall coordination of care and provides the young person and their family with a point of contact for information, support and advice throughout the whole cancer trajectory (Smith et al. 2016). This promotes a level of continuity of care, which further enhances the establishment of therapeutic relationships (Vindrola-Padros et al. 2016).

A holistic approach to AYA care is imperative to meet the unique psychosocial needs of this population (Kwak et al. 2013; NICE 2014; McCarthy et al. 2016). A holistic needs assessment (HNA) and care planning are useful tools the CNS can use to help identify and address any concerns shared by the young person. The HNA is a vital element of the recovery package and should be offered to patients who have a cancer diagnosis at specific time points in the patient journey (National Cancer Survivorship Initiative [NCSI] 2013). The Recovery Package initiative was set up in the UK to improve outcomes for individuals with cancer with recommendations that promote holistic, person-centred and integrated care through interventions such as HNA, treatment summaries, cancer care review, and health and well-being events (NCSI 2013). The output of the HNA is a person-centred care plan focusing on empowerment and promoting self-management, with signposting and/or referral to other organisations that can provide support. The care plan should be made available to other key professionals, such as the general practitioner (GP)/primary physician, to ensure that all are aware of the specific holistic needs of the individual. Identifying these needs early and introducing appropriate support mechanisms has been associated with increased quality of life during treatment and beyond (Osborn et al. 2019).

Various HNA tools have been created specifically for AYAs that aim to identify psycho-social and emotional needs distinct to this age group. One example is the Integrated Assessment Map (IAM) tool (TCT 2020b). AYAs can access the IAM tool remotely via a digital app that enables users to carry out a self-assessment of any concerns they may be experiencing based on 10 specific domains, such as education and work, sex, sexuality and fertility, and thoughts and feelings. Links to information specific to their concerns are available, and the young person has the option to share their assessment with an AYA professional (TCT 2020b). This information enables the AYA CNS to open a discussion and facilitate understanding of the young person's specific concerns, such as education, family relationships, sexuality, body image and emotional wellbeing (Smith et al. 2016). These tools can be particularly useful in initiating conversations on perhaps more sensitive topics such as sexual health, which may be difficult for some healthcare professionals to address, by providing an opportunity for the professional to introduce a discussion based on the needs identified by the individual (Albers et al. 2020).

13.6 Multidisciplinary Working

Due to the potential complexity of psycho-social needs of young people, close collaborative working with other allied professionals is crucial (Osborn et al. 2019). The AYA CNS usually works as part of a multidisciplinary team (MDT) of specialist AYA staff, which may include social workers, youth workers, a champion or lead clinician and a psychologist (NICE 2005, 2014; Osborn et al. 2019). Each member of the team provides different strengths and skillsets, enhancing AYA care (Knott et al. 2013; Lea et al. 2019). Close teamworking amongst the AYA MDT with shared learning opportunities alongside an ethos where professionals support one another has been associated with positive care delivery outcomes (Knott et al. 2013; Vindrola-Padros et al. 2016).

The AYA CNS should encourage early referral to relevant allied professionals, such as AYA social workers and youth workers, as this is crucial in reducing distress and improving coping mechanisms (Osborn et al. 2019). Additionally, AYAs can face many mental health concerns, which may continue into later life; therefore, early involvement of psychology services is advocated when appropriate. However, access to specialist AYA psychology or counselling services can be difficult in some areas throughout the UK (TCT 2021). Whilst some areas have established psychology services specifically for AYAs, many areas rely on services open to the general cancer population, which are facing increasing demands whilst managing limited resources. During the COVID-19 pandemic, TCT surveyed young people with cancer and found that 53% reported difficulties accessing emotional and psychological support (TCT 2020a). The AYA CNS has a vital role in providing one-to-one emotional support to young people, which can be a crucial source of support, as well as developing links with local psychology and counselling services to help promote early referral and intervention, when appropriate.

It is recommended that AYAs be discussed at both a cancer site-specific MDT meeting and an AYA MDT meeting, with the aim of combining disease-specific and age-specific expertise as well as incorporating holistic care to improve outcomes for patients (The National Cancer Peer Review Team – National Cancer Action Team 2011; NICE 2014). Throughout the UK, the AYA MDT is often called the multidisciplinary advisory team (MDaT) to distinguish it from the site-specific MDT, whose primary aim is diagnosis and treatment decision-making. The AYA CNS presents AYAs at the MDaT to facilitate holistic discussions regarding young people at diagnosis and end of treatment, and during the transition between services or any other significant events such as relapse. In NI, treatment-related decisions currently remain with the site-specific MDTs, and where possible, the AYA CNS attends site-specific MDT meetings. As recommended by Osborn et al. (2019), such visibility in MDT meetings facilitates the development of relationships and wider networks, early referral and awareness of the AYA service.

Within NI, alongside established AYA referral processes, the teenage and young adult cancer service have established a screening system for red flag referrals in the AYA age group, which facilitates the CNS to identify newly diagnosed AYAs at an early stage. Many UK MDaTs now incorporate the HNA programme, the IAM portal that feeds directly into the MDaT (TCT 2020b). As previously discussed, this allows young people to access a programme remotely, identifying their own concerns and further enhancing the patient's voice within the MDaT.

13.7 Healthcare Professional Knowledge

It is recognised that AYAs benefit from healthcare professionals with expertise in both their cancer and treatment as well as developmental, psycho-social and practical considerations (Bleyer and Barr 2016; Bibby et al. 2017; Lea et al. 2018). Professionals who demonstrate a passion for AYA care are reported as desirable by young people (Gibson et al. 2012; Lea et al. 2018). However, specialist AYA professionals make up a small workforce, and with young people presenting across many different settings, access to specialist staff can be challenging (TCT 2014). TCT (2014) developed competencies specifically for nurses involved in the care of AYAs, which have been endorsed by the Royal College of Nursing (RCN). These competencies aim to increase the skills, competence and knowledge of any nursing staff working with AYAs, setting out proposed training and skills based on three levels. These levels commence with being competent and progress to experienced/proficient and finally to being an expert. However, implementing such a framework can be challenging due to difficulty in releasing staff to attend relevant courses and training.

As the numbers of AYAs with cancer are small, many healthcare professionals rarely have the opportunity to care for young people in their practice, which can result in a lack of experience and awareness of the unique needs of young people. Therefore, the AYA CNS's role is paramount in facilitating education and awareness of AYA issues with other key multidisciplinary staff, which may be facilitated through formal education sessions or study days or on an informal basis when working directly with other staff.

13.8 Adolescent and Young Adult Clinical Nurse Specialist Leadership Skills

AYA teams cut across many teams and services throughout primary and secondary care. Working across settings in this manner can bring its own challenges, as each setting has its own leaders and leadership approaches. The AYA CNS may benefit from adopting a collective transformational leadership approach, inspiring and influencing others within the organisation to take ownership of shared goals and vision to improve outcomes, quality of care and patient satisfaction (Alloubani et al. 2019; De Vries and Curtis 2019; Anselmann and Mulder 2020; Bush et al. 2020). Establishing local steering groups and other such forums can also be useful in providing a platform to help promote a shared vision and successes across teams (Eckert et al. 2014).

Within NI, a teenage and young adult cancer regional clinical reference group (CRG) is well-established, with membership that includes clinicians, AYA professionals, and management from across all HSCTs in NI, as well as a young person representative. The aim of this regional group is to oversee and lead on the development of the NI teenage and young adult service, offering expertise and guidance with an aim to ensure high-quality, age-appropriate equitable care to AYAs throughout NI. The establishment of a strategic advisory board has been shown to be a strong enabler for improving AYA services (Osborn et al. 2019).

13.9 Communication with Adolescents and Young Adults

Young people have expressed benefits from being kept well-informed throughout their cancer journey (Lea et al. 2018). This involves professionals providing timely, honest, age-appropriate communication (Osborn et al. 2019). It is important that information is consistent and accurate across all professionals (Mulhall et al. 2004). Much of the age-appropriate written information is available from the AYA-specific non-statutory/charitable organisations, which can help support verbal conversations. Unmet information needs have been associated with distress and decreased quality of life in the healthcare needs of young people (DeRouen et al. 2015; Bibby et al. 2017), highlighting the fundamental requirement to focus on assessing and meeting the holistic needs of the young person by skilled professionals who are competent in providing care and supporting AYAs.

A study by Bibby et al. (2017) that focused on AYAs' preferred communication styles suggested that young people prefer healthcare professionals to exhibit both expertise and knowledge alongside communication skills in providing emotional support to a young person. Other studies suggest that young people appreciate friendly, kind professionals who offer support and take time to listen (Gibson et al. 2012; Vindrola-Padros et al. 2016). Supportive, honest, open communication is key to building therapeutic relationships with young people (Darby et al. 2014; Lea et al. 2020). By adopting these skills, the AYA CNS can act as a role model for other healthcare professionals who may not be as comfortable communicating with young people. The CNS can also advocate for the importance of establishing professional boundaries with young people, as given the nature of AYA care and the close relationships that can evolve, there can be a risk of blurring boundaries. This can be difficult particularly for more inexperienced or younger staff members; signs of potential blurring of boundaries, such as oversharing of personal information or spending time with a young person outside of work, should be observed for and discouraged and appropriate support provided to the relevant staff member (Smith et al. 2016).

The AYA CNS can empower the young person by providing all necessary information to facilitate independent decision-making and autonomy concerning treatment choices and plans (Gibson et al. 2012; Knott et al. 2013). However, this must be balanced with providing advocacy and support where appropriate, encouraging young people to have an active voice in their care, as some will require support from both families and professionals in decision-making (Coyne et al. 2014). Information-giving should be tailored to the age, personality, developmental stage and stage of treatment of the young person, as needs will vary across the cancer trajectory (Lea et al. 2019; Osborn et al. 2019).

Smith et al. (2016) state that AYAs with cancer may demonstrate regressive or childlike behaviours, persistent egocentrism and risk-taking behaviours. Such behaviours can be intensified by illness, which may result in communication challenges or treatment concordance difficulties. Behaviours may fluctuate, and the communication styles of the CNS must be responsive to these variations.

Text messaging can be a useful tool for the CNS when communicating with young people, to encourage engagement and concordance with treatment regimens (Smith et al. 2016). Wijeratne et al. (2021) completed a systematic review that included 18 papers related to text messaging in cancer supportive care. Whilst they conclude that more research is required to identify what is needed for a successful text messaging initiative, they outline benefits related to text messaging, which include cost-effectiveness, patient satisfaction and benefits in promoting medication concordance. Text messaging is considered to be particularly appealing to young people with cancer, given that this age group tend to use this mode of communication frequently (Psihogois et al. 2019).

AYAs live in a digital world, with most having access to computers or other devices, so virtual and digital methods of communication must be considered (Moody et al. 2014; Abrol et al. 2017). A cross-sectional survey on communication preferences of young people by Abrol et al. (2017) suggested that AYAs aged 19–25 years preferred digital availability of clinical information as well as online counselling. Within the NHSCT, the TYA CNS and wider team have piloted communication with young people using WhatsApp and Zoom, which has received positive feedback from patients. Various digital self-management programmes have been established; however, barriers and challenges such as governance considerations can exist in implementing online interventions (Moody et al. 2014). It is recommended that young people should be offered a choice between face-to-face and virtual alternatives (Abrol et al. 2017), with a recommendation that in-person contact should be available to support any digital interventions (Moody et al. 2014).

13.10 Age-Appropriate Environments

Providing an age-appropriate environment is a key priority for AYA care (NICE 2005; Smith et al. 2016). Young people may feel out of place in adult care settings, finding the environment intimidating, isolating and distressing and associating it with boredom (Marshall et al. 2018; Osborn et al. 2019). Across the UK, many bespoke AYA units have been established within AYA principle treatment centres (PTCs). These units have been shown to improve the experience of young people by providing a social space to bring young people together, along with access to specialist staff and resources such as music, activities, internet and provision for family members to stay overnight (Taylor et al. 2011; Darby et al. 2014; Vindrola-Padros et al. 2016). However, there is no such AYA unit in NI, and it is estimated that up to two-thirds of AYAs throughout the UK do not have access to a specialised unit (Birch et al. 2014).

The AYA CNS can encourage interventions to promote an age-appropriate ethos, such as flexibility of visiting and appointments, support from AYA teams, opportunities for peer support, access to Wi-Fi, provisions of electronic or gaming devices, or timing of medical review or medication rounds to allow a later wake-up for the young person whilst an inpatient (Smith et al. 2016; Lea et al. 2018; Marshall et al. 2018). The BRIGHTLIGHT study, which surveyed experiences of AYAs in England, UK, suggested that quality of life was measured higher by those AYAs treated outside of the AYA PTC (Taylor et al. 2020). Precise reasons for this are unclear, although one possible rationale provided is that patients prefer having treatment closer to home, allowing for as normal life as possible. Promoting normality is advocated by encouraging young people to keep in touch with peers, continuing education where appropriate and encouraging as normal a routine as possible (Marris et al. 2011; Smith et al. 2016; Lea et al. 2018). Young people also benefit from as much time at home as possible (Smith et al. 2016), although this can be challenging when patients are required to be in hospital for lengthy treatments. The AYA CNS can promote flexible access for families and friends to visit, which can help reduce loneliness that may be experienced during admissions (Lea et al. 2019).

AYA teams evolve individually in how to best improve the environment and services they provide to young people in their context (Osborn et al. 2019). The AYA CNS is well placed to explore opportunities to improve the environment, such as securing and decorating an area specifically for young people (Osborn et al. 2019).

13.11   Adolescent and Young Adult Peer Support

Peer support is another key element of AYA care, shown to be crucial for improving the experience of AYAs (Smith et al. 2016; Lea et al. 2018). It is well-documented that young people benefit from meeting others of a similar age and shared experience (Knott et al. 2013; Lea et al. 2019). The AYA CNS and wider AYA team are well-placed to encourage opportunities for peer support (Lea et al. 2019). Thinking of alternative interventions and collaborative working can help to develop approaches for peer support. Outside of AYA units, it is not uncommon for a young person with cancer to never meet another young person with cancer of a similar age whilst receiving treatment.

Within the NHSCT, the TYA CNS is undertaking a pilot scheme entitled 'TYA chemo clinic' to facilitate young people attending the clinic on a set day, opening up the opportunity for peer support during treatment. AYA teams in NI have established many diverse peer support groups for young people. Examples include exercise groups, games nights, drama or crafts workshops, bowling and make-up groups; groups with a practical focus, such as fatigue management, employment, finance and education concerns; and an interactive laboratory workshop where young people with a diagnosis of lymphoma were given the opportunity to be taken through interactive stations in a laboratory at the NHSCT, NI, demonstrating every step of the diagnostic process. Additionally, in the context of the UK, AYAs have access to national peer support groups such as TCT's Find Your Sense of Tumour conference in England, UK.

13.12   Adolescent and Young Adult Treatment Priorities

Best treatment is a priority for AYAs and requires the availability of appropriate specialists, treatment choices, place of treatment and opportunities for AYAs to engage in clinical trials that provide access to novel treatments and optimal care

(NICE 2005, 2014; Lea et al. 2018). The use of clinical trials has been linked to higher survival rates amongst childhood cancers (Hart et al. 2020); however, access to trials is challenging for AYAs across the UK and beyond (Osborn et al. 2019). Reasons include age-restrictive eligibility, the rarity of AYA cancers, scarcity of resources, lengthy difficult processes in setting up trials, inappropriate design for AYAs and trials being restricted to certain treatment centres (Fern et al. 2014; Hart et al. 2020). Therefore, ways to promote AYA trials must be explored, including re-configuration of trials, review of trial eligibility criteria, and research and administration for clinical trials (Hart et al. 2021). The CNS has a crucial role in advocating for and supporting young people to access clinical trials where available, working collaboratively alongside other AYA professionals. A study by Taylor et al. (2016) suggested that young people value information and input from clinically trained professionals such as the CNS or clinician concerning clinical research, such as drug/treatment research, whilst valuing the role of other AYA professionals, such as the social worker, in relation to non-clinical research choices.

Fertility is a well-recognised priority for young people (NICE 2014; Ahmad et al. 2016; Smith et al. 2016). Fertility discussions should be facilitated at the earliest opportunity regardless of the level of fertility risk, as treatment plans can change and many treatments, particularly chemotherapy, have at least some potential to disrupt normal fertility (Ahmad et al. 2016). The AYA CNS is well placed to facilitate such discussions, which should include contraceptive advice and pregnancy risk during and after treatment (Smith et al. 2016). The AYA CNS can advocate for the young person, ensuring appropriate and timely offers of fertility cryopreservation (taking into consideration urgency to commence treatment), which may include offers of sperm banking, egg or embryo freezing, or freezing of ovarian tissue (Teenagers and Young Adults with Cancer [TYAC] 2016). The AYA CNS can raise awareness of fertility issues with medical and nursing colleagues and has a role in advocating for fertility priorities of patients as well as in creating links with fertility services and specialists (Osborn et al. 2019).

13.13 Transitional Adolescent and Young Adult Care

Transitions of care are a regular occurrence for AYAs across the various patient pathways. These may include transitions to other hospitals for specialist treatment, such as stem cell transplant or clinical trials, transferring from children's to adult services and transition from acute to survivorship or palliative care. Good working relationships across teams, along with supportive relationships with patients and families, are crucial in supporting young people through these transitions, which can be difficult and challenging (TYAC 2015). The AYA CNS is perfectly placed to support transitions of care due to well-established relationships with young people and their families and often acts as the key worker or co-ordinator throughout the transition process (Kerr 2021). The young person should be central to the transition, which should be carefully planned and ideally carried out at a pace that suits them; offers of joint clinic reviews or early visits to the new place of care can help prepare the young person and their family (TYAC 2015; Kerr 2021). Providing supportive documentation such as treatment summaries and care plans or health passports is useful in ensuring that key, relevant information is available to appropriate professionals (NICE 2014; TYAC 2015; Kerr 2021).

13.14 Living With and Beyond Cancer

End of treatment is a key transition where young people are faced with many challenges, including feelings of uncertainty, fear of relapse or mortality, body image concerns, long-term health concerns and difficulties reintegrating into their peer groups, education or the workplace (Zebrack 2011; Moody et al. 2014; Lea et al. 2020). This period can be associated with feelings of abandonment and enhanced isolation (Meneses et al. 2010). The AYA CNS and wider team have a role in enabling and supporting young people during this reintegration, which may require specialist input over several years (Smith et al. 2016; Osborn et al. 2019). Lea et al. (2020) suggest that AYAs benefit from timely, structured, accessible support at the end of treatment.

Some nurse-led models provide formalised end-of-treatment clinics or psychosocial follow-up delivered at key points following the completion of treatment. These models have been found to be beneficial in providing a forum for young people to reflect on their cancer experience, provision of information, and opportunities for holistic assessment and care planning (Baker et al. 2021). End-of-treatment summaries, healthy lifestyle advice and communication with GPs/primary physicians have been shown to help promote self-management throughout survivorship (Pugh et al. 2018; Osborn et al. 2019). The teenage and young adult cancer teams in NI have delivered a variety of workshops focusing on survivorship issues such as education, employment, fatigue management and physical recovery; however, the successful facilitation of these approaches depends on the willingness of the young person to engage and make changes. The role of the AYA CNS in encouraging and empowering young people to develop self-management skills is, therefore, crucial (Rosenberg-Yunger et al. 2013; Moody et al. 2014; Syed et al. 2016).

13.15 Late Effects of Cancer Treatment

Whilst the majority of young people will survive cancer, the combination of intensive treatments and young age at diagnosis results in an increased risk of effects later in life as a consequence of treatment or the cancer diagnosis (NICE 2005; Ahmad et al. 2016). These vary depending on treatment and cancer type but may include cardiac or pulmonary complications secondary to chemotherapy, secondary malignancy risk, fertility problems, fatigue, and cognitive and psycho-social difficulties (Woodward et al. 2011; NICE 2014). Late-effect monitoring for AYAs is recommended in NICE guidance (2005); however, there is a lack of standardised guidelines and practice for managing the late-effect risk.

The AYA CNS has a role in educating both young people and professionals, such as the GP/primary physician, about specific potential late effects, as well as providing advice on healthy lifestyle and risk factor reduction: for example, to minimise cardiovascular effects (Ahmad et al. 2016). End-of-treatment summaries should be offered to young people post-completion of treatment and include information regarding potential late effects (NICE 2005, 2014; Osborn et al. 2019). As AYA lifestyle behaviours are often reported as being poor, opportunities for healthy lifestyle advice are paramount (Pugh et al. 2018). Cancer can be a catalyst for change with regard to healthy behaviours, and the AYA CNS should actively promote healthy behaviours through a variety of interventions, including engagement with peers to enhance the uptake of healthy behaviours (Pugh et al. 2018).

13.16 Palliative Adolescent and Young Adult Care

The AYA CNS is well-placed to help support the young person during the palliative or end-of-life stage of their care. The well-established relationships that exist between the AYA CNS and the young person and families can help support difficult conversations related to end-of-life care as well as provide emotional support. The CNS has a vital role in increasing awareness of AYA needs to the wider palliative care team, advocating for the young person and helping co-ordinate care. Excellent communication is paramount, with roles and responsibilities clearly defined to avoid confusion of roles (Osborn et al. 2019).

Palliative care brings unique challenges for AYAs. Young people may be contending with the normal developmental changes of life whilst ultimately facing their own mortality (Smith et al. 2016). They may have life ambitions, goals or bucket lists they wish to achieve during this time. The AYA CNS and wider team have a role in supporting young people to meet their ambitions, which involves flexibility, thinking outside the box, risk assessment and collaboration with teams (Smith et al. 2016). It can be a complex path to navigate, as often the priorities of young people and their families may differ, and the AYA CNS must advocate, ensuring that the young person's voice is heard and supporting them to retain some element of control in a difficult and complex time.

With complex situations alongside the close relationships that develop, professionals are at risk of secondary distress (Quinal et al. 2009). Processes to support the AYA CNS and other team members, such as opportunities for clinical supervision or reflective practice, are essential (Osborn et al. 2019).

13.17 Co-production

Co-production can be a very useful tool to adopt in AYA care. Within NI, the inclusion of young people in the design of local services, initiatives, peer support groups, local AYA steering groups and the regional CRG has been very beneficial in terms of shaping the design of services. Young people have more recently been involved in creating the proposed 10-year cancer strategy for NI (2022–2032) (Department of Health NI 2022). Prior to this proposed strategy, the NI Department of Health, Social Services and Public Safety's 'Service Framework for Cancer Prevention, Treatment and Care' (2011) addressed AYA care only in two short standard statements; however, the proposed 10-year strategy reflects the needs and priorities of AYAs throughout the document. A regional AYA patient experience survey was also recently created for the first time across NI; over 100 respondents focused on the young person's overall experience of care throughout their cancer experience. Obtaining regular patient experience feedback is a requirement of the AYA peer review measures (National Cancer Peer Review Team – National Cancer Action Team 2011). Evaluation of such surveys aims to provide insight into the young person's experience throughout the whole cancer trajectory and helps ensure that the patient's voice is at the core of any future service delivery and planning.

13.18 Conclusion

AYAs are a distinct and unique population with different needs from older adults and children (Smith et al. 2016). A joint approach to care is recommended between experts in the specific cancer and those with expertise in the AYA age group (NICE 2005). Collaborative, partnership working across teams that adopts a person-centred approach has the potential to contribute to providing high-quality, age-appropriate care. The AYA CNS's role in supporting young people and their families, working collaboratively as part of a dedicated and competent AYA multidisciplinary team, is crucial in improving outcomes and patient experience, ensuring the availability of psycho-social and practical support right from the point of diagnosis (Osborn et al. 2019). The CNS has a vital role in advocating for AYAs and sharing awareness of AYA unique needs across teams and at a strategic level to further enhance the quality of care delivered to this group of patients. AYA teams develop services individually to meet the local needs, resources and environment; however, by focusing on some of the key priorities of care, such as best treatment; healthcare professional knowledge; communication, interactions and relationships; recognising individuality; empowering young people; and promoting normality and the environment (Lea et al. 2018), the AYA CNS has an opportunity to improve the experience of young people right across the cancer trajectory, leading to improved outcomes for this diverse and unique patient population.

References

Abrol, E., Groszmann, M., Pitman, A. et al. (2017). Exploring the digital technology preferences of teenagers and young adults (TYA) with cancer and survivors: a cross-sectional service evaluation questionnaire. *Journal of Cancer Survivorship* 11: 670–682.

Ahmad, S.S., Reinius, M.A.A., Hatcher, H., and Ajithkumar, T. (2016). Anticancer chemotherapy in teenagers and young adults: managing long term side effects. *British Medical Journal* 354: i4567.

Albers, L.F., Bergsma, F.B., Mekelenkamp, H. et al. (2020). Discussing sexual health with adolescent and young adults with cancer: a qualitative study among healthcare providers. *Journal of Cancer Education* 371: 137–140.

Alloubani, A., Akhu-Zaheya, L., Abdelhafiz, I., and Almatari, M. (2019). Leadership styles influence on the quality of nursing care. *International Journal of HealthCare Quality Assurance* 32 (6): 1022–1033.

Anselmann, V. and Mulder, R. (2020). Transformational leadership, knowledge sharing and reflection, and work teams' performance: a structural equation modelling analysis. *Journal of Nursing Management* 28 (7): 1627–1634.

Baker, L., Foxhall, M., Hulbert, J. et al. (2021). Life beyond cancer: exploring the value of end-of-treatment clinics for teenagers and young adults. *Cancer Nursing Practice* 20 (6): 30–35.

Barr, R.D., Holowaty, E.J., and Birch, J.M. (2006). Classification schemes for tumors diagnosed in adolescents and young adults. *Cancer* 106 (7): 1425–1430.

Bibby, H., White, V., Thompson, K., and Anazodo, A. (2017). What are the unmet needs and care experiences of adolescents and young adults with cancer? A systematic review. *Journal of Adolescent and Young Adult Oncology* 6 (1): 6–30.

Birch, R.J., Morris, E.J.A., Stark, D.P. et al. (2014). Geographical factors affecting the admission of teenagers and young adults to age-specialist inpatient cancer care in England. *Journal of Adolescent and Young Adult Oncology* 3 (1): 28–36.

Bleyer, A. and Barr, R. (2016). *Cancer in Adolescents and Young People*, 2e. Switzerland: Springer International Publishing.

Bush, S., Michalek, D., and Francis, L. (2020). Perceived leadership styles, outcomes of leadership, and self-efficacy among nurse leaders: a hospital based survey to inform leadership development at a US Regional Medical Centre. *Nurse Leader* 19 (4): 1–5.

Cancer Research UK. (2021). Children's cancers incidence statistics. https://www.cancerresearchuk.org/health-professional/cancer-statistics/childrens-cancers/incidence#heading-Three (accessed 12 December 2021).

Carr, R., Whiteson, M., Edwards, M., and Morgan, S. (2013). Young adult cancer services in the UK: the journey to a national network. *Clinical Medicine* 13 (3): 258–262.

Coyne, L., Amory, A., Kieran, G., and Gibson, F. (2014). Children's participation in shared decision making: children, adolescents, parents and healthcare professionals' perspectives and experiences. *European Journal of Oncology Nursing* 18 (3): 278–280.

Darby, K., Nash, P., and Nash, S. (2014). Understanding and responding to spiritual and religious needs of young people with cancer. *Cancer Nursing Practice* 13 (2): 32–37.

De Vries, J.D. and Curtis, E. (2019). Nursing leadership in Ireland: experiences and obstacles. *Leadership in Health Services* 32 (3): 348–363.

Department of Health Northern Ireland. (2022). A cancer strategy for Northern Ireland 2022–2032. https://www.health-ni.gov.uk/sites/default/files/publications/health/doh-cancer-strategy-march-2022.pdf (accessed 30 July 2022).

Department of Health, Social Services and Public Safety Northern Ireland. (2011). Service framework for cancer prevention, treatment and care.

DeRouen, M.C., Smith, A.W., Tao, L. et al. (2015). Cancer-related information needs and cancer's impact over life influence health-related quality of life among adolescents and young adults with cancer. *Psycho-Oncology* 24 (9): 1104–1115.

Eckert, R., West, M., Altman, D., et al. (2014). Delivering a collective leadership strategy for health care. Center for Creative Leadership and The King's Fund. White paper. https://www.kingsfund.org.uk/sites/default/files/media/delivering-collective-leadership-ccl-may.pdf (accessed 1 December 2021).

Fern, L., Lewandowski, J., Coxon, K.M., and Whelan, J. (2014). Available, accessible, aware, appropriate and acceptable: a strategy to improve participation of teenagers and young adults in cancer trials. *Lancet Oncology* 15 (8): 341–350.

Ferrari, A. (2014). Italian pediatric oncologists and adult medical oncologists join forces for adolescents with cancer. *Pediatric Hematology and Oncology* 31 (6): 574–575.

Ferrari, A., Albrittin, K., Osborn, M. et al. (2017). Access and models of care. In: *Cancer in Adolescents and Young Adults*, 2e (ed. A. Bleyer, R. Barr, L. Gloeckler Ries, et al.), 509–547. Berlin: Springer Verlag.

Fry, R., Igielnik, R. and Patten, E. (2018). How Millennials Today Compare with their Grandparents 50 Years Ago, Washington: Pew Research Centre http://pewrsr.ch/2Dys8lr (accessed 24 October 2021).

Gibson, F., Fern, L., Whelan, J. et al. (2012). A scoping exercise of favourable characteristics of professionals working in teenage and young adult cancer care: 'thinking outside of the box'. *European Journal of Cancer Care* 21 (3): 330–339.

Ginsberg, J.P., Hobbie, W.L., Carlson, C.A., and Meadows, A.T. (2006). Delivering long-term follow-up care to paediatric cancer survivors: transition care issues. *Pediatric Blood Cancer* 46 (2): 169–173.

Hammond, C. (2017). Against a singular message of distinctness: challenging dominant representations of adolescents and young adults in oncology. *Journal of Adolescent and Young Adult Oncology* 6 (1): 45–49.

Hart, R., Hallowell, N., Harden, J. et al. (2020). Clinician-researchers and custodians of scarce resources: a qualitative study of health professionals' views on barriers to the involvement of teenagers and young adults in cancer trials. *BMC Cancer* 21 (1): 67.

Hart, R., Boyle, D., Cameron, D. et al. (2021). Strategies for improving access to clinical trials by teenagers and young adults with cancer: a qualitative study of health professionals' views. *European Journal of Cancer Care* 30 (3): e13408.

Kerr, H. (2021). Best practice in the transition to adult services for young adults who had childhood cancer. *Cancer Nursing Practice* 20 (6): e1808.

Kitson, A., Marshall, A., Bassett, K., and Zeitz, K. (2013). What are the core elements of patient-centered care? A narrative review and synthesis of the literature from health policy, medicine and nursing. *Journal of Advanced Nursing* 69 (1): 4–15.

Knott, C., Brown, L., and Hardy, S. (2013). Introducing a self-monitoring process in a teenage and young adult cancer ward: impact and implications for a team culture and practice change. *International Practice Development Journal* 3 (2): 1–2.

Kwak, M., Zebrack, B.J., Meeske, K.A. et al. (2013). Trajectories of psychological distress in adolescent and young adult patients with cancer: a 1-year longitudinal study. *Journal of Clinical Oncology* 31 (17): 2160–2166.

Lea, S., Taylor, R., Martins, A. et al. (2018). Conceptualizing age-appropriate care for teenagers and young adults with cancer: a qualitative mixed-methods study. *Adolescent Health, Medicine and Therapeutics* 24 (9): 149–166.

Lea, S., Gibson, F., and Taylor, R. (2019). The culture of young people's cancer care: a narrative review and synthesis of the UK literature. *European Journal of Cancer Care* 28 (3): 1–12.

Lea, S., Martins, A., Fern, L. et al. (2020). The support and information needs of adolescents and young adults with cancer when active treatment ends. *BMC Cancer* 20 (1): 697.

Marris, S., Morgan, S., and Stark, D. (2011). Listening to patients: what is the value of age-appropriate care to teenagers and young adults with cancer? *European Journal of Cancer Care* 20 (2): 145–151.

Marshall, S., Grinyer, A., and Limmer, M. (2018). The 'lost tribe' reconsidered: teenagers and young adults treated for cancer in adult settings. *European Journal of Oncology Nursing* 33: 85–90.

McCarthy, M., McNeill, R., Drew, S. et al. (2016). Psych-social distress and post-traumatic stress symptoms in adolescents and young adults with cancer and their parents. *Journal of Adolescent and Young Adult Oncology* 5 (4): 322–329.

Meneses, K., McNees, P., Azuero, A., and Jukkala, A. (2010). Development of the fertility and cancer project: an internet approach to help young cancer survivors. *Oncology Nursing Forum* 37 (2): 191–198.

Moody, L., Turner, A., Osmond, J. et al. (2014). Web-based self-management for young cancer survivors: consideration of user requirements and barriers to implementation. *Journal of Cancer Survivorship* 9 (2): 188–200.

Morgan, S. and Yoder, L.H. (2012). A concept analysis of person-centred care. *Journal of Holistic Nursing* 30 (1): 6–15.

Mulhall, A., Kelly, D., and Pearce, S. (2004). A qualitative evaluation of an adolescent cancer unit. *European Journal of Cancer Care* 13 (1): 16.

National Cancer Peer Review Team – National Cancer Action Team. (2011). Manual for cancer services: teenage and young adult measures, Version 1.0.

National Cancer Survivorship Initiative. (2013). The recovery package.

National Institute for Health and Care Excellence. (2005). Guidance on cancer services: improving outcomes in children and young people with cancer.

National Institute for Health and Care Excellence. (2014). Cancer services for children and young people. https://www.nice.org.uk/guidance/qs55/chapter/List-of-quality-statements (accessed 12 November 2021).

NHS England. (2013/2014). NHS standard contract for cancer: teenagers and young adults. https://www.england.nhs.uk/wpcontent/uploads/2013/09/b17.pdf (accessed 12 December 2021).

Osborn, M., Johnson, R., Thompson, K. et al. (2019). Models of care for adolescent and young adult cancer programs. *Pediatric Blood Cancer* 66 (12): e27991.

Psihogois, A.M., Li, Y., Butler, E. et al. (2019). Text message responsivity in a 2-way short message service pilot intervention with adolescent and young adult survivors of cancer. *JMIR mHealth and uHealth* 7 (4): e12547.

Public Health England. (2021). Children, teenagers and young adults UK cancer statistics report 2021. https://www.ncin.org.uk/cancer_type_and_topic_

specific_work/cancer_type_specific_work/cancer_in_children_teenagers_and_young_adults (accessed 11 December 2021).

Pugh, G., Hough, R., Gravestock, H. et al. (2018). The lifestyle information and intervention preferences of teenage and young adult cancer survivors. A qualitative study. *Cancer Nursing* 41 (5): 389–398.

Quinal, S., Harford, S., and Rutledge, D. (2009). Secondary traumatic stress in oncology staff. *Cancer Nursing* 32 (4): e1–e7.

Rosenberg-Yunger, Z., Klassen, A., Amin, L. et al. (2013). Barriers and facilitators of transition from pediatric to adult long-term follow-up care in childhood cancer survivors. *Journal of Adolescent and Young Adult Oncology* 2 (3): 104–111.

Sansom-Daly, U.M., Lin, M., Robertson, E.G. et al. (2016). Health literacy in adolescents and young adults: an updated review. *Journal of Adolescent and Young Adult Oncology* 5 (2): 106–118.

Smith, S., Mooney, S., Cable, M., and Taylor, R. (ed.) (2016). *The Blueprint of Care for Teenagers and Young Adults with Cancer*, 2e. London: Teenage Cancer Trust.

Stark, D., Bowen, D., Dunwoodie, E. et al. (2015). Survival patterns in teenagers and young adults with cancer in the United Kingdom: comparisons with younger and older age groups. *European Journal of Cancer* 51 (17): 2643–2654.

Syed, I., Nathan, P., Barr, R. et al. (2016). Examining factors associated with self-management skills in teenage survivors of cancer. *Journal of Cancer Survivorship* 10 (4): 686–691.

Taylor, R., Fern, L., Whelan, J. et al. (2011). Your place or mine?' Priorities for a specialist teenage and young adult (TYA) cancer unit: disparity between TYA and professional perceptions. *Journal of Adolescent and Young Adult Oncology* 1 (2): 145–151.

Taylor, R.M., Solanki, A., Aslam, N. et al. (2016). A participatory study of teenagers and young adults views on access and participation in cancer research. *European Journal of Oncology Nursing* 20: 156–164.

Taylor, R., Fern, L., Barber, J. et al. (2020). Longitudinal cohort study of the impact of specialist cancer services for teenagers and young adults on quality of life: outcomes from the BRIGHTLIGHT study. *British Medical Journal Open* 10 (11): e038471.

Teenage Cancer Trust. (2014). Caring for teenagers and young adults with cancer: a competence and career framework for nursing. https://www.teenagecancertrust.org/sites/default/files/Nursing-framework.pdf (accessed 10 October 2021).

Teenage Cancer Trust. (2020a). Cancer x coronavirus: The impact on young people. https://www.teenagecancertrust.org/sites/default/files/2021-12/Cancer-coronavirus-report-June-2020-Teenage-Cancer-Trust.pdf (accessed 21 October 2020).

Teenage Cancer Trust. (2020b). Welcome to IAM. https://www.iamportal.co.uk (accessed 23 March 2021).

Teenage Cancer Trust. (2021). Inadequate specialist mental health support risks derailing young cancer patients' lives, say experts. https://www. teenagecancertrust.org/media-centre-and-press-releases/inadequate-specialist-mental-health-support-risks-derailing-young (accessed 13 January 2022).

Teenagers and Young Adults with Cancer. (2015). Transition: TYAC best practice statement for health professionals.

Teenagers and Young Adults with Cancer. (2016). Fertility: TYAC best practice statement for healthcare professionals. https://www.tyac.org.uk/downloads/good-practice-guides/fertlitytyacbestpracticeguide-(1).pdf (accessed 14 December 2021).

Vindrola-Padros, C., Taylor, R.M., Lea, S. et al. (2016). Mapping adolescent cancer services: how do young people, their families, and staff describe specialised cancer care in England? *Cancer Nursing* 39 (5): 358–366.

Wijeratne, D.T., Bowman, M., Sharpe, I. et al. (2021). Text messaging in cancer-supportive care: a systematic review. *Cancers (Basel)* 13 (14): 1–16.

Wilhelm, M., Dirkson, U., Bielack, S.S. et al. (2014). ENCCA WP17-WP7 consensus paper on teenagers and young adults (TYA) with bone sarcomas. *Annals of Oncology* 25 (8): 2561–2568.

Woodward, E., Jessop, M., Glaser, A., and Stark, D. (2011). Late effects in survivors of teenage and young adult cancer: does age matter? *Annals of Oncology* 22: 2561–2562.

World Health Organisation. (2017). Global accelerated action for the health of adolescents (AA-HA!): guidance to support country implementation. https://www. who.int/publications/i/item/WHO-FWC-MCA-17.05. (accessed 18 December 2021).

Zebrack, B. (2011). Psychological, social and behavioural issues for young adults with cancer. *Cancer* 117 (10): 2289–2294.

14

COVID-19 and the Clinical Nurse Specialist

Stephanie Todd and Helen Kerr

Abstract

This chapter discusses the impact of the COVID-19 pandemic on healthcare, with a focus on the role of the clinical nurse specialist (CNS) in cancer services. The chapter will commence with a brief introduction to COVID-19 and then outline its impact on the delivery of health services and frontline workers. There will be a reflection on the role of the CNS prior to the COVID-19 pandemic, along with a discussion that highlights the changes to this role as a result of COVID-19. The chapter will conclude with a discussion on the way forward for the CNS and healthcare services post-pandemic.

14.1   Introduction

From an early stage, it was evident that COVID-19 would interrupt the spectrum of cancer care, particularly in relation to delays with diagnoses and treatment disruption (Richards et al. 2020) and possible cessation of treatments. The impact on cancer care inevitably caused a paradigm shift in the role of the clinical nurse specialist (CNS), not only within cancer services but also in other areas of healthcare. The World Health Organisation (WHO) (2020) states that the coronavirus (COVID-19) 'is an infectious disease caused by the SARS-CoV-2 virus'. Initially, this was as much information as was known from a cluster of cases in China in December 2019. As the world listened to the news reports, the magnitude of the impact of this virus became apparent, as the rapid increase in the number of cases led to a distorted normality on a global scale. It quickly became evident that COVID-19 showed no prejudice and that all individuals were vulnerable to the uncertainty of the virus and its impact. The media coverage of COVID-19 escalated as the virus and its whirlwind nature became a stark reality and threat to everyone's way of life. Over time, the unfolding of further information revealed why COVID-19 was so infectious, which was due to the transmissibility of the disease as it 'spread from person to person through droplets released when an infected person coughs, sneezes, or talks' (National Cancer Institute 2020). To minimise COVID-19 transmission, government restrictions including social distancing, reducing population footfall and closing public facilities were all implemented shortly after the potential destruction of the virus became evident. In the context of the United Kingdom (UK), the first official 'lockdown' was announced on 23 March 2020, where the public were required to 'stay at home' to save lives. This approach was mirrored in most countries around the globe at different times.

The first author, Stephanie Todd, is a CNS for individuals with a lung cancer diagnosis in a hospital in Northern Ireland (NI). The multiple components of this role include providing care from diagnosis through treatment, symptom management and end-of-life care. The first author will draw on her experiences in this role to outline the impact COVID-19 had on the delivery of healthcare services to individuals with a cancer diagnosis and their families and friends. The second author, Dr Helen Kerr, is a senior lecturer at a School of Nursing and Midwifery at a university in NI, with a clinical background in cancer and palliative care.

14.2 Impact on Healthcare Services and Frontline Healthcare Workers

Due to the infectious nature of COVID-19, rapid and unprecedented changes in healthcare had to be implemented globally to survive the potential tsunami effect this virus imposed on already-overwhelmed and fragile health systems. It was evident, with vast media coverage, that enforced continual changes in healthcare would be essential at a global, national and regional level to sustain the services provided by healthcare systems. The foresight of European and national experience of the virus supported regions to mirror changed practices such as dedicating units to help manage the COVID-19 crisis and maintaining essential services in separate areas. These approaches were tailored to local healthcare services globally.

From very early on, it was clear how these events could potentially impact patients and staff and the need to reassure patients regarding their own vulnerability to the virus with no endpoint in sight. The reassurance provided to patients by healthcare staff was in addition to staff managing and masking their personal fears, which included their own mortality. Newman et al. (2021) reported that frontline healthcare workers were more likely to report psychological burden, fear and anxiety due to increased exposure to COVID-19 treatment and care. Professionally, healthcare workers endeavoured to be proactive in a reactive situation whilst dealing with their own personal, physical and psychological safety through the ongoing uncertainty.

Staff who frequently worked long shifts with high death exposure due to COVID-19 were reported to experience higher levels of work-related stress, with a profound impact on their mental health (Neto et al. 2020).

In the context of the first author's area of work, two of the three main hospitals in the context of NI were designated as COVID-19 centres. These designated centres were referred to as 'Nightingale hospitals' locally and throughout the UK: they were aptly named after Florence Nightingale, who was known to reduce the mortality rate of the British Army during the Crimean War and use the analysis of data and statistics to revolutionise the organisation of the British Army barracks, Victorian workhouses and hospitals (Bradshaw 2017). Two crucial aspects of healthcare during the COVID-19 pandemic were respiratory medicine and intensive care units (ICUs), and within the first author's area of work, these were both relocated to the Nightingale hospitals.

14.3 Impact of COVID-19 on Cancer Services

Cancer services were affected by various changes to the healthcare system as a whole and also how cancer treatments were utilised through the pandemic in regards to the downturn of surgical services, increased use of radiotherapy and modified use of systemic anti-cancer therapy (SACT). This resulted in the reorganisation of oncology services to continue providing essential and time-critical modalities of treatment for an often-unpredictable disease whilst maintaining safety from the relatively unknown virus. Unfortunately, in addition to shouldering the burden of a cancer diagnosis, patients were also more vulnerable to COVID-19 infection. This greater susceptibility was attributed to the systemic immunosuppressive state from the malignancy itself and also was a result of SACTs: for example, chemotherapy, which is an anti-cancer drug treatment known to lower a person's white blood cell count, leaving them more susceptible to infection (Kamboj and Sepkowitz 2009). A prospective cohort study by Liang et al. (2020) observed individuals with cancer to have a greater risk of severe events from the COVID-19 virus, including the need for ventilator support and higher mortality rates than those without cancer, with reports of a 39% increase in severe complications from COVID-19 in individuals with cancer compared to those without cancer.

Richards et al. (2020) describe the public's heightened awareness of the high transmissibility of the virus resulting in a reluctance of individuals with possible signs or symptoms of cancer to present to healthcare services, resulting in a late presentation in terms of cancer diagnosis juxtaposed with the suspension of cancer screening and diagnostic services as a whole. In March 2020, in the context of the UK, the Welsh and Scottish governments announced a decision to suspend cancer-screening programmes, followed by England and NI in April 2020 (Department of Health 2020). This was mirrored globally; Waterhouse et al. (2020)

discuss the disruptions brought by COVID-19 on all aspects of cancer control and care, including cancelled cancer screening services in the United States of America (USA). This was a concern, as long-term survival is reflective of early screening in cancers such as colorectal, breast and prostate (Hanna et al. 2020).

Understandably, the public's priority was keeping safe and well at home. Reluctance to present to hospitals stemmed from fear of self-exposure to the virus as well as causing a burden to an already-overwhelmed healthcare system. With over one-quarter of cancers reported to be diagnosed through emergency routes in the context of NI (McPhail et al. 2022) and a marked decrease in emergency department (ED) attendance, the outcome of delayed diagnoses was inevitable. Furthermore, fewer people attended their general practitioner/primary physician for conditions unrelated to COVID-19 (Limb 2021), again resulting in missed diagnostic opportunities. Richards et al. (2020) describe a downturn in diagnostic investigations such as endoscopies, as these were classified as aerosol-generating procedures and associated with a higher risk of COVID-19 transmission. In Australia, investigations such as colonoscopies and sigmoidoscopies decreased by 55% between March and May 2020 (Luo et al. 2022). Macmillan Cancer Support (2020) estimate that there were 1000 fewer cancer diagnoses in NI between March and July 2020, unfortunately leading to a substantial backlog of patients. In England, UK, there was a 33% decrease in the diagnoses of early-stage cancer during the first wave of the pandemic in 2020 (Limb 2021). Many diagnostic appointments were delayed or postponed completely as healthcare services were reduced to ensure all available resources were aimed at treating individuals with COVID-19 (Macmillan Cancer Support 2020).

The relocation of some services produced an unavoidable impact on the delivery of cancer treatments ranging from surgery and radiotherapy to the delivery of SACT. Richards et al. (2020) describe the reduction in capacity for surgery during COVID-19 as due to the increased need for theatre space and ventilators to be used for individuals with COVID-19. Bhangu et al. (2021) note that surgery is the main modality of cure for most solid cancers; therefore, its downturn not only had the potential to affect patient survival outcomes but also affected the use of treatment services such as radiotherapy or hormonal therapy as therapeutic modalities (Richards et al. 2020). The ramifications of these changes resulted in both physical and psychological aspects, as the risk of cancer progression or hospital admissions arising from treatment complications was not to be underestimated. Within lung cancer, it has been established that delayed surgery may lead to disease progression with tumours that are no longer operable, resulting in worse outcomes and poorer overall survival (Shankar et al. 2020).

Patients attending for SACT or radiotherapy treatments were at a higher risk of contracting the virus due to the immunosuppressive side effect of systemic treatment, in addition to the frequent hospital attendances to have treatment, thereby increasing their potential exposure to the virus. Cancer multidisciplinary teams (MDTs) were challenged with often-difficult decisions on how best to optimally manage treatment options for patients. Vrdoljak et al. (2020) describe the fear of under-treatment bias faced by oncologists, especially in the setting of metastatic disease or adjuvant therapy. The risk versus benefit of patients embarking on treatment had to be very carefully considered on an individual basis. This was more profound for individuals with a cancer diagnosis such as small-cell lung cancer where commencement of treatment is required promptly, as often the response and symptom relief is rapid due to the initial sensitivity of the disease to chemotherapy (Sandler 2003).

14.4   The Role of the Clinical Nurse Specialist Prior to the COVID-19 Pandemic

In 2014, Balsdon and Wilkinson (2014) stated that the role of the CNS has continued to develop over the last two decades, which appears to be the continuing trajectory. Adopting and adapting are within the CNS ethos, and these skills were required during the COVID-19 pandemic. Kerr et al. (2021) conducted an integrative literature review to evaluate the role of the CNS in cancer care, with their findings highlighting the integral role the CNS occupies within the MDT in supporting and developing cancer services.

As far back as 2003, it has been shown that the CNS is fundamental in meeting targets in relation to prompt diagnosis and treatment (Corner 2003). The cancer pathway can often be difficult for patients to navigate, especially while psychologically managing the challenges that a cancer diagnosis may bring. Therefore, having a key worker from diagnosis to advocate and provide holistic support has proven beneficial for patients. (The key worker role is the focus of Chapter 5 in this book.) Although CNSs are reported to improve patients' experience of care, continual service evaluation from both service users and providers is recommended (Macmillan Cancer Support 2015). A CNS has an advanced scope of practice and provides expert clinical advice and care and may also be involved in the diagnosis and treatment of a health condition (International Council of Nurses [ICN] 2020). Additionally, a CNS provides symptom management, expert and evidence-based clinical advice and guidance to patients and healthcare providers to ensure optimal care within their specialised field (ICN 2020).

The CNS role in cancer services has undoubtedly transformed, with many aspects of treatment and care formally carried out by medical staff now within the job role of the specialist nurse (Henry 2015). Nurse-led clinics (the focus of Chapter 11 in this book) and contributions to innovations in practice are embedded within the CNS role in cancer care, and many have professionally developed and enhanced their level of assessment and review skills by achieving qualifications such as non-medical prescribing (Henry 2015). The CNS is ideally placed to practice as a non-medical prescriber in cancer services (Osborne and Kerr 2021).

Additionally, within cancer services, the CNS is the point of contact for patients with access to the multidisciplinary cancer team. Patients benefit from this with seamless and prompt service, particularly regarding symptom management and expediting review with the oncologist if required (Alessy et al. 2022).

The first author's day-to-day pre-COVID-19 role as a lung CNS involved multiple components in relation to caring for individuals with lung cancer, such as involvement with patients at diagnosis, through various elements of treatment, symptom management and end-of-life care. It is a varied role inclusive of respiratory, oncology and palliative care. The first author is also a non-medical prescriber with health assessment skills, which has enriched the role further to provide a holistic and specialised level of care to individuals with lung cancer. The role extends to individuals in the inpatient and outpatient settings, with well-established relationships with community staff to whom onward referrals are often completed by the CNS to ensure ongoing continuity of care for patients.

The role is valued by the MDT and is regarded as functioning at an advanced level within the scope of lung cancer services. Education of nursing staff and healthcare professionals is a vital aspect of the role to enhance the level of care that individuals with lung cancer receive. As captured by LaSala et al. (2007), the CNS influences the professional development of staff, acts as a mentor and helps to identify learning needs. The CNS plays a pivotal role in service improvement, quality care and cost-effectiveness (Salamanca et al. 2017). Tod et al. (2015) completed qualitative research on the nature of the lung cancer nurse specialist role and how it was operationalised with the patient and MDT to expedite access to treatment. Their findings concluded how vital the lung cancer nurse specialist was within the MDT, especially in extraditing access to treatment for patients through assessment, symptom management and emotional and psychological support. These authors discuss the benefit of patients being able to access the lung cancer CNS at any stage through the whole cancer pathway. Tod et al. (2015) also discuss the benefit of swift, accurate prescribing for symptoms such as pain and breathlessness, which helps improve patient quality of life and may also improve their suitability for treatment. Research on the benefits of the CNS role in multiple areas of healthcare has highlighted how integral it has become over the recent decades, and the agility of the specialist nurse proved paramount during the pandemic.

14.5 Devolvement of Staff over the COVID-19 Pandemic

The increased volume of patients admitted to hospital due to COVID-19, especially within ICUs, outweighed pre-existing staff capacity (Vera San Juan et al. 2022). Hospitals were therefore compelled to optimise staff allocation to ensure safe patient care. Healthcare workers from other clinical areas and services, who were deemed non-essential during the global pandemic, were assigned to units such as intensive care to complete key tasks of care such as patient hygiene (Doyle et al. 2020). Appropriate induction and training are required when any staff member commences a new role; however, enabling this during COVID-19 proved challenging. The swiftness with which events unfolded during COVID-19 was phenomenal. Time constraints and stringent infection control measures challenged normal training delivery (Vera San Juan et al. 2022). In some countries, such as the UK, healthcare professionals were re-deployed to areas outside their speciality to support staff in caring for individuals with COVID-19. This resulted in the COVID-19 pandemic creating an urgent need for staff development (Zuo and Miller Juve 2020). It was not unnoticed that redeployment affected healthcare staff with regards to their mental well-being, heightened fears of contracting the virus and potentially infecting their loved ones at home (Vera San Juan et al. 2022).

Within the clinical guidelines for the management of the surge during the COVID-19 pandemic, the National Health Service (NHS) in the context of England, UK, detail how redeployment was dictated by the stage of the pandemic and individual care facilities from a geographical and population context (NHS England 2020). Within the first author's area of work, many medical and nursing staff were re-deployed from outpatient and surgical wards to other areas such as ICUs and respiratory medicine, and re-deployed staff experienced fear and anxieties due to feeling that they received inadequate training and support, along with a lack of experience working within these intense and specialised areas. This echoes the findings of Khajuria et al. (2021), who conducted an international cross-sectional study on workplace factors associated with the mental health of healthcare workers during the COVID-19 pandemic. They found that factors such as lack of adequate support and training, access to adequate levels of personal protective equipment (PPE) and last-minute changes to rota shifts all contributed to heightened anxiety and stress of re-deployed staff. Contrary to this, Danielis et al. (2021) reported some re-deployed healthcare workers using the opportunity positively to change their way of thinking when faced with challenging and difficult situations.

14.6 Impact of COVID-19 on the Clinical Nurse Specialist Role and Patient Care

With the evolving practices of healthcare areas and disciplines during the pandemic, the CNS was not left untouched. This role was integral for patients and families as a contact and key worker, providing advice, co-ordinating care and being an invaluable source of support at a distressing time. The first author's role within lung cancer services and the management of patients with extreme breathlessness, cough and respiratory distress also aligned with the management of the symptoms individuals experienced with COVID-19. It became apparent that the skills and knowledge of the lung cancer CNS were transferable to managing COVID-19 patients. The first author's day-to-day role changed to incorporate both maintaining the lung CNS service and educating staff on the management and treatment of individuals with COVID-19 and support and guidance within COVID-19 care. Mamais et al. (2022, p. 104) describe agile CNSs during the COVID-19 pandemic and their 'unique contributions within three spheres of impact: patient, organisation and nurse'. The first author was involved in educating medical and nursing staff on managing symptoms experienced by individuals with COVID-19. Education addressed the symptom management of patients still receiving active management and those sadly dying from COVID-19.

The first author, in their daily role, also provided support and guidance to staff involved in difficult conversations, using advanced communication skills. Significant barriers to communication with patients were experienced due to staff wearing personal protective equipment (PPE) and the restriction on family and friends visiting, meaning telephone and virtual platforms were used for discussions with family and loved ones instead of face-to-face discussions. A qualitative descriptive study by Green et al. (2022) focusing on the communication challenges and strengths of nurses working in ICUs during the first two pandemic waves highlights the frustration and difficulties experienced when communicating with patients due to PPE and the patients' medical condition. This was echoed by Houchens and Tipirneni (2020), who reported the barriers to communication experienced by healthcare staff due to PPE impeding the ability to express and recognise emotional cues from patients. This was a challenge to healthcare workers; the inability to communicate directly to family members was against the ethos of communicating face-to-face with individuals, especially for distressing conversations.

Many guidelines and acronyms have been developed to educate healthcare staff on breaking bad news, such as SPIKES (Baile 2000), which discusses setup, perception, invitation, knowledge, empathy and strategy and summary. Each of these headings has recommendations and suggestions to facilitate breaking bad news; unfortunately, aspects of this guidance could not be completed during COVID-19 – especially allowing patients to have a friend or family member present, choosing an appropriate environment and being able to observe people's reactions and emotions – due to face masks or a virtual environment. In ICUs and COVID-19 wards, the use of virtual platforms became one of the main ways to communicate to patient's families and loved ones, for both patients and healthcare staff. Rose et al. (2021) describe both the benefits and barriers to virtual visiting. They discuss the positives that ICU staff felt from virtual visiting, including promoting patient physical and psychological recovery and enhancing person-centred care. Furthermore, some family members and friends experienced difficulties accessing video platform technology;

connectivity issues and lack of staff time and training were highlighted as challenges to engaging in virtual visiting.

As previously outlined, within cancer services, CNSs were frequently re-deployed to clinical areas of need to directly support the COVID-19 workload, with those remaining within cancer care having to significantly change their routine practices (Forster et al. 2022). During the first months of COVID-19, the first author worked in the lung cancer CNS role with rotation into COVID-19 clinical areas when required to provide education and support to staff in the management and treatment of COVID-19 symptoms and communicating and providing support to families and healthcare staff. The CNS role also adapted to using virtual platforms as a new means of communicating during COVID-19 within their daily role and also within the areas they were re-deployed to. These digital approaches developed out of a need to ensure that vulnerable patients who were shielding continued to do so for staff protection and maintaining social distancing (Robbins et al. 2020).

It was vital that face-to-face outpatient clinics continued functioning for patients when required, especially when patients were receiving difficult or bad news (O'Reilly et al. 2021). When patients presented with complex symptoms and required specific assessment and treatment, it was often deemed necessary for a face-to-face consultation to be conducted (Royal College of Nursing 2020). These appointments were carried out with special measures and precautions in place to protect patients and staff and were often accompanied by a telephone call the day preceding the appointment to ensure that the patient was not experiencing any signs of COVID-19, as recommended by the European Society for Medical Oncology (2020). Therefore, those patients that required physical attendance to hospital were able to access it; but for the majority of patients, telephone and virtual consultations were used.

The CNS was often pivotal in the initial triaging process in assessing patients as to the appropriate means of consultation depending on their individual circumstances. Many CNSs had experience with telephone clinics before COVID-19 and were therefore in an ideal position to conduct many of these online consultations. Research has shown the positive impact of nurse-led virtual clinics in terms of cost-effectiveness and efficient delivery of care (Almeida and Montayre 2019). The first author did experience an increase in the number of telephone calls from patients daily compared to pre-pandemic. Many of these interactions required additional time to discuss patient fears and concerns about COVID-19 and the assessment of complex symptoms for which patients were delaying seeking medical attention, with worries of attending hospital or a healthcare facility and potential exposure to the virus. Forster et al. (2022) conducted a cross-sectional survey into the impact of COVID-19 on CNSs and individuals with cancer, with their findings also reporting that encounters with patients took an average of between 5 and 20 minutes longer due to patients requesting to discuss COVID-19.

Within the first author's area of practice, the use of virtual platforms was also developed in order to maintain communication between clinical teams and keep abreast of important changes daily (digital health is the focus of Chapter 15 in this book). All staff meetings were undertaken via virtual platforms, and the number of staff and team interactions increased to ensure that adequate and safe services were provided to meet patient needs. The first author was involved in developing a virtual clinic for individuals with lung cancer undergoing respiratory follow-up who were felt to be too vulnerable to attend hospital at the height of the COVID-19 pandemic. A standard operating procedure (SOP) for the virtual clinic was developed by lung cancer CNSs, providing guidance on how the virtual clinic should operate. As a CNS who conducts virtual clinics, the first author was assured that if, following remote consultation with the patient, the CNS felt it was necessary that they attend hospital for medical review, this was easily organised for the patient. This was an important foundation of the virtual clinic and was established with medical approval before initiation of the remote consultations. For this vulnerable group of patients, having the option to attend hospital for a clinic appointment reassured them and provided a sense of relief, knowing the CNS conducting the remote consultation could access this if required.

Hospital location and demographics dictated the first author's day-to-day working. This required working across various hospital sites depending on patient needs and service requirements. Mamais et al. (2022) describe how the CNS influenced changes within the spheres of patients, nurses and the organisation. They discuss the impact the CNS had through creating SOPs, developing policies to guide clinicians on how to safely facilitate visitation to a dying patient and the implementation of training of MDT members.

14.7 The Future of Healthcare Services Post-COVID-19 Pandemic

Healthcare services have inevitably transformed and developed during COVID-19, given the vast changes that occurred to daily clinical practice to keep patients and staff safe. With change, there are often both positive and negative outcomes. Nelson (2020) describes the positive effects of the sudden change in human behaviour as a response to COVID-19: for example, lower rates of crime, fewer car crashes and a fall in the number of other infectious diseases. Balanced with this was the downside of the sudden rise in patients presenting to ED with strokes, heart attacks and other conditions, confirming that patients delayed seeking appropriate and timely medical attention due to a fear of contracting the virus (Grady 2020).

Doherty et al. (2020) discuss the technological advances and shifts in standards of care treatment as a result of COVID-19 and ask the question of what patient safety now means within a virtual context. Many healthcare facilities have developed guidelines concerning the use of virtual platforms for patient consultations to ensure that patient safety is maintained. In a systematic review, Moynihan et al. (2021) highlighted the positive outcomes of the disruption to healthcare services and the use of telemedicine, with patients being spared unnecessary treatment. Within the first author's area of work, the use of virtual platforms has been welcomed positively and has become a permanent change on the premise that those patients who require a face-to-face clinic appointment will have this facilitated. With this in mind, it is also important to remember patient preference and suitability for virtual consultation, as shown by a survey conducted by Byrne et al. (2022): the results concluded that over half of patients and clinicians had a positive response to remote consultations but would prefer face-to-face consultations to return in the future.

Remote training, education and staff meetings have also continued, with the use of online platforms allowing attendance at multiple meetings and minimising the cost and time spent travelling to and from meeting facilities and conferences (Scarlat et al. 2020). It must also be acknowledged that utilising technology can amplify inequities such as generational differences and those who are not information technology (IT) literate, so technology must be implemented with this in mind (Zuo and Miller Juvé 2020). Within healthcare, the future is taking on a virtual persona for some aspects of clinical care whilst also continuing to return to pre-pandemic functioning. Within healthcare settings, COVID-19 precautions such as PPE and social distancing continue acting as a subtle reminder that the virus continues to exist and is the 'new normal' within healthcare, which is still a process for all to adjust to (Khanduja and Scarlat 2020).

14.8 Conclusion

The COVID-19 pandemic changed the world on an epic scale, and the post-pandemic landscape continues to evolve, so it remains premature to fully determine the impact of these changes (Scarlat et al. 2020). Within healthcare, frequent changes to practice had to be implemented in response to COVID-19. Despite different countries being at different 'pandemic stages', maintaining patient and staff safety remains at the forefront, and adaptation to healthcare workers' roles, including that of the CNS, proved vital in contributing to this. Changes to roles, upskilling and using new technology ensured remote assessment and management of patient needs (Gray and Saunders 2020). Research demonstrates that the transferable skills of the CNS have been pivotal in ensuring ongoing patient management throughout COVID-19, whether clinically involved in the care of patients or completing education, training and support to healthcare staff. At present, some adaptations to practice have remained; however, the full scale of the repercussions of the pandemic is yet to be actualised and will invariably have an impact on healthcare, patient outcomes and the role of the CNS for a long time to come.

References

Alessy, S.A., Davies, E., Rawlinson, J. et al. (2022). Clinical nurse specialists and survival in patients with cancer: the UK National Cancer Experience Survey. *British Medical Journal Supportive and Palliative Care* 1–17.

Almeida, S. and Montayre, J. (2019). An integrative review of nurse-led virtual clinics. *Nursing Praxis in New Zealand* 35 (1): 18–28.

Baile, W.F. (2000). SPIKES – A six-step protocol for delivering bad news: application to the patient with cancer. *The Oncologist* 5 (4): 302–311.

Balsdon, H. and Wilkinson, S. (2014). A trust-wide review of clinical nurse specialists' productivity. *Nursing Management* 21 (1): 33–37.

Bhangu, A., Glasbey, J., Manick, J. et al. (2021). Effect of COVID-19 pandemic lockdowns on planned cancer surgery for 15 tumour types in 61 countries: an international, prospective, cohort study. *Lancet Oncology* 22 (11): 1507–1517.

Bradshaw, N.-A. (2017). Florence Nightingale (1820–1910): A pioneer of data visualisation. In: *Women in Mathematics: Celebrating the Centennial of the Mathematical Association of America* (ed. J.L. Beery, S.J. Greenwald, J.A. Jensen-Vallin, and M.B. Mast), 197–217. Springer https://doi.org/10.1007/978-3-319-66694-5_11.

Byrne, H., Roslan, F., Kasbia, H. et al. (2022). The new Normal? A survey of patients' and clinicians' satisfaction of remote consultations during the COVID-19 pandemic. *British Journal of Surgery* 109 (Supplement 1).

Corner, J. (2003). The role of nurse-led care in cancer management. *The Lancet Oncology* 4 (10): 631–636.

Danielis, M., Peressoni, L., Piani, T. et al. (2021). Nurses' experiences of being recruited and transferred to a new sub-intensive care unit devoted to COVID-19 patients. *Journal of Nursing Management* 29: 1149–1158.

Department of Health Northern Ireland. (2020). Cancer screening programmes. https://www.health-ni.gov.uk (accessed 22 March 2022).

Doherty, G.J., Goksu, M., and de Paula, B.H.R. (2020). Rethinking cancer clinical trials for COVID-19 and beyond. *Nature Cancer* 1 (6): 568–572.

Doyle, J., Smith, E.M., Gough, C.J. et al. (2020). Mobilising a workforce to combat COVID-19: an account, reflections, and lessons learned. *Journal of the Intensive Care Society* 23 (2): 177–182.

European Society for Medical Oncology. (2020). Cancer patient management during the COVID-19 pandemic. http://www.esmo.org/guidelines/cancer-patient-management-during-the-covid-19-pandemic (accessed 29 August 2022).

Forster, A.S., Zylstra, J., von Wagner, C. et al. (2022). The impact of COVID-19 on clinical nurse specialists and patients with Cancer. *Clinical Nurse Specialist* 36 (5): 272–277.

Grady, D. (2020). The pandemic's hidden victims: sick or dying, but not from the virus. *New York Times.* https://www.nytimes.com/2020/04/20/health/treatment-delays-coronavirus.html (accessed 13 September 2022).

Gray, R. and Sanders, C. (2020). A reflection on the impact of COVID-19 on primary care in the United Kingdom. *Journal of Interprofessional Care* 34 (5): 672–678.

Green, G., Sharon, C., and Gendler, Y. (2022). The communication challenges and strength of nurses' intensive Corona Care during the two first pandemic waves: a qualitative descriptive phenomenology study. *Healthcare* 10 (5): 837.

Hanna, T.P., King, W.D., Thibodeau, S. et al. (2020). Mortality due to cancer treatment delay: systematic review and meta-analysis. *British Medical Journal* 371: 1–11.

Henry, R. (2015). The role of the cancer nurse specialist. *Nursing in Practice.* https://www.nursinginpractice.com/clinical/cancer/the-role-of-the-cancer-specialist-nurse (accessed 30 March 2022).

Houchens, N. and Tipirneni, R. (2020). Compassionate communication amid the COVID-19 pandemic. *Journal of Hospital Medicine* 15 (7): 437–439.

International Council of Nurses. (2020). Guidelines of advanced practice nursing 2020.

Kamboj, M. and Sepkowitz, K.A. (2009). Nosocomial infections in patients with cancer. *The Lancet Oncology* 10 (6): 589–597.

Kerr, H., Donovan, M., and McSorley, O. (2021). Evaluation of the role of the clinical nurse specialist in cancer care: an integrative literature review. *European Journal of Cancer Care* 30 (3): 1–13.

Khajuria, A., Tomaszewski, W., Liu, Z. et al. (2021). Workplace factors associated with mental health of healthcare workers during the COVID-19 pandemic: an international cross-sectional study. *BMC Health Services Research* 21 (1): 1–11.

Khanduja, V. and Scarlat, M.M. (2020). Reaching a new 'normal' after COVID pandemic and orthopaedic implications. *International Orthopaedics* 44 (8): 1449–1451.

LaSala, C.A., Connors, P.M., Pedro, J.T., and Phipps, M. (2007). The role of the clinical nurse specialist in promoting evidence-based practice and effecting positive patient outcomes. *The Journal of Continuing Education in Nursing* 38 (6): 262–270.

Liang, W., Guan, W., Chen, R. et al. (2020). Cancer patients in SARS-CoV-2 infection: a nationwide analysis in China. *The Lancet Oncology* 21 (3): 335–337.

Limb, M. (2021). Covid-19: early stage cancer diagnoses fell by third in first lockdown. *British Medical Journal* https://www.bmj.com/content/373/bmj.n1179.

Luo, Q., O'Connell, D.L., Yu, X.Q. et al. (2022). Cancer incidence and mortality in Australia from 2020 to 2044 and an exploratory analysis of the potential effect of treatment delays during the COVID-19 pandemic: a statistical modelling study. *The Lancet Public Health* 7 (6): 537–e548.

Macmillan Cancer Support. (2015). Cancer clinical nurse specialists. https://www. macmillan.org.uk/documents/aboutus/research/impactbriefs/ clinicalnursespecialists2015new.pdf (accessed 22 January 2022).

Macmillan Cancer Support. (2020). The forgotten 'c'? The impact of COVID-19 on cancer care. https://www.macmillan.org.uk/assets/forgotten-c-impact-of-covid-19-on-cancer-care.pdf (accessed 30 January 2022).

Mamais, F., Jasdhaul, M., Gawlinski, A. et al. (2022). The agile clinical nurse specialist. *Clinical Nurse Specialist* 36 (4): 190–195.

McPhail, S., Swann, R., and Barclay, M. (2022). Risk factors and prognostic implications of diagnosis of cancer within 30 days after an emergency hospital admission (emergency presentation): an international Cancer benchmarking partnership (ICBP) population-based study. *Lancet Oncology* 23: 587–600.

Moynihan, R., Sanders, S., Michaleff, Z.A. et al. (2021). Impact of COVID-19 pandemic on utilisation of healthcare services: a systematic review. *British Medical Journal Open* 11 (3): e045343.

National Cancer Institute. (2020). COVID-19. https://www.cancer.gov/publications/ dictionaries/cancer-terms/def/covid-19 (accessed 13 September 2022).

Nelson, B. (2020). The positive effects of covid-19. *British Medical Journal* 369. https://www.bmj.com/content/369/bmj.m1785/rr.

Neto, M.L.R., Almeida, H.G., Esmeraldo, J.D. et al. (2020). When health professionals look death in the eye: the mental health of professionals who deal daily with the 2019 coronavirus outbreak. *Psychiatry Research* 288: 112972.

Newman, K.L., Jeve, Y., and Majumder, P. (2021). Experiences and emotional strain of NHS frontline workers during the peak of the COVID19 pandemic. *International Journal of Social Psychiatry* 68 (4): 1–9.

NHS England. (2020). Other resources. https://www.england.nhs.uk/coronavirus/ secondary-care/other (accessed 29 August 2022).

O'Reilly, D., Carroll, H., Lucas, M. et al. (2021). Virtual oncology clinics during the COVID-19 pandemic. *Irish Journal of Medical Science* 190: 1295–1301.

Osborne, J. and Kerr, H. (2021). The role of the clinical nurse specialist as a non-medical prescriber in managing the palliative care needs of individuals with advanced lung cancer. *International Journal of Palliative Nursing* 27 (4): 334–341.

Richards, M., Anderson, M., Carter, P. et al. (2020). The impact of the COVID-19 pandemic on cancer care. *Nature Cancer* 1 (6): 565–567.

Robbins, T., Hudson, S., Ray, P. et al. (2020). COVID-19: a new digital dawn? *Digital Health* 6.

Rose, L., Yu, L., Casey, J. et al. (2021). Communication and virtual visiting for families of patients in intensive care during COVID-19: a UK National Survey. *Annals of the American Thoracic Society* 18 (10): 1685–1692.

Royal College of Nursing. (2020). Remote consultations guidance under COVID-19 restrictions. https://www.rcn.org/Professional-Development/publications/rcn-remote-consultations-guidance-under-covid-19-restrictions-pub-009256 (accessed 30 May 2020).

Salamanca-Balen, N., Seymour, J., Caswell, G. et al. (2017). The costs, resource use and cost-effectiveness of clinical nurse specialist–led interventions for patients with palliative care needs: a systematic review of international evidence. *Palliative Medicine* 32 (2): 447–465.

Sandler, A. (2003). Chemotherapy in small cell lung cancer. *Seminars in Oncology* 30 (1): 9–25.

Scarlat, M.M., Sun, J., Fucs, P.M.B. et al. (2020). Maintaining education, research and innovation in orthopaedic surgery during the COVID-19 pandemic. The role of virtual platforms. From presential to virtual, front and side effects of the pandemic. *International Orthopaedics* 44 (11): 2197–2202.

Shankar, A., Saini, D., Bhandari, R. et al. (2020). Lung cancer management challenges amidst COVID-19 pandemic: hope lives here. *Lung Cancer Management* 9 (3): 1–6.

Tod, A.M., Redman, J., McDonnell, A. et al. (2015). Lung cancer treatment rates and the role of the lung cancer nurse specialist: a qualitative study. *British Medical Journal Open* 5 (12): e008587.

Vera San Juan, N., Clark, S.E., Camilleri, M. et al. (2022). Training and redeployment of healthcare workers to intensive care units (ICUs) during the COVID-19 pandemic: a systematic review. *British Medical Journal Open* 12 (1): e050038.

Vrdoljak, E., Sullivan, R., and Lawler, M. (2020). Cancer and coronavirus disease 2019; how do we manage cancer optimally through a public health crisis? *European Journal of Cancer* 132: 98–99.

Waterhouse, D.M., Harvey, R.D., Hurley, P. et al. (2020). Early impact of COVID-19 on the conduct of oncology clinical trials and long-term opportunities for transformation: findings from an American Society of Clinical Oncology survey. *JCO Oncology Practice* 16 (7): 417–421.

World Health Organisation. (2020). Coronavirus disease (COVID-19). https://www.who.int/health-topics/coronavirus (accessed 13 September 2022).

Zuo, L. and Miller Juvé, A. (2020). Transitioning to a new era: future directions for staff development during COVID-19. *Medical Education* 104–107.

15

Digital Health

Amy Vercell and Sarah Hanbridge

Abstract

Achieving long-term sustainability of health and social care services will require investment in both people and technology. It is paramount to ensure that digital health systems and processes are implemented robustly, promoting interoperability between systems. Adequate education and support for healthcare workers accessing these systems must be provided, ensuring that they are clinically meaningful for the patient population to which they are directed. The cancer clinical nurse specialist plays a pivotal role in delivering cancer care; providing a point of access, often in a key worker role; ensuring that information needs are met; and delivering specialist holistic care to patients. Supporting nurses to be digitally literate to deliver digitally enabled care is crucial. This chapter explores the history of digital health, provides current examples of digital nursing and looks to the future of digital innovation.

15.1   Introduction

The first author, Amy Vercell, is a chief clinical information officer (CCIO) for Nursing and Allied Health Professionals with protected time for research; she completed a National Institute for Health and Care Research Pre-Doctoral Fellowship last year and is now working towards a doctoral application. She also works as an acute oncology advanced nurse practitioner (ANP) one day each week. Previous experience has been varied across oncology and haematology services and included working on an inpatient haematology ward and as unit sister in outpatient systematic anti-cancer therapy (SACT) delivery, acute oncology clinical nurse specialist (CNS), lead nurse for cancer of unknown primary (CUP), moving to acute oncology ANP upon completion of a master's qualification. The second author, Sarah Hanbridge, is a CCIO at

Leeds Teaching Hospital, England, United Kingdom (UK). Previous to this, Sarah worked at The Christie National Health Service (NHS) in Greater Manchester (a cancer specialist hospital) as the CCIO, and was the regional chief nursing information officer (CNIO) for the Northwest of England. Sarah has predominantly worked in acute care in clinical, operational, educational and digital roles.

With an ever-growing public health need, healthcare providers globally are being challenged to improve patient outcomes whilst containing costs, with digital technologies now being acknowledged as a key tenet in achieving this goal. Digital health tools can potentially improve the efficiency, accessibility and quality of care delivered to patients worldwide (Fahy and Williams 2021). Digital transformation enables a more holistic view of patient health through increased access to data whilst providing the tools to improve patient autonomy and self-management (The King's Fund 2022).

Digital health refers to the use of information and communication technologies in healthcare to manage illness, reduce health risks and promote wellness (Ronquillo et al. 2022). It incorporates a broad scope of categories, including mobile health, health information technology, wearables, telehealth and telemedicine, artificial intelligence and machine learning, virtual visits and personalised medicine (Food and Drug Administration [FDA] 2020). The World Health Organisation (2021) established three key objectives to promote the adoption and scale-up of digital health and innovation: translating data, research and evidence into practice; enhancing knowledge through scientific collaborations; and systematically assessing country needs to co-develop innovations to ensure that they are fit for purpose and meet the requirements of the individual population. Digital health is perceived as a tool to improve access to healthcare, reduce inefficiencies in the healthcare system, improve care quality, lower costs and enable more personalised care to be delivered (Ronquillo et al. 2022).

Ruth May, chief nursing officer (CNO) for the NHS England, UK, emphasised the importance of digital and data, proclaiming her support for every healthcare organisation to have a CNIO, identifying that this would enable significant developments within the digital sphere. Her strategic plan for research was announced in November 2021 and complements ambitions set out in 'Saving and Improving Lives: The Future of UK Clinical Research Delivery' (Department of Health and Social Care 2021) and the NHS Long Term Plan (NHS England 2019). Ms May identified five objectives that will promote the delivery of a person-centred research environment that empowers nurses to lead, participate in and deliver research (NHS England 2021). Creating digitally enabled nurse-led research is key to delivering better outcomes for the public. This work is being supported by The Phillips Ives Review, which aims to prepare the nursing and midwifery workforce to deliver the digital future. In the context of the UK, Professor Natasha Philips is currently the national CNIO for England. *The Topol Review* (2019) provided a view of digital healthcare technologies and recommendations that will enable NHS staff to make the most of innovative technologies such as genomics, digital medicine, artificial intelligence and robotics to improve services with the projected impact on the NHS workforce over the next 12 years. This nursing-focussed review, which plans to publish its findings at the CNO Summit in 2023, will build upon Topol's findings and recommendations to determine the requirements of the nursing and midwifery workforce to deliver healthcare in the digital age during the next 5, 10 and 12 years.

15.2 The Role of the Informatics Nurse/Chief Nursing Information Officer

Until recently, nursing informatics was one of the lesser-known nursing specialties, even though it has been a recognised specialty for over 30 years (Kirby 2015). It may be surprising how nursing informatics evolved, but the concept of informatics can be traced back to Florence Nightingale during the Crimean War when she recognised the importance of documenting patient care to monitor a patient's progress. This ingenious notion may have seemed radical at the time, but we now understand the importance of documenting patient care and collecting patient data (Kirchner 2014). Clinical nurses have many opportunities to get involved during the electronic health record (EHR) selection and implementation process, and this stakeholder involvement improves engagement and acceptance. In general, phases of the process include system selection; system design and development, including current and future state validation, testing and education implementation or 'go live'; and ongoing maintenance and optimisation (Coiera 2003). Through partnerships and collaboration with other professional leaders, the CNIO can present a unified message and direction for innovation focused on safety, quality and efficiency (American Nurses Association 2015).

The Royal College of Nursing (RCN) kick-started the campaign 'Every nurse an e-nurse' during NHS Digital's Nursing Week (RCN 2018). The aim of the campaign was to transition every nurse into an e-nurse by 2020, with a focus on training for various aspects of e-nursing, including patient bedside technology, wearable technology, mobile health and data security (Stevens 2018).

15.3 Electronic Observations

Delivering healthcare is complex, and optimising quality and safety is the priority. One of the first examples of using digital technology to improve care was the introduction of electronic observations. This technology facilitates a real-time clinical assessment to be conducted at the patient's bedside, enabling prompt detection of any change in the patient's condition and allowing the required intervention to be implemented swiftly to attenuate clinical deterioration (Lang et al. 2019). Prior to electronic observations, vital signs were documented on paper observation charts, and incorrect calculation and interpretation of the Early Warning Score (as it was then), combined with poor compliance in clinical escalation protocols, had a detrimental impact on morbidity and mortality (Schmidt et al. 2015; Wong et al. 2015). Electronic observations ensure that complete data is inputted, and the National Early Warning Score 2 (NEWS2) is automatically calculated, with clinical recommendations provided based on that score, optimising outcomes (Royal College of Physicians 2017). The innovative technology allows real-time, automatic information processing with the aim of improving the efficacy of Early Warning Scores in practice and provides greater visibility of key patient data.

15.4   Electronic Health Records

Traditionally, health records were written on paper and maintained in folders divided into sections based on the type of note, with only one copy available. New computer technology developed in the 1960s and 1970s laid the foundation for the development of the EHR. The use of EHRs has not only made patients' clinical information more accessible but also changed the format of health records and, thus, changed healthcare (Evans 2016). One of the first and most successful attempts to streamline and improve the keeping of patient records was in the American problem-oriented medical record (POMR). Developed by Dr Lawrence Weed in 1968, POMR is still used by some medical and behavioural health providers today. In 1972, the first iteration of what we now know as an EHR was introduced. The Regenstrief Institute in Indianapolis enlisted the help of Clement McDonald to develop its EHR programme. McDonald set out to tackle a twofold problem: the design of the database, with multiple issues that arise when attempting to link healthcare organisations, disciplines and professions through one central records system; and allowing for the full spectrum of capabilities, such as medication ordering, laboratory tests and radiology.

By the early 1990s, most American industries had taken the plunge into automating data and transactions. Healthcare, on the other hand, was struggling to keep up. In 1991, a book titled *The Computer-Based Patient Record: An Essential Technology for Health Care* (Institute of Medicine [IoM] 1991) shook the industry out of complacency and helped drive the adoption of EHRs by breaking down challenges associated with technology. In response to advances in technology, a shift from paper-based health records to electronic records commenced in the UK

(IoM 1997; Evans 2016) as the inadequacies of paper-based health records gradually became evident in the healthcare industry (Ornstein et al. 1992).

In 2002, the UK government chose a top-down, government-driven approach to implement one EHR nationally, known as the NHS Care Records Service; this was the cornerstone of the £12.7 billion National Programme for Information Technology (NPfIT) investment (Maude 2011). This very ambitious programme required enormous resources that proposed to eliminate the challenges of interoperability between various competitive EHR systems around the UK, reforming the way the NHS uses information to improve the quality of care being delivered (Justinia 2017). However, failings became apparent early in implementation in terms of an overambitious design without the required skills and strategy to deliver, and the programme was consequently dismantled in 2011. This failing highlights the necessity to ensure that digital systems and processes meet the needs of the population they serve, emphasising culture and leadership.

15.5 Digitalisation of Blood Glucose Monitoring

One of the biggest advances in recent years regarding home blood sugar monitoring has been the introduction of the continuous glucose monitor (CGM), which is an alternative means of measuring glucose levels subcutaneously (Fain 2022). It uses a sensor placed on the upper arm and worn externally by the user, allowing glucose information to be monitored continuously. This information helps the patient and their multiprofessional team to identify what changes are needed regarding insulin administration to achieve optimal glucose control, which allows patients to quickly assess glycaemic patterns and prevent a hypoglycaemic episode. CGM devices comprehensively optimise diabetes management by reviewing activity levels, medication and insulin dosing, food intake and stress to provide patients with information about how self-care decisions affect glucose levels. This promotes patient empowerment and gives them much more control over their diabetes management.

Rather than performing capillary stabs numerous times daily to monitor glucose levels, patients with a CGM device insert a small sensor wire under the surface of their skin with an automatic applicator and secure it with an adhesive patch. A glucose-oxidase platinum electrode attached to the sensor measures the glucose concentration in interstitial fluids throughout the day and night. A transmitter sends real-time glucose readings wirelessly to a handheld receiver or compatible smart device (or insulin pump), which displays current glucose levels and trends (Fain 2022).

Personal CGM systems measure blood glucose continuously and record readings every five minutes. Unlike self-monitoring, which provides a snapshot or point-in-time glucose measurement, CGM devices report data in numerical and graph-like formats, indicating current glucose levels and possible patterns. This allows patients to respond quickly to prevent acute glycaemic episodes and make informed decisions about insulin dosing and self-management.

Corticosteroids are a key tenet within cancer services for the myriad of complications associated with anti-cancer treatments; consequently, steroid-induced hyperglycaemia and steroid-induced diabetes mellitus are becoming more frequently seen within the cancer population (Jeong et al. 2016). Blood glucose monitoring is advised when commencing patients on steroids; however, there appears to be a disparity in practice due to a lack of clear clinical guidelines (Dinn 2019). The cancer CNS plays a significant role in educating patients on symptoms associated with hyperglycaemia and how to monitor their blood sugars using the equipment that has been provided whilst liaising with the primary care team and/or endocrine team regarding any required interventions to optimise patient care.

15.6 Electronic Nurse Prescribing

There was a time when prescribing was the realm of the medical profession. In May 2006, appropriately qualified/registered nurses gained access to the full British National Formulary (BNF), giving them similar independent prescribing capabilities as medical practitioners. Now non-medical prescribing in the UK is well-established as a mainstream qualification (it is the focus of Chapter 12 in this book). The ambition behind this expansion began in July 2000, when the Department of Health published 'The NHS Plan'. It promised to create new roles and responsibilities for nurses and provide more opportunities to extend their nursing roles.

To qualify as a non-medical prescriber, nurses must undertake a recognised Nursing and Midwifery Council (NMC) accredited prescribing course through a UK university. Upon successful completion, the qualification must be registered with the professional body, such as the NMC in the UK. Evidence shows that nurse prescribing improves patient care by ensuring timely access to medicines and treatment and increasing flexibility for patients who would otherwise need to wait to see a medical doctor (Drennan et al. 2009). Electronic independent nurse prescribing has been transformational for the cancer CNS. Electronic prescribing enhances quality and safety by reducing prescribing errors, increasing efficiency and supporting healthcare costs (Porterfield et al. 2014). Similarly, cancer electronic prescribing systems enable improved access to drug reference information, warnings and alerts, with improved efficiencies for pharmacy and drug administration (NHS Transformation Directorate 2017).

15.7 Nurse Digitally Requesting Bloods

With new models of cancer care emerging and evolving, there is a clear clinical need for more effective information sharing between and across care settings. This is especially apparent in CNS roles when managing patients with complex cancer needs, to optimise clinical outcomes and improve the quality of care. Enabling nurses and other healthcare professionals to order tests and procedures electronically has been a positive step towards the future of pathology, with the overall objective of improving patient care. It has enabled clinicians to access pathology, microbiology and cytology tests and results across healthcare by receiving the right information at the right time and place, to support improved clinical decision-making and patient safety. Many cancer CNSs involved in the delivery of SACT order blood tests for patients prior to each cycle of SACT treatment. Having electronic order sets increases efficiency within the SACT pathway, as it ensures that the correct blood tests are ordered, with results displayed within the EHR to promote accessibility for the clinical team whilst illustrating any trends in blood results. This trend is of value when assessing tumour markers, for example, as rising tumour markers can indicate disease progression (Liu et al. 2021).

15.8 Remote Consultations

Prior to the COVID-19 pandemic commencing in 2019, developments in digital health had been modest. Within cancer services, the delivery of remote outpatient cancer care was being explored, but progression was impeded by system inertia and slow speeds of adoption. Several factors appear to have been at the heart of this, including a lack of integration with existing clinical systems, lack of technology validation, and lack of technology usability and technical support (Palacholla et al. 2019). Within a matter of weeks, the COVID-19 pandemic dramatically accelerated digital health uptake, with many countries adopting digital-first strategies, remote monitoring and telehealth platforms to enable the delivery of care to continue without the need for any physical interactions to minimise the risk of COVID-19 transmission (Peek et al. 2020). Almost overnight, these digital health tools moved from being perceived as a potential opportunity for service development and innovation to becoming absolute necessities to maintain cancer services (Fahy and Williams 2021). Consequently, remote monitoring and virtual consultations have become the norm within cancer care, with reported benefits including improved patient access and convenience, the facilitation of caregiver involvement and maintaining the delivery of clinical services (Lafata et al. 2021).

The cancer CNS nurse-led clinic was one of many services affected by this shift to online during the pandemic. Nurse-led cancer clinics provide psychosocial care, symptom control and information needs (Molassiotis et al. 2021). (They are the focus of Chapter 11 in this book.) It could be argued that the value of this service was even greater during this time due to patient distress, with many services being suspended when the pandemic was declared. Standard operating procedures have been written to formally illustrate how the service will be delivered, ensuring equitability and accessibility, with clear inclusion and exclusion criteria (NHS University Hospitals of Leicester 2021). An evaluation of virtual cancer clinics in Ireland (n = 104) found that most individuals with cancer were satisfied by the care they received within the virtual clinic and were very relieved to avoid a hospital visit (O'Reilly et al. 2021).

15.9 Virtual Wards

The responsibilities of the cancer CNS are vast, with specialist clinical knowledge vital to delivering high-quality, evidence-based care, as well as leadership, education and service development. Telephone clinics and support have become a valuable service provision, enabling specialist cancer support to be delivered without needing hospital attendance. A recent advancement of remote monitoring brought about as a direct consequence of the global COVID-19 pandemic is the implementation of the virtual ward. A virtual ward is defined as a safe, efficient and convenient alternative to NHS bedded care, which is enabled by technology (NHS England 2022).

Virtual wards support patients who would otherwise be in hospital to receive the acute care, monitoring and treatment they need in their own homes. Virtual wards are technology-enabled remote monitoring and patient self-management, with minimal face-to-face provision, supported by clear and robust escalation pathways. A virtual ward is not chronic disease management, home infusion services, safety netting or proactive deterioration prevention (NHS England 2022).

The conception of the virtual ward in the UK was first aimed at people with COVID-19. National Health England Service Transformation (NHSX) supported a pilot during the first wave of the pandemic whereby patients were provided with a pulse oximeter and a mobile phone 'app', meaning they could leave hospital early or avoid a hospital admission altogether (NHS England Transformation Directorate 2021). This addressed the overwhelming demand for the health service, where many patients would present to the emergency department (ED) with severe COVID-19 symptoms requiring invasive treatment and potential admission to intensive care units/high dependency units, with, unfortunately, some patients dying. The COVID-19 virtual ward was designed to avoid an unnecessary hospital admission by instigating appropriate care at the appropriate place whilst enabling earlier detection of a clinical decline, allowing required interventions to be implemented sooner to attenuate clinical deterioration (Vindrola-Padros et al. 2021).

To set up a virtual ward in an organisation, a 'ward' is created in a hospital system; an example is Careflow. This is undertaken in the same way as an inpatient ward is set up but has a dashboard with individual patient details assigned to it. The service is typically led by acute oncology teams, with a consultant overseeing care with daily ward rounds and acute oncology nurses delivering the care. For patients wearing devices such as pulse oximetry, parameters are set so that triggers are sent if readings go out of range to enable prompt detection of deterioration. Evidence of the benefits of virtual wards has been noted (Vindrola-Padros et al. 2021), which has instigated more patient cohorts being included, such as patients with pain and frailty.

Integrated care systems (ICSs) offer the opportunity to integrate health and care services across multiple settings. Interoperable digital systems are key to effective and seamless virtual wards (The King's Fund 2022). Currently, there are variations of virtual wards nationally and internationally, with limited visibility of data reflecting virtual ward activity, measures of quality, patient outcomes or experience shared. Consequently, there is a national objective in England, UK, for Health and Social Care Trusts to submit a minimum dataset of aggregate information about usage and details of the configuration of the virtual ward. This data will be used to guide remuneration and developments.

15.10   Electronic Patient-Reported Outcome Measures

The global cancer burden is predicted to reach 28.4 million cases in 2040, a 47% rise from 2020 (Sung et al. 2021). Individuals with cancer experience a wide range of symptoms, both physical and emotional, that may have a significant impact on their quality of life. These symptoms can be related to the cancer itself or toxicities related to the treatment patients are receiving for their cancer, potentially exacerbated by any existing co-morbidities. Enabling people with cancer to self-manage their symptoms and quality of life can result in more informed, autonomous patients who are partners in their own care, which can consequently reduce the burden on health services by minimising unnecessary hospital attendance (Girgis 2020). Engaging patients and caregivers in technology-enabled structured symptom collection has several benefits, particularly related to the early detection of adverse events (Oakley-Girvan et al. 2021). The use of health-related quality-of-life assessments completed by patients prior to a clinical review has been found to increase the frequency and quality of these holistic assessments, aiding clinicians in identifying patients with moderate-to-severe health concerns (Detmar et al. 2002). Electronic patient-reported outcome measures (ePROMs) – validated, digitalised health questionnaires that can promote person-centred care – have consequently become more widely utilised (Shipman and Faivre-Finn 2021).

PROMs were initially developed to provide clarity and understanding of the effect of disease and treatments on patients' daily lives, with hundreds of standardised measures developed in the last 30 years in paper form (Nelson et al. 2015). Digital versions have since been developed, with evidence showing significant benefits of ePROMs regarding patient care, such as greater patient-clinician satisfaction, improved communication and enhanced efficiency in clinics (Crockett et al. 2021).

The Christie NHS Foundation Trust is the first centre in the UK to introduce ePROMs in a routine setting on a large scale. Their use over the last two years within the Health and Social Care Trust has stratified and enhanced planned out-patient appointments and enabled the delivery of more personalised follow-up. In accordance with national and Trust strategic objectives, a priority is delivering more proactive care through a responsive service whereby ePROM alerts can be directed to and acted upon by the hospital 24-hour hotline nursing team in a timely manner, prioritising early intervention for patients reporting severe symptoms. The development of a responsive ePROM intervention will enable real-time proactive care to be delivered by hotline nurses to acutely unwell individuals who are post-SACT by notifying clinicians of changes in reported symptoms. This will address the need for earlier intervention to attenuate symptoms, reduce unnecessary hospital attendances, which are burdensome for the patient and poor use of hospital services, and minimise late SACT deferrals.

15.11 Mobile Cancer Applications

Mobile phone use has become ubiquitous, and internet users are growing at an annual rate of 4.8%, equating to more than 600 000 new users daily (DataReportal 2022). Technological advances have seen the emergence of smartphones, whose features include powerful computing technology that supports third-party applications (apps) (Bender et al. 2013). Mobile health apps are increasingly used to promote prevention, improve early detection, increase patient autonomy and provide holistic support for those living with chronic medical conditions (Jongerius et al. 2019). Apps are becoming more widely used in cancer services, with an emphasis on positively impacting self-efficacy, empowerment and improved self-management (Charbonneau et al. 2020). The exponential growth of mobile technologies has provided opportunities for advancing the delivery of healthcare (Cai et al. 2021), including self-monitoring. Patient-reported symptoms can enable subtle changes to be detected even when consultations are being conducted remotely.

The 'Plan for Digital Health and Social Care' has been published, which reveals that £2 billion has been allocated to further transform health and care with digital technology in the UK, including the NHS App (Department of Health and Social Care and NHS England 2022). According to the Department of Health and Social Care and NHS England (2022), soon NHS app users will be able to receive NHS notifications and messaging, communicate with their general practitioner (GP)/primary physician, and view and manage hospital elective care appointments.

15.12   Home Blood Monitoring

Cancer represents a major health issue and economic burden to healthcare systems worldwide. Maximising the efficiency of treatment pathways and optimising patient outcomes are key priorities (Rotter et al. 2019), with COVID-19 greatly emphasising this need. Around 28% of people diagnosed with cancer receive SACT (Public Health England 2017). SACT refers to the systemic delivery of drugs with antineoplastic effects (NHS England 2013). These drugs include traditional cytotoxic chemotherapy as well as newer biological agents such as monoclonal antibodies, targeted therapies and immunotherapy (Leach 2020). Patients receiving SACT can incur treatment toxicities, which they must navigate and manage with support from their caregivers and clinical team. Toxicities can vary in severity and require management ranging from supportive medication in an outpatient setting to hospitalisation, dose interruptions and/or dose reductions (Djebbari et al. 2018).

Prior to every administration of SACT, the patient has a clinical assessment and full blood screen to ensure that it is safe to administer treatment. This blood test either requires an additional visit to a healthcare facility within 48 hours of their intended SACT appointment or can be completed on the day of treatment administration, resulting in a longer day for the patient. Either option is burdensome to the patient (Dunwoodie 2018), and during the pandemic, these additional or longer hospital visits increased the potential risk of greater transmission of COVID-19 and increased footfall at a hospital. Neutropenia, thrombocytopaenia and anaemia are common reasons for SACT deferral. They may directly cause the patient to be acutely unwell, and therefore, related blood levels are the first indication that treatment cannot proceed.

The creation of a point-of-care device that allows the patient to self-test a capillary sample at home to provide a full blood count could revolutionise existing clinical pathways. At a time when the global COVID-19 pandemic continues to impact care delivery, utilising innovative technologies can minimise treatment interruptions whilst promoting remote and ambulatory care. Research is underway at The Christie NHS Foundation Trust, UK, in collaboration with the medical technology company Entia Ltd., who are hoping to create the world's first home blood monitoring device, called Liberty. This point-of-care device will require a patient to carry out a finger prick test in their own home, with the obtained sample subsequently being analysed to give a full blood count result. The result will provide a value for total white blood cells, neutrophils, haemoglobin and platelets, comparable to a venous full blood count result analysed in a hospital laboratory. This will enable clinicians to ascertain if the patient's full blood count is within the desired parameters to proceed with treatment without the patient leaving their home. Those patients whose full blood count is not within the required range for treatment can be assessed virtually. If this virtual assessment highlights anything of concern, a proactive review can be arranged to ascertain if any intervention is required. Prompt detection of neutropenia and the monitoring of recovery could positively impact patients' quality of life and potentially contribute to individualising SACT delivery (Dunwoodie 2018).

15.13 Artificial Intelligence

With artificial intelligence (AI) and robotic systems on the increase, combined with society's dependence on mobile technology, the internet and social media, the NHS and health systems globally have the capability to increase the telehealth service to implement new virtual models of care. Regardless of these potential advances, global challenges continue for nursing to support clinical practice and digitally enabled patient care. Many exemplars show how digital technologies already benefit nursing practice and education (Krick et al. 2019). For example, nurses are providing daily monitoring, coaching and triage of patients with several chronic diseases, which has helped reduce emergency department admissions, and the use of telehealth has been extremely beneficial (van Berkel et al. 2019). Mobile devices, in particular smartphones and health apps, enable nurses to offer remote advice on pain management to adolescent patients with cancer (Jibb et al. 2017) and supplement aspects of nursing education by providing innovative educational solutions for content delivery and remote learning opportunities (Chuang et al. 2018).

The development and application to nursing of systems based on AI are still in their infancy. AI technologies could potentially support the nursing profession with significant benefits in data analytics and advanced clinical decision support in cancer care. It is evident from the literature that further research and funding are required, with consideration to nursing leadership in this domain to help support the development of new practice policy, regulatory frameworks and ethical guidelines to guide nursing practice (Booth et al. 2021). Preliminary evidence suggests that virtual chatbots could play a part in streamlining communication with patients, and robots could increase the emotional and social support patients receive from nurses to support cancer patients through their care pathways whilst acknowledging inherent challenges such as data privacy, ethics and cost-effectiveness (Buchanan et al. 2020).

15.14 Barriers to Digital Health

It must be acknowledged that digital health technologies can potentially increase inequities between users and non-users. A cross-sectional study of 151 individuals with cancer explored barriers and enablers of patients' uptake of technology for healthcare services and found that over one-quarter did not have daily access to the internet, and nearly one-third did not own a smartphone capable of displaying mobile apps (Potdar et al. 2020). Socioeconomic disparities are evident worldwide, and research illustrates that people with lower incomes and less education are less likely to live a healthy lifestyle and access cancer screening programmes (Raghupathi and Raghupathi 2020). Thus, people from these backgrounds are seen to have increased morbidity and mortality in relation to cancer and other conditions (Clegg et al. 2009). Other barriers may pertain to usability. Technology-based interventions must be developed with consideration of how they will 'sit' within the user's day-to-day life by considering ease of use and perception of their impact on disease management and quality of life (de Ridder et al. 2017).

15.15 Conclusion

Since March 2020, the COVID-19 pandemic has dictated the health and care storyline, and technology has been at the forefront of innovation in helping nurses and healthcare professionals to engage and connect with the world. Developments in digital health have been modest over the years, with technology being perceived as a potential solution to the advancement of care. However, the pandemic expedited uptake of digital health. In the current sphere of living with COVID-19 whilst trying to recover cancer services, reducing health inequalities and fostering resilience for the future NHS, technology is the facilitator. The CNS role has been pivotal to these significant technology developments by implementing at-home monitoring and outpatient video consultations and using the EHR to document the right data to support vital clinical research into treatments that improve clinical outcomes and the patient experience.

References

American Nurses Association (2015). *Scope and Standards of Practice: Nursing Informatics*, 2e. Silver Springs, MD: Nursesbooks.org.

Bender, J.L., Yue, R.Y.K., To, M.J et al. (2013). A lot of action, but not in the right direction: systematic review and content analysis of smartphone applications for the prevention, detection, and management of cancer. *Journal of Medical Internet Research* 15 (12): e287.

Booth, R., Strudwick, G., McBride, S. et al. (2021). How the nursing profession should adapt for a digital future. *British Medical Journal* 373: n1190.

Buchanan, C., Howitt, M.L., Wilson, R. et al. (2020). Predicted influences of artificial intelligence on the domains of nursing: scoping review. *JMIR Nursing* 3 (1).

Cai, T., Huang, Y., Zhang, Y. et al. (2021). Mobile health applications for the care of patients with breast cancer: a scoping review. *International Journal of Nursing Sciences* 8 (4): 470–476.

Charbonneau, D.H., Hightower, S., Katz, A. et al. (2020). Smartphone apps for cancer: a content analysis of the digital health marketplace. *Digital Health* 6: 1–7.

Chuang, Y.H., Lai, F.C., Chang, C.C., and Wan, H.T. (2018). Effects of a skill demonstration video delivered by smartphone on facilitating nursing students' skill competencies and self-confidence: a randomized controlled trial study. *Nurse Education Today* 66: 63–68.

Clegg, L.X., Reichman, M.E., Miller, B.A. et al. (2009). Impact of socioeconomic status on cancer incidence and stage at diagnosis: selected findings from the surveillance, epidemiology, and end results: National Longitudinal Mortality Study. *Cancer Causes & Control* 20 (4): 417–435.

Coiera, E. (2003). *Guide to Health Informatics*, 2e. Boca Raton, FL: CBC Press.

Crockett, C., Gomes, F., Faivre-Finn, C. et al. (2021). The routine clinical implementation of electronic patient-reported outcome measures (ePROMs) at the Christie NHS foundation trust. *Clinical Oncology* 33 (12): 761–764.

DataReportal. (2022). Digital around the world. https://datareportal.com/global-digital-overview (accessed 5 May 2022).

de Ridder, M., Kim, J., Jing, Y. et al. (2017). A systematic review on incentive-driven mobile health technology: as used in diabetes management. *Journal of Telemedicine and Telecare* 23 (1): 26–35.

Department of Health and Social Care. (2021). Saving and improving lives: The future of UK clinical research delivery. https://www.gov.uk/government/publications/the-future-of-uk-clinical-research-delivery/saving-and-improving-lives-the-future-of-uk-clinical-research-delivery (accessed 1 July 2022).

Detmar, S.B., Muller, M.J., Schornagel, J.H. et al. (2002). Health-related quality-of-life assessments and patient-physician communication: a randomized controlled trial. *Journal of the American Medical Association* 288 (23): 3027–3034.

Dinn, G. (2019). Steroid-induced diabetes in cancer patients. *Journal of Prescribing Practice* 1 (12): 610–615.

Djebbari, F., Stoner, N., and Lavender, V.T. (2018). A systematic review of non-standard dosing of oral anti-cancer therapies. *BMC Cancer* 18 (1154): 1–15.

Drennan, J., Naughton, C., Allen, D. et al. (2009). National independent evaluation of the nurse and midwife prescribing initiative. University College Dublin. https://www.lenus.ie/handle/10147/89103 (accessed 1 July 2022).

Dunwoodie, E. (2018). Home testing of blood counts in patients with cancer. M.D. thesis, University of Leeds.

European Observatory on Health Systems and Policies, Fahy, N., and Williams, G.A. (2021). Use of digital health tools in Europe: before, during and after COVID-19. World Health Organisation. Regional Office for Europe. https://apps.who.int/iris/handle/10665/345091 (accessed 1 July 2022).

Evans, R.S. (2016). Electronic Health Records: Then, Now, and in the Future. *Yearbook of Medical Informatics* (Suppl 1): S48–S61. https://doi.org/10c.15265/IYS-2016-s006 (accessed 1 July 2022).

Fain, J. (2022). Continuous glucose monitoring: the basics. Technology aids diabetes self-management and enhances treatment planning. *American Nurse Journal* 17 (5): 6–11.

Food and Drug Administration. (2020). What is digital health? https://www.fda.gov/medical-devices/digital-health-center-excellence/what-digital-health (accessed 5 June 2022).

Girgis, A. (2020). The role of self-management in cancer survivorship care. *The Lancet Oncology* 21 (1): 8–9.

Institute of Medicine (1991). *The Computer-Based Patient Record: An Essential Technology for Health Care*. Washington, DC: The National Academies Press https://doi.org/10.17226/18459.

Institute of Medicine Committee on Improving the Patient Record (1997). *The Computer-Based Patient Record. The Computer-Based Patient Record.'* Revised Edition. Washington, DC: National Academy Press.

Jeong, Y., Han, H.S., Lee, H.D. et al. (2016). A pilot study evaluating steroid-induced diabetes after antiemetic dexamethasone therapy in chemotherapy-treated Cancer patients. *Cancer Research and Treatment* 48 (4): 1429–1437.

Jibb, L.A., Stevens, B.J., Nathan, P.C. et al. (2017). Implementation and preliminary effectiveness of a real-time pain management smartphone app for adolescents with cancer: a multicenter pilot clinical study. *Pediatric Blood Cancer* 64: 1–9.

Jongerius, C., Russo, S., Mazzocco, K., and Pravettoni, G. (2019). Research-tested Mobile apps for breast Cancer care: systematic review. *JMIR mHealth and uHealth* 7 (2): e10930.

Justinia, T. (2017). The UK's National Programme for IT: why was it dismantled? *Health Services Management Research* 30 (1): 9.

Kirby, S.B. (2015). Informatics leadership: the role of the CNIO. *Nursing* 45: 21–22.

Kirchner, R.B. (2014). Introducing nursing informatics. *Nursing* 44 (9): 22–23.

Krick, T., Huter, K., Domhoff, D. et al. (2019). Digital technology and nursing care: a scoping review on acceptance, effectiveness and efficiency studies of informal and formal care technologies. *BMC Health Services Research* 19: 400.

Lafata, J., Smith, A.B., Wood, W.A. et al. (2021). Virtual visits in oncology: enhancing care quality while designing for equity. *JCO Oncology Practice* 17 (5): 220–223.

Lang, A., Simmonds, M., Pinchin, J. et al. (2019). The impact of an electronic patient bedside observation and handover system on clinical practice: mixed-methods evaluation. *Journal of Medical Internet Research Medical Informatics* 7 (1): e11678.

Leach, C. (2020). Complications of systemic anti-cancer treatment. *Medicine (United Kingdom)* 48 (1): 48–51.

Liu, Z., Wang, Y., Shan, F. et al. (2021). Combination of tumor markers predicts progression and pathological response in patients with locally advanced gastric cancer after neoadjuvant chemotherapy treatment. *BMC Gastroenterology* 21 (1): 1–14.

Maude, F. (2011). Major projects authority programme assessment review of the national programme for IT. https://assets.publishing.service.gov.uk/government/uploads/system/uploads/attachment_data/file/62256/mpa-review-nhs-it.pdf (accessed 16 September 2022).

Molassiotis, A., Liu, X.L., and Kwok, S.W. (2021). Impact of advanced nursing practice through nurse-led clinics in the care of cancer patients: a scoping review. *European Journal of Cancer Care* 30 (1): e13358.

National Health Service England. (2019). The NHS long term plan. https://www.longtermplan.nhs.uk (accessed 10 June 2022).

National Health Service England. (2021). Chief nursing officer for England's strategic plan for research. https://www.england.nhs.uk/wp-content/uploads/2021/11/B0880-cno-for-englands-strategic-plan-fo-research.pdf (accessed 10 May 2022).

Nelson, E.C., Eftimovska, E., Lind, C. et al. (2015). Patient reported outcome measures in practice. *British Medical Journal* 350: 1–3.

NHS England. (2013). 2013/14 NHS standard contract for cancer: chemotherapy (adult). B15/S/a. https://www.england.nhs.uk/wp-content/uploads/2013/06/b15-cancr-chemoth.pdf (accessed 10 June 2022).

NHS England. (2022). Virtual ward including hospital at home. https://www.england.nhs.uk/wp-content/uploads/2021/12/B1207-i-supporting-guidance-virtual-ward-including-hospital-at-home.pdf (accessed 1 July 2022).

NHS England Transformation Directorate. (2017). Oncology electronic prescribing integrated with an electronic patient record – cancer digital playbook. https://www.nhsx.nhs.uk/key-tools-and-info/digital-playbooks/cancer-digital-playbook/oncology-electronic-prescribing-integrated-with-an-electronic-patient-record (accessed 1 July 2022).

NHS England Transformation Directorate. (2021). Digital home care for people with coronavirus. https://transform.england.nhs.uk/blogs/digital-home-care-for-people-with-coronavirus (accessed 1 July 2022).

NHS University Hospitals of Leicester. (2021). UHL Gynaecology Governance Committee SOP for clinical nurse specialist led virtual clinics for gynaecology oncology patients. https://secure.library.leicestershospitals.nhs.uk/PAGL/Shared%20Documents/Gynaecology%20Oncology%20Virtual%20Nurse%20Led%20Clinic%20Standard%20Operating%20Procedure%20UHL%20Gynaecology%20Guideline.pdf (accessed 4 July 2022).

Oakley-Girvan, I., Davis, S.W., Kurian, A. et al. (2021). Development of a mobile health app (TOGETHERCare) to reduce cancer care partner burden: product design study. *JMIR Formative Research* 5 (8): e22608.

O'Reilly, D., Carroll, H., Lucas, M. et al. (2021). Virtual oncology clinics during the COVID-19 pandemic. *Irish Journal of Medical Science* 190 (4): 1295–1301.

Ornstein, S.M., Oates, R.B., and Fox, G.N. (1992). The computer-based medical record: current status. *Journal of Family Practice* 35 (5): 556–565.

Palacholla, R.S., Fischer, N., Coleman, A. et al. (2019). Provider and patient-related barriers to and facilitators of digital health technology adoption for hypertension management: scoping review. *JMIR Cardio* 3 (1): e11951.

Peek, N., Sujan, M., and Scott, P. (2020). Digital health and care in pandemic times: impact of COVID-19. *BMJ Health and Care Informatics* 27 (1): e100166.

Porterfield, A., Engelbert, K., and Coustasse, A. (2014). Electronic prescribing: improving the efficiency and accuracy of prescribing in the ambulatory care setting. *Perspectives in Health Information Management* 11 (Spring), 1g: 1–10.

Potdar, S., Ianevski, A., Mpindi, J.P. et al. (2020). Breeze: an integrated quality control and data analysis application for high-throughput drug screening. *Bioinformatics* 36 (11): 3602–3604.

Public Health England. (2017). National cancer registration and analysis service short report: chemotherapy, radiotherapy and surgical tumour resections in England: 2013–2014 v2. https://www.ncin.org.uk/cancer_type_and_topic_specific_work/topic_specific_work/main_cancer_treatments (accessed 10 May 2022).

Raghupathi, V. and Raghupathi, W. (2020). The influence of education on health: an empirical assessment of OECD countries for the period 1995–2015. *Archives of Public Health* 78 (1): 20.

Ronquillo, Y., Meyers, A., and Korvek, S.J. (2022). *Digital Health.* Treasure Island (FL): StatPearls Publishing LLC.

Rotter, T., de Jong, R., Lacko, S. et al. (2019). *Improving healthcare quality in Europe: characteristics, effectiveness and implementation of different strategies. Copenhagen (Denmark): European Observatory on Health Systems and Policies. Health Policy Series* 53 (12): https://www.ncbi.nlm.nih.gov/books/NBK549262.

Royal College of Nursing. (2018). Every nurse an e-nurse: insights from a consultation on the digital future of nursing.

Royal College of Physicians. (2017). National Early Warning Score (NEWS) 2: Standardising the assessment of acute-illness severity in the NHS. Updated report of a working party.

Schmidt, P.E., Meredith, P., Prytherch, D.R. et al. (2015). Impact of introducing an electronic physiological surveillance system on hospital mortality. *BMJ Quality and Safety* 24 (1): 10–20.

Shipman, L.A. and Faivre-Finn, C. (2021). 1748 electronic patient reported outcome measures – next generation Cancer patient monitoring? *Children's Cancer and Leukaemia Group* 106 (Suppl 1): A475–A476.

Stevens, L. (2018). NHS Digital endorses 'Every nurse an e-nurse' campaign. https://www.digitalhealth.net/2017/08/nhs-digital (accessed 4 July 2022).

Sung, H., Ferley, J., Siegel, R. et al. (2021). Global Cancer statistics 2020: GLOBOCAN estimates of incidence and mortality worldwide for 36 cancers in 185 countries. *CA: a Cancer Journal for Clinicians* 71 (3): 209–249.

The King's Fund. (2022). Digital health care. https://www.kingsfund.org.uk/projects/positions/digital-health-care (accessed 10 May 2022).

The Topol Review. (2019). Preparing the healthcare workforce to deliver the digital future. An independent report on behalf of the Secretary of State for Health and Social Care. https://topol.hee.nhs.uk/wp-content/uploads/HEE-Topol-Review-2019.pdf (accessed 1 July 2022).

van Berkel, C., Almond, P., Hughes, C. et al. (2019). Retrospective observational study of the impact on emergency admission of telehealth at scale delivered in community care in Liverpool, UK. *British Medical Journal Open* 9: e028981.

Vindrola-Padros, C., Singh, K.E., Sidhu, M.S. et al. (2021). Remote home monitoring (virtual wards) for confirmed or suspected COVID-19 patients: a rapid systematic review. *eClinicalMedicine* 37: 1–8.

Wong, D., Bonnici, T., Knight, J. et al. (2015). SEND: a system for electronic notification and documentation of vital sign observations. *BMC Medical Informatics and Decision Making* 15 (68).

World Health Organisation. (2021). Global strategy on digital health 2020–2025.

16

Future Direction of the Clinical Nurse Specialist in Cancer Care

Barry Quinn and Helen Kerr

Abstract

This chapter explores and examines the future direction and possible trends in practice and care delivery for clinical nurse specialists (CNS)s working in cancer services. There will be an emphasis on the continuing central role of caring within this specialist role. Mindful that the CNS is required to work within a context that is rapidly changing and within health care services that must be able to respond to these changing needs, there will be an exploration of some of the current skills required of the CNS and how these skills may need to change and develop to meet current and future needs. CNSs working within cancer teams and alongside people living with cancer will have an important leadership role in helping to redesign services that are more inclusive and can better respond to diverse needs of those with cancer. Finally, to continue achieving the core components of this vital role in nursing and health care, the chapter will focus on the importance of learning from practice through encouraging structured reflection.

A patient is the most important person in our hospital. They are not an interruption to our work; they are the purpose of it. They are not an outsider in our hospital; they are a part of it. We are not doing a favour by serving them; they are doing us a favour by giving us an opportunity to do so.

(Adapted from Mahatma Gandhi)

16.1 Introduction

This chapter will consider the future evolvement of the clinical nurse specialist (CNS) role in cancer care. The chapter will commence with a brief overview of the emergence and development of the CNS role to provide a background to the current global context. The vision for the direction of travel of the CNS role will predominately focus on the clinical component of the CNS role; however, as the role is supported with leadership, education and other components, these important factors will be explored. The chapter will delineate some of these key principles related to the CNS role, including caring, knowledge, skills and the ability to respond to diverse needs to ensure greater inclusivity and fairness. Case studies from practice will be used to illustrate the continuing and central role of the CNS in advancing practice.

Today, the role of the CNS continues to grow, and the CNS is recognised as a key contributor, core to the delivery of quality nursing practice in cancer services. The first author of this chapter, Barry Quinn, has worked for over 30 years in cancer and palliative care as a specialist nurse, researcher, author and leader in a number of teaching hospitals in London, United Kingdom (UK) and is currently a senior lecturer at Queen's University Belfast. The second author, Helen Kerr, is a senior lecturer at the School of Nursing and Midwifery, Queen's University Belfast, with a clinical background in cancer and palliative care nursing.

Although the concept of nursing care has been present in most societies from ancient times, nursing as a profession has more recently developed in a range of global contexts over the last century. Since nursing was inducted as a profession in the early twentieth century, the profession has been developing in response to the changing needs of diverse populations. This has required leadership, adaptability and a range of innovations that adequately meet society's changing needs. Nursing is reported to be one of the most trusted professions (International Council of Nurses (ICN) 2020a), evidencing the population's perspectives of the nursing profession's approach to these changing needs. In addition to these developments, nursing has evolved to be the profession with the greatest number of healthcare professionals, accounting for 59% of health professions with an estimated 27 million nurses globally (ICN 2020b).

One of the developments in the nursing profession relates to advancing nurses' roles beyond initial registration (East et al. 2015). Advancing nursing practice is one of the profession's approaches to meeting the changing healthcare needs of individuals, groups, communities and populations. One aspect of advanced nursing practice is the availability of advanced nursing roles, given the reported growing need for nurses working at an advanced level (Kleinpell et al. 2014), with one international study identifying 52 different advanced nursing roles in 26 countries (Heale and Buckley 2015). Bryant-Lukosius and Martin-Misener (2016) report that the CNS role is one of the two most common denominations of advanced practice nurse roles, along with the nurse practitioner. The ICN (2020c) state, 'the CNS provides healthcare services based on advanced specialised expertise when caring for complex and vulnerable patients or populations. In addition, nurses in this capacity provide education and support for interdisciplinary staff and facilitate change and innovation in healthcare systems' (p. 12).

Advanced practice nurse roles, including the CNS, contribute to better care for people, improved health for populations and lower healthcare costs (Bryant-Lukosius and Martin-Misener 2016). In cancer care, the CNS role is reported to enhance patient outcomes through improved symptom management, greater information provision, better psychological support, improved service coordination and increased patient satisfaction (Kerr et al. 2021). It has been argued that quality graduate education is fundamental to the success of advanced nurse practice roles (Bryant-Lukosius and Martin-Misener 2016), with a minimum educational requirement for the CNS role recommended as a master's qualification (ICN 2020c). However, due to contextual variations across the globe, it is recognised that this may not be the standard across all countries.

16.2   The Role of Caring and the Clinical Nurse Specialist

The way nursing and, more specifically, nursing as a profession has been delivered and developed over time has changed (Quinn 2020a); however, the actual presence of nursing within societies has consistently played a role among ancient cultures and communities throughout the world (ICN 2020a). The seeds of nursing and nursing practice can be seen in many of these ancient cultures, including within the First Nations of Africa, Canada, Australia and New Zealand. As nursing changed in response to each generation's needs, nursing was acted out within different contexts, i.e. in response to wars across Europe and Asia, during times of plague and famine, and through the major religious communities who felt called to respond to the poor and to those in need (Quinn et al. 2021). Through the ground-breaking work of individuals such as Mary Seacole and Florence Nightingale, nursing gradually began to be recognised as a profession, with a growing focus on health promotion and preventing illness (Thompson et al. 2020).

Within each of these historic and modern-day developments, and at the heart of all nursing practice, is the ability to care for another person in need (Quinn 2017). Some years ago, Brykczynska (1997), in her book *Caring: The Compassion and Wisdom of Nursing*, suggested that to consider nursing without caring is similar to thinking of nursing without a soul. This ability to care continues to be a core aspect of the CNS role. Jean Watson (2005), in exploring the meaning of nursing, spoke of the central role of caring in nursing practice. Watson (2005) believed that it was through the caring relationship between the nurse and the patient (one in need) that healing took place, and both the nurse and the one being cared for were enriched. More recently, Johns (2004) linked the concept of care to easing the suffering of others as people faced advanced disease and the reality of death. Karlsson and Pennbrant (2020) suggest that it is through this caring relationship, paying attention and treating the individual as a person with respect, that nurses can support the person's sense of well-being and self-worth. The concept of caring has been examined by numerous writers over the centuries and has recently been

Table 16.1 Compassion in healthcare.

Presence: The ability to listen with fascination
Understanding distress: Aware of one's own and the other's distress
Feelings response: Ability to empathise without being overwhelmed
Impulse to help: Remembering why one came into healthcare and nursing

---

Source: Adapted from West and Chowla (2017).

described as the ability to be actively present to someone in need, with a willingness to help and support (West and Chowla 2017) (Table 16.1).

The activity of caring requires the CNS to actively engage with the other by being fully present in all aspects of nursing care and practice. In the context of delivering expert and advanced nursing care, the CNS role models this long-held notion at the heart of nursing of compassionate care while responding to current global, local and individual needs.

16.3 Developing Skills for Today and the Future

The ICN (2020c) clearly state that nurses working in specialist roles require a diverse range of skills enabling them to provide safe and competent person-centred care with a strong base within nursing education. Each CNS uses a range of highly developed clinical and humanity-based skills to respond to the spiritual, social, emotional and physical needs of those who, for a temporary or a permanent period, require the support of another (Table 16.2) (Johns 2004; Quinn 2020b). These skills are acted out in the daily practice of the CNS, who may be required to explain to a person living with cancer that their cancer has advanced despite undergoing cancer treatments, and gently and sensitively explain what this means for the person whilst maintaining hope. Closely aligned to this concept of humanity-based practice is a CNS workforce that is highly skilled in a number of important elements of clinical nursing practice. These may be referred to as the

Table 16.2 Clinical and humanity based skills.

Assessing and responding to each person's:
- Physical needs – prescribing drugs and treatments, delivering nurse led treatment clinics, managing side effects of disease and treatments
- Emotional needs – addressing hope, joy, relief, fear, anxiety, stress, isolation, depression, loss
- Social needs – supporting concerns with inability to work, returning to work, financial concerns, adjusting to life after treatment, living with limitations
- Spiritual needs – exploring beliefs, values, hopes, dreams, future

---

Source: Quinn (2017, 2022).

four core pillars of the CNS role: nurses who can deliver evidence-based expert nursing practice, who are able to teach and role-model expert nursing practice and care for others, who are actively engaged in relevant research and forward planning of services, and who have the ability to lead others in the delivery of care (Quinn 2003; Quinn 2017; ICN 2020c).

However, for the CNS to continue working in this specialist role requires a high level of clinical expertise (Royal College of Nursing (RCN) 2018; ICN 2020c). Each CNS is required to demonstrate, maintain and update the competencies and agreed standards, which are reviewed in the light of global and national changes in health and social care (RCN 2018). This means every CNS must be committed to their ongoing learning and professional development. CNSs are required to provide leadership and insight in response to the global, social, political, economic and technological realities of health and social care needs (ICN 2020a).

16.4   Leadership

An important but sometimes overlooked component of the CNS role is the ability to use a combination of management and leadership skills in daily practice and interactions with others. While some CNSs may feel competent in using management skills to plan, ensure patient safety, support colleagues and deliver care, others may be more effective in using their skills to motivate and mentor colleagues, role-model expert practice, provide leadership and promote a vision of what clinical nursing can be (Quinn 2017). While both sets of skills are central to all nurses in health and social care, working in the role of a CNS places them in an ideal position to promote leadership in all aspects of clinical practice and service delivery (Storey and Holti 2013). This requires the CNS to adapt to the changing nature of cancer treatments and the settings in which these treatments may be delivered.

People with cancer require a CNS who can articulate a vision of care and support that places the patient at the heart of any new and developing service, who is able to work with and influence the team in creating services that exclude no one, and who has the ability to plan for future needs. Govier and Nash (2009) suggest that nurses in these leadership positions have a responsibility to help create a caring environment for patients, families and colleagues. If staff feel supported and cared for, they too will be able to pass on that care and support to people living with cancer (Govier and Nash 2009). Recognising multiple demands, the CNS has an important advocacy role in ensuring that those in power provide the resources necessary to deliver care, listening to their colleagues' needs and not allowing patient care to be diminished (Quinn 2017). This means the CNS has to be engaged with the decision-making process, ensuring that they are at the decision-making table, engaging with education providers and influencing regional and national

Table 16.3 Quality and skills for leadership.

- Credible
- Inclusive
- Listens and hears
- Courageous
- Engaging
- Empowering
- Visible
- Self-reflection/self-care
- Leads from a place of compassion

Source: Adapted from Quinn (2017).

agendas (RCN 2018). CNSs use their expert knowledge and skills to learn from those they care for, influence healthcare discussions and advocate for the needs of patients and their families, including guiding where resources might need to be allocated. Alongside this reality, the CNS needs to be compassionate, visible and credible; have the courage to influence change; and role-model the importance of reflection in practice and self-care (Table 16.3).

Although each CNS may have their preferred approach to leadership, influenced by their personal life and professional experiences, a variety of approaches and a willingness to adapt are required. In an emergency situation, the CNS working in an autocratic manner may reduce morbidity and prevent death, while being with someone who is receiving a new cancer diagnosis or facing death requires the approach of one who serves (Quinn 2020b). The notion of the serving leader, first described by Greenleaf (1970, 1997), is an approach that the CNS may find helpful in their goal to deliver care that focuses on the person (McCormack 2020). Similarly, Alimo-Metcalfe and Alban-Metcalfe (2008) describe a partnership approach, where the leader (the CNS), as a servant, ensures that the person living with cancer, their family and the wider team are invited to participate in treatment choice and care planning. The partnership approach corresponds well with the principle of good leadership as outlined in the National Health Service (NHS) Leadership Academy (Storey and Holti 2013) in the context of the UK. The CNS who is willing to serve and show empathy and compassion is crucial to improving the lives of those living with illness and advanced disease (Cornwell and Goodrich 2009; Quinn 2017).

With the focus on person-centred care, the Department of Health (2013) reported that in the UK, the majority of people living with cancer had been given an opportunity to talk about their needs and had an individualised plan of care, one based on a holistic response to the person's need. In contrast, Guldhav et al. (2017) and Hill-Kayser et al. (2011) found that many older people with cancer were excluded from taking part in their care planning and treatment options. Each CNS has an important leadership role within the broader team delivering the person's care, working to ensure that the person's needs are heard, assessed, addressed, responded to and monitored (Guldhav et al. 2017). The Department of Health report (2013) stated that to implement a more holistic needs assessment and care planning approach, members of the cancer team, including the CNS, need to have more confidence in their leadership and clinical practice, develop better communication skills and help to create a collaborative teamworking culture, placing the person in need at the centre (Department of Health 2013).

Effective leadership requires thinking differently to deliver care that is inclusive of all and exclusive of none. This involves engaging with people whose voices are not always heard in healthcare settings, including those with dementia, mental health conditions and learning disabilities; older people; lesbian, gay, bisexual and transgender people; refugees; and ethnic and religious minorities.

16.5 Equality, Diversity and Inclusion in the Role of the Clinical Nurse Specialist

The ability of each CNS to continually adapt their practice is fundamental to the growing and changing needs of a diverse and often transient population. This includes both opportunities and challenges in delivering a fairer global health and social care system for all (ICN 2020a) (Table 16.4). In his book *Falling Upwards, Reflecting on Spirituality and Getting Old*, Rohr (2013) reminds the reader that it people who are on the edges of society or do not conform to what society might define as normal or acceptable often have the most to teach us. Yet he goes on to say that we, as a society, have a pattern of excluding such people from many aspects of life (Rohr 2013). This exclusion can also exist within cancer services and practices, where people can be judged consciously or unconsciously by their age (ageism), race (racism), gender (chauvinism), ability/disability, mental health, sexuality (homophobia), religion or cultural background. The CNS and, indeed, all those working in cancer services must be more mindful of creating services

Table 16.4 Equity, diversity and inclusion.

- Equity in healthcare means equal opportunities and fairness for every individual in need.
- Inclusion is based on the belief that all people in society are entitled to share in society's benefits and resources (people who in the past have been placed at the margins of society should live as part of their communities).
- Diversity means recognising and celebrating our differences as individuals, but also recognises the common needs that unite us, including the need for good health and social care services.

Source: Adapted from RCN (2018).

that include and do not exclude those who are perceived differently. Recent research has demonstrated that many people over 65 years living with cancer have not always been included in important conversations and decisions about their treatment and care plans. In some cases, people have been over-treated with minimal benefits or, in some cases, have not been offered treatments that would have benefited them (Fitch et al. 2015; Noordman et al. 2017).

The Nursing and Midwifery Council (NMC 2021), the Royal College of Nursing (RCN 2018) and the General Medical Council (2022) of the UK, similar to other professional bodies globally, are committed to the idea that patients are people. Each person has a right to be treated fairly, with dignity and respect, regardless of their age, gender, ethnic origin, sexual preference, economic status or religious beliefs (or non-beliefs). This means moving away from the notion of one size fits all to one that is person-centred and at the heart of all good nursing practices. The focus requires the CNS to use their knowledge, expertise and leadership to create and deliver inclusive and adaptable services, ensure that people get fair access to health and social care, and ensure that justice is achieved. This requires the CNS taking a leading role, working with colleagues and services to challenge attitudes, cultures and activities that exclude others; working to ensure a more inclusive and integrated healthcare and social system and focusing on people with the greatest level of need to reduce the ongoing stark health inequalities that exist. This includes promoting and influencing the better commissioning of services that are respectful of diversity and inclusion. The following case study 1 provides an example of potential unconscious bias.

Case Study 1

Nora (she/her), a 74 year old lady, had previously been diagnosed and treated for colorectal cancer. Norah was admitted to the ward with a persistent cough, tiredness and weight loss. Following multiple tests, the team, the oncologist, a junior doctor and the CNS have come to tell Norah that despite her treatment, the cancer has spread to her lungs. Before beginning the conversation, the CNS asks Norah if she would like anyone with her. Nora says she would like her partner to be present. The CNS asks Nora what her partner's name is and whether she would like her to call him. Norah smiles and says her partner's name is Grace (she/her), and yes, she would like her partner to be there.

This simple case helps to illustrate how an unconscious bias (Norah's partner must be male) can get in the way of person-centred care. By being mindful of the diversity that exists and using more inclusive language, the health and social care team can make it easier for people in need to express what is important to them.

16.6 New Ways of Working

As the CNS and the wider health and social care team respond to the changing needs of a global community, how and where cancer services will be delivered now and in the future needs to be considered (ICN 2020a; Quinn 2022). As many of the chapters within this book have demonstrated, the global context in which the CNS operates and where health and social care is being delivered is changing (Table 16.5). In many parts of the world today, due to developments in diagnosing, treating and responding to cancer and other illnesses, more people are living longer, often with multiple co-morbidities and needs. Alongside this reality is the ongoing need for the CNS and health and social care services to respond and adapt to these growing and diverse needs and issues.

In recognition that people spend most of their lives living in their own homes, neighbourhoods and communities, there is an increasing need to plan health and social care with a more community-based focus. This means re-allocating limited resources to innovative ways of working and services delivered closer to where people want to live and be cared for and supported, and where they can live with advancing illness and their social care needs are addressed (Quinn et al. 2021). This will require not only a more critical approach to how resources are used but also finding new and creative ways of delivering care and new ways of working. The CNS workforce in cancer services will need to be prepared with an even broader range of clinical skills, including the ability to clinically assess, prescribe and lead clinics as well as deliver these services and skills beyond the hospital setting, and to work within a range of community settings. This will also require continuing to move beyond a one-dimensional model of care, largely based on a medical model, to one that puts the person at the heart of health and social care delivery (McCormack 2020). Such as model could include the CNS delivering nurse-led/multiprofessional clinics in more community-based settings, including

Table 16.5 The role of the clinical nurse specialist in a changing world.

- Increasing ageing population
- People living longer with multiple co-morbidities
- Increased focus on a community approach to care delivery
- Further integration of health and social care
- Inequitable access to support and services
- Workforce challenges – recruitment and retention
- Workforce opportunities – nurse-led services and new ways of working
- Extending scope of nursing practice (including independent prescribing)

Source: The King's Fund (2012), Quinn et al. (2021).

general practice (GP)/primary physician services, local pharmacies and local neighbourhood meeting places.

This will mean moving beyond a limited Monday to Friday, 09.00–17.00 service to a broader, consistent, more inclusive and seamless, seven-day service that meets the needs of all (ICN 2020a). Such an increasingly person-centred approach is perhaps in recognition of what Quinn (2020b) was referring to when he described individuals having to live with their personal experience of illness, seeing beyond the medical diagnosis to the reality of illness that disrupts their ability to engage with the world around them. It is this person-centred reality that the CNS, with their diverse range of clinical skills and advanced practice, strives to respond to.

The changing needs of people living with cancer and other co-morbidities mean the CNS will be required not only to be a nursing expert in their own field of cancer practice but also to be knowledgeable in a range of other illnesses and co-morbidities. With a growing emphasis on the individual rather than simply the disease (cancer) or condition, the CNS will require a diverse range of knowledge and skills to support the person in need, traversing hospital and community-based practice. The following case study 2 provides an example of how the CNS can be involved in the development of community cancer services.

The role of the CNS, like any healthcare professional, includes recognising their skills and limitations while seeking out opportunities for further learning, support and supervision. This means being held to account and taking responsibility

---

Case Study 2

Jim (he/him) has been a CNS in cancer for seven years, having undertaken post-registration training in cancer, non-medical prescribing and assessment. Many of the people Jim supports are older people living with cancer and other co-morbidities. To avoid people having to travel long distances to the hospital, Jim delivers an innovative community support service for people living with cancer based on a local GP/primary physician service. Local GP and community nursing teams can refer patients living with cancer in the local area to Jim's clinic. People living with cancer have an opportunity to talk to Jim about their symptoms relating to their disease and the side effects of treatment and to voice their worries and concerns.

Anna (she/her) is part of a community-based outreach cancer team. Anna visits people in their own homes following any of the following: a new diagnosis of cancer, a change in treatment plan, advancing disease or completion of treatment. Anna has found that completing a holistic needs assessment (HNA) in this environment has enabled her to learn much more about people's needs and concerns.

for one's own clinical judgements, actions and omissions. As the CNS role continues to adapt to need, it is important that the governance required to protect the patient, nurse and organisation are in place. This means each CNS job description and job plan reflects all aspects of the CNS role, including support of the extended roles nurses are required to undertake. Each CNS needs to work with their organisation and service to ensure that every aspect of the role is clearly understood and reflected in all relevant local policies and procedures.

16.7 Self-Reflection

Abore et al. (2006), writing in their book *When Professionals Weep*, discuss the impact of being exposed to others in times of need and suffering. They clearly describe the impact this daily exposure can have on healthcare professionals and the huge demands this places on their psyches, their souls and who they are as a person. Unless a CNS finds a way to care for themselves, it is difficult to see how they can continue to care for and effectively support another, which may lead to their expert role being diminished (Quinn 2003). Benner (2000) has stated that the expert nurse is one who is able to reflect on and learn from their own clinical practice. However, in another study focusing on nurses supporting people living with cancer, nurses spoke of the importance of learning not only from reflecting on clinical practice but also from reflecting on their own life experiences (Quinn 2003). This study showed that life experience is also important in effective nursing care and expertise. Part of the CNS role is to role-model and promote the importance of reflecting on and learning from clinical practice and other aspects of life.

An individual's ability to reflect on their life experiences and clinical practice is an important component of being an effective practitioner. Johns (2002) has demonstrated the benefits of reflective practice in healthcare in supporting clinical practice and nursing leadership. Johns' work reported that the healthcare system in which many nurses operate did not acknowledge the pressures facing nursing colleagues. However, Johns (2002) went on to stress that an important aspect of the reflection process for all expert nurses was learning to care for themselves. This will become increasingly important as CNSs continue to adapt and evolve in response to changing societal needs.

16.8 Conclusion

The important role of the CNS is changing within the world of health and social care and, more specifically, in supporting people with cancer. The CNS will continue to play a key role in the individual's care and treatment, including at the time of diagnosis, during treatment, and when facing recovery or, in some cases, the death of an individual. The key is for each CNS to critically consider all aspects of their expert role and how they may need to adapt to changing needs while not compromising the heart of nursing care. The role of nurses working within these expert roles is not simply to follow others but to play a key role in leading a more inclusive approach to care and treatment delivery. While the CNS will continue to deliver clinical expertise in practice, lead, teach, role-model and be part of future planning, this is best undertaken when the focus is on the individual and not simply a disease. Mindful of the increasing number of people living with cancer and other co-morbidities, the CNS will need to continue their commitment to their own professional development and developing skills that respond to the holistic needs of people living with cancer. The CNS will continue to play a vital role in delivering expert nursing practice within and across multiple community and hospital-based settings.

References

Abore, P., Katz, R.S., and Johnson, T.A. (2006). Suffering and the caring professional. In: *When Professionals Weep* (ed. R.S. Katz and T.A. Johnson), 13–26. New York: Routledge.

Alimo-Metcalfe, B. and Alban-Metcalfe, J. (2008). *Engaging Leadership: Creating Organisations that Maximise the Potential of their People*. London: Chartered Institute of Personnel and Development.

Benner, P. (2000). *From Novice to Expert: Excellence and Power in Clinical Nursing Practice*. Upper Saddle River, NJ: Prentice Hall.

Bryant-Lukosius, D. and Martin-Misener, R. (2016). *ICN Policy Brief Advanced Practice Nursing: An Essential Component of Country Level Human Resources for Health*. Geneva: ICN.

Brykczynska, G. (1997). A brief view of the epistemology of caring. In: *Caring: The Compassion and Wisdom of Nursing* (ed. G. Brykczynska and M. Jolley), 1–9. London: Arnold.

Cornwell, J. and Goodrich, J. (2009). Exploring how to ensure compassionate care in hospital to improve patient experience. *Nursing Times* 105 (15): 14–16.

Department of Health. (2013). Living with and beyond cancer: taking action to improve outcomes. https://assets.publishing.service.gov.uk/government/uploads/system/uploads/attachment_data/file/181054/9333-TSO-2900664-NCSI_Report_FINAL.pdf (accessed 1 August 2022).

East, L., Knowles, K., Pettman, M., and Fisher, L. (2015). Advanced level nursing in England: organisation challenges and opportunities. *Journal of Nursing Management* 23: 1011–1019.

Fitch, M.I., McAndrew, A., and Harth, T. (2015). Perspectives from older adults receiving cancer treatment about the cancer-related information they receive. *Asia-Pacific Journal of Oncology Nursing* 2 (3): 160–168.

General Medical Council. (2022). Equality, diversity and inclusion targets and priorities. https://www.gmc-uk.org/-/media/documents/equality--diversity-and-inclusion---targets---progress-and-priorties_pdf-89470868.pdf (accessed 1 July 2022).

Govier, I. and Nash, S. (2009). Examining transformational approaches to effective leadership in healthcare settings. *Nursing Times* 105 (18): 24–27.

Greenleaf, R.K. (1970). *The Servant as Leader*. Atlanta GA: The Greenleaf Center for Servant Leadership.

Greenleaf, R.K. (1997). *Servant Leadership: A Journey into the Nature of Legitimate Power and Greatness*. New York: Paulist Press.

Guldhav, K.V., Jepsen, R., Ytrehus, S., and Grov, E.K. (2017). Access to information and counselling older cancer patients' self- report: a cross-sectional survey. *BMC Nursing* 16: 18.

Heale, R. and Buckley, C. (2015). An international perspective of advanced practice nursing regulation. *International Nursing Review* 62: 421–429.

Hill-Kayser, C.E., Vachani, C., Hampshire, M.K. et al. (2011). The role of internet-based cancer survivorship care plans in care of the elderly. *Journal of Geriatric Oncology* 58–63.

International Council of Nurses. (2020a). Nurses: a voice to lead nursing the world to health.

International Council of Nurses. (2020b). State of the world's nursing.

International Council of Nurses. (2020c). Guidelines on advanced practice nursing.

Johns, C. (2002). *Guided Reflection: Advancing Practice*. Oxford: Blackwell Publishing.

Johns, C. (2004). *Being Mindful Easing Suffering: Reflection on Palliative Care*. London: Jessica Kingsley Publishers.

Karlsson, M. and Pennbrant, S. (2020). Ideas of caring in nursing practice. *Nursing Philosophy* 21 (4): 1–5.

Kerr, H., Donovan, M., and McSorley, O. (2021). Evaluation of the role of the clinical nurse specialist in cancer care: an integrative literature review. *European Journal of Cancer Care* 30 (3): 1–13.

Kleinpell, R., Scanlon, A., Hibbert, D. et al. (2014). Addressing issues impacting advanced nursing practice worldwide. *The Online Journal of Issues in Nursing* 19 (2).

McCormack, B. (2020). The person-centred nursing and person-centred practice frameworks: from conceptual development to programmatic impact. *Nursing Standard* 35 (10): 86–89.

Noordman, J., Driesenaar, J.A., Henselmans, I. et al. (2017). Patient participation during oncological encounters: barriers and need for supportive interventions experienced by elderly cancer patients. *Patient Education and Counseling* 2262–2268.

Nursing and Midwifery Council. (2021). Equality, diversity and inclusion. https://www.nmc.org.uk/about-us/equality-diversity-and-inclusion (accessed 2 August 2022).

Quinn, B. (2003). 'An exploration of the nurses' experience of supporting a cancer patient in their search for meaning. *European Journal of Oncology Nursing* 7 (3): 164–171.

Quinn, B. (2017). Role of nursing leadership in providing compassionate care. *Nursing Standard* 32 (16–19): 53–63.

Quinn, B. (2020a). Using Patricia Benner's model of clinical competency to promote nursing leadership. *Nursing Management* 27 (2): 33–40.

Quinn, B. (2020b). Living with uncertainty and the reality of death. *International Journal of Palliative Care Nursing* 26 (6): 278–283.

Quinn. B. (2022). How should nurses assess and manage pain in a person with cancer? Cancer Nursing Practice. https://rcni.com/cancer-nursing-practice/evidence-and-practice/practice-question/how-should-nurses-assess-and-manage-pain-a-person-cancer-183851 (accessed 28 July 2022).

Quinn, B., O'Donnell, S., and Thompson, D. (2021). Gender diversity in nursing: time to think again. *Nursing Management* 29 (2): 20–24.

Rohr, R. (2013). *Falling Upwards. A Spirituality for Two Halves of Life.* London: SPCK Publishing.

Royal College of Nursing. (2018). Advanced level nursing practice section 2: advanced level nursing practice competencies.

Storey, J. and Holti, R. (2013). *Towards a New Model of Leadership for the NHS.'* NHS Leadership Academy. London: Open University Business School.

The King's Fund. (2012). Leadership and engagement for improvement in the NHS: together we can.

Thompson, D., Quinn, B., and Watson, R. (2020). Getting more men into nursing: an urgent priority (too little, too late). *Journal of Nursing Management* 28: 1463–1464.

Watson, J. (2005). Caring science as a sacred science. In: *Theoretical Basis for Nursing* (ed. M. McEwen and E. Wills). USA: Lippincott Williams and Wilkins.

West, M. and Chowla, R. (2017). Compassionate leadership for compassionate health care. In: *Compassion: Concepts, Research and Applications* (ed. P. Gilbert), 237–257. London: Routledge.

Index

The Role of the Clinical Nurse Specialist in Cancer Care, First Edition. Edited by Helen Kerr.
© 2024 John Wiley & Sons Ltd. Published 2024 by John Wiley & Sons Ltd.
Companion website: www.wiley.com/go/kerr

Printed and bound by CPI Group (UK) Ltd, Croydon, CR0 4YY

10/10/2024

14571743-0001